MANUAL OF PEDIATRIC PARENTERAL NUTRITION

MANUAL OF PEDIATRIC PARENTERAL NUTRITION

EDITED BY

John A. Kerner, Jr., M.D.
Assistant Professor of Pediatrics
Director of Pediatric Gastroenterology
Coordinator of Pediatric Nutritional Support Services
Stanford University Medical Center
Stanford, California

A WILEY MEDICAL PUBLICATION
JOHN WILEY & SONS
New York • Chichester • Brisbane • Toronto • Singapore

Library of Congress Cataloging in Publication Data:

Main entry under title:

Manual of pediatric parenteral nutrition.

  (A Wiley medical publication)
  Includes index.
  1. Parenteral feeding for children—Handbooks,
manuals, etc. I. Kerner, John A. II. Series.
[DNLM: Parenteral feeding—In infancy and childhood—
Handbooks. WB 410 M294]
RJ53.P37M36 1983   615.8′55   82-20264
ISBN   0-471-09291-6

Printed in the United States of America

10 9 8 7 6 5 4 3 2 1

To Dr. Philip Sunshine and Dr. John D. Johnson, for stimulating my interest in parenteral nutrition and for their personal and professional support; to my wife, Louise, for her tireless help with this manual and for her encouragement and love; and to all of our patients at Stanford University Medical Center and the Children's Hospital at Stanford.

Contributors

Michael D. Amylon, M.D.
Assistant Professor of Pediatrics
Stanford University Medical Center
Stanford, California
Staff Hematologist/Oncologist
Children's Hospital at Stanford
Palo Alto, California

Amy S. Andolina, R.N., B.S.N.
Nutritional Support Nurse
Department of Pharmacy Services
Stanford University Medical Center
Stanford, California

Jo Ann Tatum Hattner, R.D., M.P.H.
Pediatric Nutrition Specialist
Department of Dietetics
Stanford University Medical Center
Stanford, California

John A. Kerner, Jr., M.D.
Assistant Professor of Pediatrics
Director of Pediatric Gastroenterology
Coordinator of Pediatric Nutritional Support Services
Stanford University Medical Center
Stanford, California

Louise Poirier-Kerner, R.N.
Pediatric Oncology Nurse
Department of Nursing Services
Children's Hospital at Stanford
Palo Alto, California

Nick Mackenzie, M.D.
Department of Anesthesia
Stanford University Medical Center
Stanford, California

Alice I. Morrow, R.N., M.S.N.
Supervisor, Pediatric Intensive Care Unit
Children's Medical Center
Dallas, Texas

Robert L. Poole, Pharm. D.
Supervisor, Pediatrics/Nursery
Satellite Pharmacy
Stanford University Medical Center
Stanford, California

M. Eileen Walsh, R.N., C.P.N.P., M.S.N.
Pediatric Gastroenterology Nurse Specialist
Department of Pediatrics and
    Department of Nursing Services
Stanford University Medical Center
Stanford, California

Foreword

Since the late 1960s, when the techniques for appropriate intravenous nutrition were developed, there has been an almost exponential increase in knowledge of and experience with the use of parenteral nutrition. Although several manuals have been developed concerning adults and older children, Dr. Kerner and his associates have written a handbook that is oriented specifically to the management of patients in the pediatric age group. The *Manual of Pediatric Parenteral Nutrition* was developed and written by the members of the nutritional support team at Stanford University Medical Center who deal with infants and children. The manual approaches the problems from a multidisciplinary standpoint and offers practical as well as theoretical approaches to the use of parenteral nutrition in infants and children.

The manual contains an extensive and thorough discussion of nutritional assessments and indications for the use of parenteral nutrition, as well as specific requirements for the various nutrients, especially protein, fats, and trace elements. In fact, the review of intravenous fats is probably the most complete and extensive that has been written to date.

The practical applications and techniques of preparing and delivering the parenteral nutrition solution are lucidly described; the complications, both technical and metabolic, are clearly delineated; and the mechanisms and approach to the transition from parenteral to enteral nutrition are presented in a practical manner. An important chapter is devoted to the psychological aspects of providing care for the patient receiving intravenous nutrition and the family involved. Many previously written treatises unfortunately have not even mentioned this important aspect of patient care.

Valuable tables in Chapter 20 list the analysis of various formulas and enteral products. These tables are complete and current and can be found in no other text. The appendices contain helpful information as well.

Finally, there is a chapter on the use of computers, and Appendix V contains a complete computer program for the use of parenteral nutrition in infants and children.

In a rapidly changing field, in which new information is constantly being generated, and whose techniques can be applied to greater numbers of patients both in hospital and at home, Dr. Kerner and his associates have performed a valuable service by bringing the science and art of parenteral nutrition up to date for those who care for pediatric patients. For this service I am deeply indebted and appreciative.

PHILIP SUNSHINE, M.D.
Harold K. Faber Professor of Pediatrics
Director of Newborn Nurseries
Stanford University Medical Center
Stanford, California

Preface

This *Manual of Pediatric Parenteral Nutrition* is designed to be a practical guide to the use of central and peripheral parenteral nutrition in infants and children. It is based on our clinical and research experience at Stanford University Medical Center and the Children's Hospital at Stanford over the last 10 years. It includes significant contributions from our pharmacist, nutritionist, and nursing staff that enable the text to be helpful to all health professionals who care for pediatric patients.

The manual contains "cookbook" style guidelines for the actual mechanics of parenteral nutrition, with many valuable tables that summarize our recommendations. In addition, there are detailed discussions of necessary background information for the novice as well as thorough reference lists at the end of each chapter for those who desire an in-depth review.

The text is divided into five parts. The first discusses the indications for parenteral nutrition in pediatrics and the techniques of nutritional assessment in infants and children. The subsequent parts include specific nutrient requirements, complications of parenteral nutrition, practical aspects, and special considerations.

Parenteral nutrition is a therapy in evolution, and no manuscript can be entirely current. Nevertheless, we have attempted to review the literature thoroughly through March, 1982. The reader should be cautioned that nutritional products and the recommendations for their use may change with time; therefore, current publications should be referred to for new information.

JOHN A. KERNER, JR.

Acknowledgments

I would like to express my deep appreciation for the superb editorial assistance I received from Carole Poole; Robert Poole, Pharm. D.; Philip Sunshine, M.D.; Peggy Richardson, R.D.; and Claudia Rupp, Pharm. D. In addition, I would like to thank each author who contributed to this unique manual.

I wish to thank the Mead Johnson Nutritional Division for its support of several of the research studies discussed in this manual. Finally, I would like especially to acknowledge the excellent secretarial assistance of Beth Sunshine and Helen Wada.

JOHN A. KERNER, JR.

Contents

Part I
Introduction to Pediatric Parenteral Nutrition

1
Indications for Parenteral Nutrition in Pediatrics

John A. Kerner, Jr.

Nearly four decades have elapsed since the first report of the successful use of total parenteral nutrition (TPN) in an infant (1). Helfrick and Abelson infused hypertonic dextrose, a casein hydrolysate, and a homogenized emulsion of olive oil and lecithin in an alternating manner to a marasmic infant for five days. They were able to demonstrate a significant improvement in the child's nutritional status. During the next 20 years parenteral nutrition (PN) in infants and children was unsuccessful, largely due to the inability of peripheral veins to tolerate the hyperosmolar infusates. Significant side effects, including allergic manifestations and marked elevations of body temperature, further complicated attempts at PN. Often there was inadequate provision of calories to allow the nitrogen to be utilized efficiently.

A group of surgeons at the University of Pennsylvania developed the techniques that provided the stimulus for the current widespread use of TPN. Dudrick, Wilmore, Vars, and Rhoades demonstrated in beagle puppies, and later in an infant, that the continuous intravenous infusion of hypertonic dextrose and amino acids through deep venous catheters could provide adequate caloric intake and allow normal growth and development (2–5). They found that with slow infusions, the rapid blood flow through the superior vena cava diluted the hypertonic infusate, thereby preventing phlebitis and thrombosis.

The development of a safe intravenous fat preparation, Intralipid, was another major advance in PN. Earlier fat emulsions had not gained significant acceptance because of their serious toxic side effects. Fat emulsions now offer the dual advantage of high caloric density and isotonicity, thereby meeting caloric requirements without damaging peripheral veins.

With the availability of fat emulsions and the technical advance of central venous nutrition, the physician now has alternatives for providing nutritional support to infants and children who cannot or should not be fed enterally. The spectrum of parenteral nutritional support in pediatrics ranges from the provision of single nutrients—to meet either partial or total daily requirements—to the delivery of *total* parenteral nutrition.

3

Combination parenteral/enteral nutrition provides some nutrients enterally (those that can be digested and absorbed by the gastrointestinal tract) and the remainder parenterally (6). Such a regimen is advantageous for the following patients: low birth weight infants, who are able to tolerate limited enteral feedings; infants with intractable diarrhea, for whom the provision of small amounts of nutrients enterally stimulates the recovery of certain intestinal enzymes; and patients being "weaned" from TPN to a program of complete enteral nutrition (e.g., the infant with short bowel syndrome).

Although PN is a potentially life-saving therapy and is now an accepted practice, increasing experience has demonstrated metabolic, mechanical, and infectious complications (see Chapters 11–14). Therefore, candidates for PN should be selected carefully and the indications considered diligently. The principal indications for PN are listed in Table 1.

PN is supportive therapy for some illnesses and primary therapy for others. PN is supportive for burn patients, patients with protracted diarrhea and malnutrition, and patients with congenital gastrointestinal anomalies. Studies have documented its worth as primary therapy for patients with gastrointestinal fistulas, the short

Table 1 Indications for Parenteral Nutrition in Pediatric Patients (6–11)

Condition	Examples
Surgical gastrointestinal disorders	Gastroschisis, omphalocele, tracheoesophageal fistula, multiple intestinal atresias, meconium ileus and peritonitis, malrotation and volvulus, Hirschsprung's disease with enterocolitis, diaphragmatic hernia
Intractable diarrhea of infancy	
Inflammatory bowel disease	Crohn's disease, ulcerative colitis
Short bowel syndrome	
Serious acute alimentary diseases	Pancreatitis, pseudomembranous colitis, necrotizing enterocolitis
Chronic idiopathic intestinal pseudoobstruction syndrome	
Gastrointestinal fistulas	
Hypermetabolic states	Severe burns and trauma
Renal failure	
Intensive care of low birth weight infants	
Special circumstances	Anorexia nervosa, cystic fibrosis, cardiac cachexia, hepatic failure, sepsis, cancer
Rare disorders	Chylothorax and chylous ascites, congenital villous atrophy, *Cryptosporidium*[a]-induced secretory diarrhea

[a] Cryptosporidium is a protozoal parasite that rarely infects humans; it can produce a secretory diarrhea.

bowel syndrome, renal failure, and Crohn's disease. In addition, PN is now being suggested for use in malnourished oncology patients, patients with hepatic failure, malnourished patients before major surgery, patients with cardiac cachexia, and patients requiring prolonged respiratory support. Nutritional repletion in these patients has been associated with an apparent reduction in the incidence of sepsis, with proper wound healing, and with a return of normal skin test reactivity (7).

PN is indicated for most patients who are unable to tolerate enteral feedings for a significant period of time (8). Four or five days without adequate oral nutrition is usually sufficient indication for instituting some form of PN. Even 2–3 days without adequate nutritional intake for very low birth weight infants or infants with pre-existing nutritional depletion is likely to result in significant depletion of their limited endogenous stores.

Although PN is used to replete the malnourished child, it may be started prophylactically in clinical situations in which prolonged starvation is expected (e.g., as postoperative support) (9). Other general indications for PN include a recent loss of more than 10% of lean body weight with a concomitant inability to ingest sufficient nutrients to reverse this state or those patients with marginal nutritional reserves who would be unable to ingest sufficient calories to prevent further negative nitrogen balance.

Infants receiving central vein TPN retain nitrogen and grow as well as normal infants fed either human milk or standard formulas. TPN has been directly credited with improving the survival of certain infants (10). The mortality of patients with gastroschisis and intractable diarrhea has decreased to approximately 10% today from 75-90% before the development of TPN (8). This drop in mortality has occurred without major changes in the medical aspects of therapy in these conditions and seems to be due solely to the prevention of starvation (8). TPN is "supportive" therapy in these infants, providing normal nutrition until the gastrointestinal tract is capable of functioning on its own.

Surgical Gastrointestinal Disorders

No controlled studies exist on the efficacy of TPN in infants requiring surgery on their intestinal tract, but the data overwhelmingly argue in its favor. In surgical gastrointestinal disorders, congenital anomalies prevent the use of the alimentary tract. TPN supplies the patient's nutritional needs until recuperation from the corrective surgical procedure occurs (11). Heird and Winters (12) studied infants with surgical gastrointestinal disorders for at least 12 months postoperatively; all 21 received TPN. At follow-up, 15 of the 21 patients had normal gastrointestinal function, two had special dietary requirements, and the remaining four had died. Their results were dramatic in a group of patients that before the advent of TPN would have had an extremely high mortality. Dudrick et al. described 18 infants who received TPN following surgery for ruptured omphalocele or gastroschisis (13). None of their patients died, and without TPN, they would have predicted a 60-80% mortality. Other investigators have demonstrated similar positive responses to the use of TPN in major gastrointestinal tract surgery (14–20).

Intractable Diarrhea

Determining the cause of intractable diarrhea is often difficult, if not impossible, because of the secondary effects of malabsorption and malnutrition. The malnutrition leads to caloric, protein, vitamin, and ion deficiencies that create adverse changes in the mucosa, flora, and motility of the gastrointestinal tract. Therefore, determining the primary etiology may be impeded. In addition, the diagnostic work-up may exacerbate the diarrhea and further weaken the patient. The initial medical approach involves correction of the secondary effects by providing adequate calories, protein, fluid, and electrolytes for restoration and regeneration of the intestinal tract; this approach usually requires the use of TPN (21).

Greene and co-workers (22) showed that nutritional support with PN for infants with intractable diarrhea may be enhanced by adding continuous feeding of a dilute elemental diet. Their infants receiving the combined parenteral/enteral regimen had a more rapid return of important intestinal activity of the disaccharidases sucrase and maltase as compared to the group of infants receiving strictly TPN.

Inflammatory Bowel Disease

In the management of inflammatory bowel disease (IBD), two questions remain incompletely answered: (1) Is TPN a useful adjunct to therapy for IBD? and (2) What roles does TPN have as primary therapy for IBD? In response to the first question, the consensus in the literature is an overwhelming *yes* (23).

Bowel rest—the complete elimination of enteral intake—has been a mainstay in the treatment of symptomatic exacerbations of IBD for many years (24–26). Standard intravenous fluid therapy, however, results in nutritional depletion and compromises patient recovery. TPN has been advocated because it provides adequate nutritional support while allowing the damaged intestinal mucosa to heal. The presence of nutrients in the gut results in an increase in intestinal blood flow, stimulation of biliary and pancreatic secretion, release of enteric hormones, mucosal growth, and formation of stool bulk. In patients with IBD it seems logical to place the bowel "at rest" to reduce the irritation of the inflamed mucosa and to reduce the workload of the intestine in order to allow healing (24–26). Clinical experience has demonstrated that avoidance of regular oral intake diminishes the diarrhea and abdominal pain of patients with IBD (26).

PRIMARY THERAPY

PN is being used as primary therapy during severe exacerbations of Crohn's disease. PN can be particularly beneficial when instituted early in the management of disease "flares," before drug therapy has failed and the disease has become "intractable." Enterocutaneous fistulas are another indication for protracted intravenous support. PN has also been recommended for the reversal of growth retardation in patients with Crohn's disease. In many situations primary therapy is currently being attempted with defined formula diets to avoid the placement of central venous lines.

TPN as Primary Therapy for Medical Relapse.   Rosenberg (26) summarized the data of eight reported series of ulcerative colitis patients (27–34) and nine reported series of Crohn's disease patients without fistulas (27–29, 31–33, 35–38). In all of these patients, TPN was used as "primary therapy for failure of medical treatment" (26). Nutritional repletion was achieved in 61% (31 of 51) of the ulcerative colitis patients, and clinical remission in the hospital was achieved in 35%. Colectomy was uncommonly averted in patients with uncontrolled disease. In contrast, 100% (85/85) of the Crohn's disease patients underwent successful nutritional repletion; 81% had a clinical remission in the hospital, and 61% were in full remission or successfully managed as outpatients for at least 3 months. When oral intake was reinstituted relapses occurred with variable frequency. Careful comparisons of treatment of Crohn's colitis versus ulcerative colitis have not been reported (25).

TPN as Primary Therapy for Fistulas in Crohn's Disease.   The use of TPN and bowel rest for fistulas in Crohn's disease has had variable results. Symptomatic relief, nutritional repletion, and diminished fistula drainage frequently occur. Medication plus nutritional support may enhance healing. Greenberg et al. observed spontaneous closure of fistulas for at least 2 years in six of seven patients who received both TPN and corticosteroids, but in only one of seven who received TPN alone (37). In addition, TPN plus metronidazole appears to be promising therapy for perianal fistulas associated with Crohn's disease (26).

In Rosenberg's summary (25) of eight reported series in which TPN was given for Crohn's with fistulas, 43% of patients with fistulas healed in the hospital and 30% had long-term closure (more than 3 months). There have been reports of fistula closure with home TPN when conventional inpatient TPN with bowel rest and/or surgical attempts at fistula closure had failed (38,39). Defined formula diet has produced results comparable to those achieved by TPN.

PN as Primary Therapy for Growth Retardation.   Retarded skeletal growth and delayed onset of puberty sometimes occur in young patients with IBD, particularly in those with Crohn's disease. The work of Kelts et al. (40) attributes this growth failure to prolonged inadequate caloric intake, which accompanies the anorexia of the disease.

To reestablish skeletal growth, nutritional requirements must be met. Sulfasalazine and/or corticosteroid therapy, preferably given on alternate days, may provide substantial symptomatic relief so that adequate dietary intake to achieve growth can be restored. Oral formula supplements are frequently needed to achieve calorie–protein goals. Patients who fail to respond to a carefully designed oral regimen may require more intensive nutritional support either by enteral tube feeding or with TPN (26).

Recent studies have confirmed that treatment of growth retardation in Crohn's disease with adequate nutritional intake—either with TPN (38,41), PN plus oral feedings (40), or vigorous enteral feedings (42,43)—may reestablish skeletal growth. The effects of nutritional therapy for growth retardation related to ulcerative colitis have not been studied (26).

ADJUNCTIVE THERAPY

In any severely malnourished patient with IBD who must undergo surgery or diagnostic evaluation, TPN can be used to achieve nutritional repletion. Preoperative and postoperative TPN in such patients may improve surgical risk. For the patient with resultant short bowel syndrome, TPN can be used in the immediate postoperative period as well as for prolonged nutritional support at home until intestinal adaptation again allows enteral nutrition. There has also been an increasing use of defined formula diets (see chapter 20) to achieve "partial" bowel rest as an alternative to TPN (24–26).

CONTROLLED TRIAL

Recently, a controlled and prospective trial of TPN and bowel rest was described in a group of 36 patients with IBD. Dickinson et al. (34) concluded that TPN offered no primary therapeutic effect on the course of IBD. The study's small number of patients (nine patients with Crohn's disease) does not allow us to draw definitive conclusions. A controlled prospective study is currently underway at the University of Chicago Pritzker School of Medicine and at two other medical centers to help define the role of bowel rest and TPN in Crohn's disease.

Short Bowel Syndrome

Total parenteral nutrition has had a dramatic effect on the lives of those who have lost large amounts of small bowel (23). In the acute stage after an abdominal catastrophe (e.g., necrotizing enterocolitis) and major intestinal resection, TPN permits the maintenance of fluid and electrolyte balance while preventing nutritional depletion (26). After the initial postoperative, hypersecretory period, TPN supplies the patient's nutritional needs until the remaining intestine can compensate for the rapid transit and inadequate absorptive surface (11). A gradual transition from parenteral to enteral feedings can then begin. This transition may take months or years, depending on the amount and location of the remaining bowel. The nutritional management of pediatric short bowel patients has been discussed in detail (11,44–48).

Serious Acute Alimentary Disorders

In patients with severe pancreatitis, the immediate goal is to place the pancreas "at rest" to decrease the secretion of proteolytic enzymes. TPN is used in some cases to prevent further nutritional deterioration while nasogastric suction is instituted (26). TPN has not been shown to reduce the incidence of complications from pancreatitis when compared to conventional management, but it has been shown to a useful adjunct for nutritional support in this illness (49). Peripheral vein TPN has been used with excellent results in three children with serious pancreatic injuries, including severe pancreaticoduodenal injury with obstructive jaundice, continuing pancreatitis with pseudocyst, and severe pancreatic trauma associated with major abdominal and neurologic injuries (50). In pseudomembranous colitis and necrotizing enterocolitis (51), the use of TPN permits bowel rest and nutritional support while the intestine recovers.

Chronic Intestinal Pseudo-obstruction

Patients with idiopathic chronic intestinal pseudoobstruction may suffer from malnutrition because they are unable to maintain adequate oral intake without the development of obstructive symptoms. TPN has been used in such patients both on a short-term and long-term (home hyperalimentation) basis (52,53). TPN can provide adequate nutrition until normal bowel function returns or until definitive therapy for this chronic disease is found (52).

Gastrointestinal Fistulas

In the past, the treatment of gastrointestinal fistulas has been associated with a morbidity and mortality rate ranging from 40–60% (54). The severe catabolic state, tissue breakdown, septic complications, and renal failure all contributed to morbidity, particularly in the absence of intensive nutritional support (54).

With the use of TPN and total bowel rest, MacFayden et al. (55) observed spontaneous closure in 70.5% of 62 patients who had 78 enterocutaneous fistulas; on the average, closure occurred 34.9 days after initiation of TPN. Following successful closure, 94% of the patients eventually underwent surgery (55). The overall mortality in the series was 6.67%. Similar data were reported by Deitel, using TPN and complete bowel rest in 100 patients with gastrointestinal fistulas (56).

MacFayden (54) believes that the management of patients with gastrointestinal fistulas should include early institution of TPN, which should be continued for at least 4 weeks. If there is no evidence of spontaneous fistula closure at that time, surgical intervention should be considered.

Hypermetabolic States

The discussion of the management of severe burns and trauma is beyond the scope of this text. Nutritional support in these disease states is well discussed in several recent articles (57–61).

Renal Failure

Abel and co-workers (62) demonstrated that the recovery from acute renal failure (ARF) in adults was improved with the use of an experimental intravenous mixture. In their study, an experimental group received a solution of hypertonic dextrose with essential amino acids (EAA) while the control group received an isocaloric amount of only hypertonic dextrose. Complications during ARF (e.g., pneumonia, sepsis, and gastrointestinal hemorrhage) were tolerated significantly better by the group receiving the experimental solution. Baek et al. (63) studied 129 consecutive adult patients with ARF, giving 66 hypertonic dextrose alone and 63 hypertonic dextrose plus fibrin hydrolysate. The mortality rate was significantly lower in the group receiving the added protein.

Abitbol and Holliday described six anuric children who received TPN (64). An increase in nonprotein (glucose) calories from 20 cal/kg/day to 70 cal/kg/day progressively reduced body protein catabolism; nitrogen balance improved. When an EAA solution was added, net urea production decreased and nitrogen balance became positive. They concluded that TPN with EAA improved the nutritional status of severely ill anuric children and might influence recovery.

More recently, Holliday et al. (65) compared the use of EAA to general amino acids (GAA), which provide more nitrogen, in restoring nutritional well-being to anuric undernourished children. They found that an EAA formulation in a ratio of 1 g/100 cal or a GAA formulation of 2 g/100 cal would induce retention of nitrogen as body protein. Nitrogen retention appeared to be greater when larger doses of nitrogen were given as GAA, but they felt that their finding was tentative because of limited data.

The use of EAA hyperalimentation for ARF in children has resulted in hyperammonemia and hyperchloremic metabolic acidosis associated with an abnormal plasma aminogram (66). Initial infusion of GAA and reintroduction of GAA solution after the EAA trial resulted in progressive amelioration of or complete recovery from these metabolic disturbances. The nephrologist on the TPN committee at Stanford feels that there are not adequate data showing benefit from the two commerically available EAA solutions (67) as compared to standard GAA solutions. Therefore, since EAA solutions are significantly higher in cost than GAA solutions, they are not recommended for patients with renal failure. Additional guidelines for the use of TPN in patients with renal failure are described by Miller (68).

Intensive Care of Low Birth Weight Infants

RESPIRATORY DISTRESS SYNDROME (RDS)

A controlled study (69) of peripheral TPN (consisting of casein hydrolysate, dextrose, and soybean emulsion) in 40 premature infants with RDS showed that TPN neither favorably altered the course of RDS nor worsened an infant's pulmonary status. Infants under 1500 g with RDS had an increased survival rate compared to controls if they received TPN (71% survival versus 37%). Further controlled studies are needed.

VERY LOW BIRTH WEIGHT INFANTS

Yu and co-workers (70) performed a controlled trial of TPN on 34 preterm infants with birth weights under 1200 g. Infants in the TPN group had a greater mean daily weight gain in the second week of life and regained birth weight sooner than did control infants. Four infants in the milk-fed control group developed necrotizing enterocolitis, whereas none did in the TPN group.

As a rule, premature infants who are unable to tolerate enteral feedings for more than 3 days are candidates for parenteral nutrition (71). Providing nutritional support early is imperative because of the premature infant's limited stores of essential nutrients. Under conditions of total starvation, the full-term infant has sufficient reserves to survive for approximately 1 month, the 2000 g infant has reserves to survive for approximately 12 days, and the 1000 g infant has reserves for only 4.5 days (72). Daily provision of glucose intravenously (semistarvation) will prolong survival (72).

In addition, the most concentrated critical period of brain growth occurs between the thirtieth week of gestation and the fifth month of life (73). Studies of laboratory animals have shown that nutritional compromise during this period of growth may result in decreased brain growth that cannot be reversed, despite future implementation of adequate nutrition (73–78).

Very low birth weight infants often have major medical problems that limit their ability to ingest and absorb adequate calories (79), such as respiratory distress, cardiovascular immaturity, hemorrhagic tendencies, and an immature renal system, in addition to a relatively immature digestive system. These infants lack the ability to digest fat, starches, and protein (80) appropriately. Incompetence of the gastroesophageal sphincter, delayed gastric emptying, poor coordination of intestinal motility, and a reduced gastrointestinal immune response all tend to make the provision of adequate calories by the enteral route a formidable challenge. The development of stasis and abdominal distention coupled with a propensity for infection also leads to the infant's vulnerability when initiation of enteral feeding is attempted. Thus, there is a need to provide calories intravenously while the intestinal tract is gradually adapting to extrauterine life (79). Many medical centers supplement oral feedings with peripheral PN until a premature infant can tolerate all required calories enterally (81).

Special Circumstances

ANOREXIA NERVOSA

In anorexia nervosa, the malnutrition can be effectively treated with TPN; however, the central venous catheter is a potential focus for manipulative behavior (23). There is no evidence that enteral administration of diets through feeding tubes is any less effective than TPN in this condition (23,82–84).

CYSTIC FIBROSIS

A 21-day period of nutritional supplementation with PN in twelve problem cystic fibrosis (CF) patients resulted in improved growth and nutrition as well as improved clinical and respiratory status (85). The use of intravenous fat in the treatment of the essential fatty acid deficiency of CF is discussed in detail in Chapter 7. Since there are several nutritional deficiencies associated with CF (86), nutritional support is essential. Controlled studies are needed to document the benefit of nutritional support using PN as opposed to vigorous enteral supplementation.

SEPSIS AND HEPATIC FAILURE

Abnormal serum amino acid patterns have been documented in septic patients. The infusion of a branched-chain amino acid solution to septic patients resulted in normalization of the serum amino acids and in clinical improvement (87). In hepatic failure, solutions rich in branched-chain amino acids and deficient in aromatic acids have been shown to result in positive nitrogen balance with recovery from hepatic encephalopathy (88). In this way, adequate nitrogen for protein conservation and synthesis can be provided without aggravating hepatic encephalopathy (23).

OTHER CONDITIONS

The use of parenteral nutrition in pediatric oncology patients is described in Chapter 24 of this manual. TPN has been shown to be of benefit in both traumatic and refractory chylous ascites (89,90).

Preshaw and co-workers (91) in a controlled trial found that the provision of TPN for 24 hours before and for five days after surgery had no effect on colonic wound healing. This finding is comparable to another study in which healing of esophageal anastomoses was not influenced by TPN. TPN does not appear to be of benefit in improving healing of gastrointestinal tract anastomoses (92).

Route of Administration—Central Versus Peripheral Vein

Ziegler and co-workers (93) compared the complication rates among children receiving central and peripheral nutrition. Their findings are summarized in Table 2. Although infectious complications occurred in approximately 10% of the central vein group and in none of the peripheral vein group, morbidity related to solution administration was more prevalent in the peripheral vein group. The peripheral vein group suffered primarily soft tissue sloughs, whereas such complications as pleural effusions and thrombosis occurred in the central vein group. The overall complication rate was greater in the central vein group, but the complication rate per day of parenteral nutrition was not (Table 2). Thus, while the complications encountered in the central vein group were more serious, the assumed safety of peripheral vein delivery can be questioned.

Ziegler and co-workers (93) acknowledge that the problem of venous accessibility is a deterrent to central venous nutrition in small children. Their experience with percutaneous subclavian vein cannulation suggests that this technique is safe, allows repeated cannulation of the central venous system, and can be used in very low birth weight infants. Their data implies that *caloric need* is the primary determining factor for selecting the route of nutritional support. Peripheral vein nutrient solu-

Table 2. Complications of TPN

Determinant	Central Vein	Peripheral Vein
Number of patients	200	385
Mean duration (days)	33.7	11.4
Therapy days	6629	4389
Percent who maintained or gained weight	82.5%	63%
Complications		
Infectious	21	0
Administration	7	32
Metabolic	12	3
Complication rate		
Total number	40(20%)	35(9.08%)
Per patient day	0.604%	0.79%

SOURCE: Ziegler M, Jakobowski D, Hoelzer D, et al: Route of pediatric parenteral nutrition: Proposed criteria revision. *J Pediatr Surg* 15:472, 1980.

tions are less calorically dense than central vein solutions; therefore, centrally alimented patients can potentially receive more calories and gain more weight on a daily basis. Further, with frequent peripheral vein infiltrations, the amount of calories actually infused is often less than ordered (94). Thus, if minimal stress is present and only a brief course of maintenance therapy, without full growth and development, is the therapeutic goal, the peripheral route is appropriate. In the stressed, growing child, for whom prolonged therapy is projected, central venous nutrition is the treatment of choice (93,95).

References

1. Helfrick FW, Abelson NM: Intravenous feeding of a complete diet in a child. *J Pediatr* 25:400, 1944.
2. Dudrick SJ, Wilmore DW, Vars HM: Long-term total parenteral nutrition with growth in puppies and positive nitrogen balance in patients. *Surg Forum* 18:356, 1967.
3. Dudrick SJ, Wilmore DW, Vars HM, et al: Long-term total parenteral nutrition with growth, development and positive nitrogen balance. *Surgery* 64:134, 1968.
4. Wilmore DW, Dudrick SJ: Growth and development of an infant receiving all nutrients exclusively by vein. *JAMA* 203:140, 1968.
5. Dudrick SJ, Vars HM, Rhoades JE: Growth of puppies receiving all nutritional requirements by vein. *Fortschritte der Parenteralen Ernährung.* Symposium of International Society of Parenteral Nutrition, Munich, Pallas Verlag, 1967, p 2.
6. Coran AG: *Profiles in Nutritional Management: The Infant Patient.* Chicago, Medical Directions, Inc, 1980, p 3.
7. Reimer SL, Michener WM, Steiger E: Nutritional support of the critically ill child. *Pediatr Clin North Am* 27:647, 1980.
8. Levy JS, Winters RW, Heird WC: Total parenteral nutrition in pediatric patients. *Pediatrics in Review* 2:99, 1980.
9. Filler RM: Parenteral support of the surgically ill child, in Suskind RM (ed): *Textbook of Pediatric Nutrition.* New York: Raven Press, 1981, p 341.

10. Candy DCA: Parenteral nutrition in paediatric practice: A review. *J Hum Nutr* 34: 287, 1980.

11. Jewett TC Jr, Lebenthal E: Recent advances in gastrointestinal tract surgery in children, in Gluck L (ed): *Current Problems in Pediatrics.* Chicago, Yearbook Medical Publishers, 1978, vol 9, no 2, p 15.

12. Heird WC, Winters RW: Total parenteral nutrition: The state of the art. *J Pediatr* 86:2, 1975.

13. Dudrick SJ, Copeland EM III, MacFadyen BV Jr: Long-term parenteral nutrition: Its current status. *Hosp Pract* 10:47, 1975.

14. Wagner CW, Parrish RA: Gastroschisis. *Am Surg* 47:174, 1981.

15. Firor HV: Technical improvements in the management of omphalocele and gastroschisis. *Surg Clin North Am* 55:129, 1975.

16. Zerella JT, Martin LW: Jejunal atresia with absent mesentery and a helical ileum. *Surgery* 80:550, 1976.

17. Fraser GC, Simpson W, Pendray M, et al: Surgical treatment of congenital defects in the abdominal wall. *Ann Surg* 42:474, 1976.

18. Fonkalsrud EW: Selective repair of neonatal gastroschisis based on degree of visceroabdominal disproportion. *Ann Surg* 191:139, 1980.

19. Stothert JC Jr, McBride L, Lewis JE, et al: Esophageal atresia and tracheoesophageal fistula: Preoperative assessment and reduced mortality. *Ann Thorac Surg* 28:54, 1979.

20. Duhamel JF, Coupris L, R'evillon Y, et al: Gastroschisis: Study of a series of 50 cases from 1960 to 1976 and therapeutic indications. *Arch Fr Pediatr* 36:40, 1979.

21. Sunshine P, Sinatra FR, Mitchell CH: Intractable diarrhea of infancy. *Clin Gastroenterol* 6:445, 1977.

22. Greene HL, McCabe DR, Merenstein GB: Protracted diarrhea and malnutrition in infancy: Changes in intestinal morphology and disaccharidase activities during treatment with total intravenous nutrition or oral elemental diets. *J Pediatr* 87:695, 1975.

23. Goodgame JT Jr: A critical assessment of the indications for total parenteral nutrition. *Surg Gynecol Obstet* 151:433, 1980.

24. Rombeau JL: Parenteral nutrition and inflammatory bowel disease. *ASPEN 6th Clinical Congress,* San Francisco, California, 1982, p 117.

25. Rosenberg IH: Inflammatory bowel disease, in Postgraduate Course VI: Nutritional Support and Gastrointestinal Disease. *ASPEN 5th Clinical Congress,* New Orleans, 1981, p 25.

26. Rosenberg IH: *Profiles in Nutritional Management: The GI Patient.* Chicago, Medical Directions, Inc, 1981.

27. Reilly J, Ryan JA, Strole W, et al: Hyperalimentation in inflammatory bowel disease. *Am J Surg* 131:192, 1976.

28. Fischer JE, Foster GS, Abel RM, et al: Hyperalimentation as primary therapy for inflammatory bowel disease. *Am J Surg* 125:165, 1973.

29. Cohen MI, Boley SI, Daum F, et al: The role and effect of parenteral nutrition on the liver and its use in chronic inflammatory bowel disease in childhood, in Bode HH, Warshaw JB (eds): *Advances in Experimental Medicine and Biology.* New York, Plenum Press, 1974, vol 46, p 214.

30. Stanchev P: Parenteral nutrition in the treatment of ulcerohaemorrhagic colitis, in Romieu C, Solassal C, Joyeux H, et al (eds): *International Congress on Parenteral Nutrition,* France, University of Montpelier, 1974, p 501.

31. Franklin FA, Grand RJ: Parenteral nutrition for inflammatory bowel disease in childhood and adolescence, in Romieu C, Solassal C, Joyeux H, et al (eds): *International Congress on Parenteral Nutrition,* France, University of Montpelier, 1974, p 583.

32. Vogel CM, Corwin TR, Baue AE: Intravenous hyperalimentation in the treatment of inflammatory diseases of the bowel. *Arch Surg* 108:460, 1974.

33. Elson CO, Layden TJ, Nemchausky BA, et al: An evaluation of total parenteral nutrition in the management of inflammatory bowel disease. *Dig Dis Sci* 25:42, 1980.

34. Dickinson RJ, Ashton MG, Axton ATR, et al: Controlled trial of intravenous hyperalimentation and total bowel rest as an adjunct to routine therapy of acute colitis. *Gastroenterology* 79:1199, 1980.

35. Anderson DL, Boyce HW Jr: Use of parenteral nutrition in treatment of advanced regional enteritis. *Am J Dig Dis* 18:633, 1973.

36. Marshall F II: Hyperalimentation as a treatment of Crohn's disease. *Am J Surg* 128:652, 1974.

37. Greenberg GR, Haber GB, Jeejeebhoy KN: Total parenteral nutrition (TPN) and bowel rest in the management of Crohn's disease. *Gut* 17:828, 1976.

38. Strobel CT, Byrne WJ, Ament ME: Home parenteral nutrition in children with Crohn's disease: An effective management alternative. *Gastroenterology* 77:272, 1979.

39. Byrne WJ, Burke M, Fonkalsrud EW, et al: Home parenteral nutrition: An alternative approach to the management of complicated gastrointestinal fistulas not responding to conventional medical or surgical therapy. *JPEN* 3:355, 1979.

40. Kelts DG, Grand RJ, Shen G, et al: Nutritional basis of growth failure in children and adolescents with Crohn's disease. *Gastroenterology* 76:720, 1979.

41. Layden T, Rosenberg J, Nemchausky B, et al: Reversal of growth arrest in adolescents with Crohn's disease after parenteral alimentation. *Gastroenterology* 70:1017, 1976.

42. Morin CL, Roulet M, Roy CC, et al: Continuous elemental enteral alimentation in children with Crohn's disease and growth failure. *Gastroenterology* 79:1205, 1980.

43. Kirschner BS, Klich JR, Kalman SS, et al: Reversal of growth retardation in Crohn's disease with therapy emphasizing oral nutritional restitution. *Gastroenterology* 80:10, 1981.

44. Bohane TD, Haka-Ikse K, Biggar WD, et al: A clinical study of young infants after small intestinal resection. *J Pediatr* 94:552, 1979.

45. Feldman FJ, Dowling RH, McNaughton J, et al: Effect of oral versus intravenous nutrition on intestinal adaptation after small bowel resection. *Gastroenterology* 70:712, 1976.

46. Tepas JJ III, MacLean WC Jr, Kolback S, et al: Total management of short gut secondary to midgut volvulus without prolonged total parenteral alimentation. *J Pediatr Surg* 13:622, 1978.

47. Buhrdel P, Beyreiss K, Scheerschmidt G, et al: Therapeutic problems in the "short-bowel-syndrome." *Zentralbl Chir* 103:1062, 1978.

48. Rickham PP: Clinical results of an extensive gut resection in newborn infants. *Paediatr Paedol* Suppl 3:41, 1975.

49. Goodgame JT, Fischer JE: Parenteral nutrition in the treatment of acute pancreatitis: Effect on complications and mortality. *Ann Surg* 186:651, 1977.

50. Cummins GE, Grace AEN, Beardmore HE: Supportive use of total parenteral alimentation in children with severe pancreatic injuries. *J Pediatr Surg* 11:961, 1976.

51. Gregory JR, Campbell JR, Harrison MW, et al: Neonatal necrotizing enterocolitis: A 10 year experience. *Am J Surg* 141:562, 1981.

52. Faulk DL, Anuras S, Freeman JB: Idiopathic chronic intestinal pseudo-obstruction: Use of central venous nutrition. *JAMA* 240:2075, 1978.

53. Byrne WJ, Cipel L, Euler AR, et al: Chronic idiopathic intestinal pseudo-obstruction syndrome in children—Clinical characteristics and prognosis. *J Pediatr* 90:585, 1977.

54. MacFayden BV Jr: The role of IVH in gastrointestinal diseases. *Clinical Consultations in Nutritional Support* 2(1):1, 1982.

55. MacFayden BV Jr, Dudrick SJ, Ruberg RL: Management of gastrointestinal fistulas with parenteral hyperalimentation. *Surgery* 74:100, 1973.

56. Deitel M: Nutritional management of external small bowel fistulas. *Can J Surg* 19:505, 1976.

57. Solomon JR: Nutrition in the severely burned child. *Prog Pediatr Surg* 14:63, 1981.

58. Long JM III: Planning metabolic and nutrition support for severely burned patients. *ASPEN Update* 3(5):1, 1981.

59. Derganc M: Parenteral nutrition in severely burned children. *Scand J Plast Reconstr Surg* 13:195, 1979.

60. Wilmore DW: Parenteral nutrition in burn patients, in Greep JM, Soeters PB, Wesdorp RIC, et al (eds): *Current Concepts in Parenteral Nutrition*. The Hague, Nijhoff Medical Division, 1977, p 227.

61. Woolfson AMJ, Heatley RV, Allison SP: Insulin to inhibit protein catabolism after injury. *N Engl J Med* 300:14, 1979.

62. Abel RM, Beck CH Jr., Abbott WM, et al: Improved survival from acute renal failure following treatment with intravenous L-amino acids and glucose. *N Engl J Med* 288:695, 1973.

63. Baek S, Makabali GG, Bryan-Brown CW, et al: The influence of parenteral nutrition on the course of acute renal failure. *Surg Gynecol Obstet* 141:405, 1975.

64. Abitbol CL, Holliday MA: Total parenteral nutrition in anuric children. *Clin Nephrol* 5:133, 1976.

65. Holliday MA, Wassner S, Ramirez J: Intravenous nutrition in uremic children with protein-energy malnutrition. *Am J Clin Nutr* 31:1854, 1978.

66. Motil KJ, Harmon WE, Grupe WE: Complications of essential amino acid hyperalimentation in children with acute renal failure. *JPEN* 4:32, 1980.

67. Martin DJ: Comparison of commercial EAA solutions for renal failure. *Nutritional Support Services* 1(3):35, 1981.

68. Miller DG: Use of total parenteral nutrition in patients with renal failure. *Nutritional Support Services* 1(2):14, 1981.

69. Gunn T, Reaman G, Outerbridge EW: Peripheral total parenteral nutrition for premature infants with the respiratory distress syndrome: A controlled study. *J Pediatr* 92:608, 1978.

70. Yu VYH, James B, Hendry P, et al: Total parenteral nutrition in very low birthweight infants: A controlled trial. *Arch Dis Child* 54:653, 1979.

71. Sutphen JL: Nutritional support of the pediatric patient. *Clinical Consultations in Nutritional Support* 1(4):1, 1981.

72. Heird WC, Driscoll JM Jr, Schullinger JN, et al: Intravenous alimentation in pediatric patients. *J Pediatr* 80:351, 1972.

73. Denson SE: Nutritional considerations of IV support of the neonate, in Coran AG, Denson SE, Fletcher AB, et al (eds): *The Compromised Neonate*. New York, Pro Clinica, 1980, p 10.

74. Dobbing J: The later development of the brain and its vulnerability, in Davis JA, Dobbing J (eds): *Scientific Foundations of Pediatrics*. Philadelphia, WB Saunders Co, 1974, p 565.

75. Dickerson JWT, Dobbing J, McCance RA: The effect of undernutrition on the postnatal development of the brain and cord in pigs. *Proc R Soc Lond (Biol)* 166:396, 1966–67.

76. Winick M, Noble A: Cellular response in rats during malnutrition at various ages. *J Nutr* 89:300, 1966.

77. Winick M, Rosso P: The effect of severe early malnutrition on cellular growth of human brain. *Pediatr Res* 3:181, 1969.

78. Rosso P, Hormazabol J, Winick M: Changes in brain weight, cholesterol, phospholipid and DNA content in marasmic children. *Am J Clin Nutr* 23:1275, 1970.

79. Kerner JA Jr, Sunshine P: Parenteral alimentation. *Semin Perinatol* 3:417, 1979.

80. Grand RJ, Watkins JB, Torti FM: Development of the human gastrointestinal tract: A review. *Gastroenterology* 70:790, 1976.

81. Cashore WJ, Sedaghatian MR, Usher RH: Nutritional supplements with intravenously administered lipid, protein hydrolysate, and glucose in small premature infants. *Pediatrics* 56:8, 1975.

82. Mueller KJ: Anorexia nervosa. *Clinical Nutrition Newsletter.* December 1981, p 1.

83. Perl M: TPN and the anorexia nervosa patient. *Nutritional Support Services* 1(6):13, 1981.

84. Pertschuk MJ, Forster J, Buzby G, et al: The treatment of anorexia nervosa with total parenteral nutrition. *Biol Psychiatry* 16:539, 1981.

85. Shepherd R, Cooksley WGE, Cooke WDD: Improved growth and clinical, nutritional, and respiratory changes in response to nutritional therapy in cystic fibrosis. *J Pediatr* 97:351, 1980.

86. Chase HP, Long MA, Lavin MH: Cystic fibrosis and malnutrition. *J Pediatr* 95:337, 1979.

87. Freund HR, Ryan JA Jr, Fischer JE: Amino acid derangements in patients with sepsis: Treatment with branched chain amino acid rich infusions. *Ann Surg* 188:423, 1978.

88. Fischer JE, Rosen HM, Ebeid AM, et al: The effect of normalization of plasma amino acids on hepatic encephalopathy in man. *Surgery* 8:77, 1976.

89. Asch MJ, Sherman NJ: Management of refractory chylous ascites by total parenteral nutrition. *J Pediatr* 94:260, 1979.

90. Viswanathan U, Putnam TC: Therapeutic intravenous alimentation for traumatic chylous ascites in a child. *J Pediatr Surg* 9:405, 1974.

91. Preshaw RM, Attisha RP, Hollingsworth WJ, et al: Randomized sequential trial of parenteral nutrition in healing of colonic anastomoses in man. *Can J Surg* 22:437, 1979.

92. Jeejeebhoy KN: TPN and wound healing. *Gastroenterology* 80:621, 1981.

93. Zeigler M, Jakobowski D, Hoelzer D, et al: Route of pediatric parenteral nutrition: Proposed criteria revision. *J Pediatr Surg* 15:472, 1980.

94. Faubion WC, Wesley JR, Coran AG: Calories ordered versus calories received in 20 neonates on peripheral parenteral nutrition. *JPEN* 4:592, 1980.

95. Heird WC: Panel report on nutritional support of pediatric patients. *Am J Clin Nutr* 34:1223, 1981.

2

Nutritional Assessment of the Pediatric Patient

Jo Ann Tatum Hattner
John A. Kerner, Jr.

Because nutrition is such an essential component of normal growth and development, nutritional assessment has traditionally been a part of pediatric care. Assessment of growth, using the measurements of weight, length, and head circumference plotted on growth grids, is routine practice in the pediatrician's office. The clinical examination of children normally includes an evaluation of the physical effects of the child's nutrition. The pediatrician then utilizes the growth grid and the clinical exam to evaluate the child's health status, and when it becomes apparent that growth and development potential are not being attained, further assessment is initiated. Nutritional assessment is not foreign ground in pediatrics; in fact, one might conclude that its roots are in pediatrics.

However, in the early 1970s an increased awareness of the significance of nutritional assessment developed as a result of Butterworth's emphasis on the recognition of iatrogenic (physician induced) malnutrition (1). The further identification of hospitalized adult patients who were malnourished, either as a result of their primary disease process or secondary to treatment of their underlying condition, was reported by clinicians Bistrian and Blackburn (2). With the subsequent development of nutritional assessment methods (3), nutritional assessment attained a new status in medicine. Merritt and Suskind then reported evidence of acute malnutrition in one third of the pediatric inpatient population in Boston (4). This brought attention to the problem of protein energy malnutrition in the pediatric age group.

In the last few years, the nutritional assessment process has become more sophisticated, nutritional support teams have evolved, and numerous articles have been written on the beneficial effects of nutritional assessment and support on treatment responses, wound healing, shortened length of hospital stay, and decreased morbidity and mortality. Presently, nutritional assessment is routine practice for candidates for nutritional support therapy, and the nutritional support teams are fulfilling a needed role in clinical medicine.

The application of the newer assessment techniques and therapies in pediatrics has been focused primarily on the hospitalized patient. The methods of assessment presented can be used in the hospital or, in some cases, in the outpatient clinic. The scope of the assessment will depend upon the individual facility, the age of the child, cost, resources, available laboratory tests, and the expertise of the staff. Critical to any form of assessment is (1) methodology, (2) standards for comparison, and (3) trained health professionals who can design and implement effective nutritional therapies.

Nutritional assessment is a tool to be used to identify the child's nutritional status. It is a mistake to think that only those children with conditions such as failure to thrive, shortness of stature, Crohn's disease, or ulcerative colitis should be assessed. Particularly in pediatrics, nutritional assessment can help determine the potential to tolerate therapies, procedures, or surgery. The rationale for assessment and nutritional monitoring for the adult and pediatric population is essentially the same:

1. To determine the nutritional status of the patient.
2. To provide baseline data to evaluate the effects of therapy.
3. To determine the patient's need for nutritional support.

Pediatric patients, compared to adults, are in a more precarious position with regard to nutritional status. Nutritional deprivation during their hospitalization or therapy may interfere with their growth and development, particularly if it is superimposed on an already poor nutritional status. Therefore, nutritional assessment for the pediatric patient is imperative.

One could argue that a good physical exam by a skilled practitioner is all that is needed to determine nutritional status in children, for children readily reflect nutritional deprivation, such as calorie and protein deficiency, with physical signs. Wasted buttocks, generalized muscle wasting, decreased adipose tissue, and edema are easily recognized. However, although one may document a "normal" physical exam in a child, the diet history may identify potential inadequacies or laboratory investigation may reveal subclinical signs of malnutrition. Anthropometric measurements may provide evidence of depleted adipose or lean tissue stores before depletion is physically apparent. The four facets of the assessment are (1) medical history and clinical exam, (2) diet history and evaluation, (3) anthropometric measurements, and (4) laboratory assessment; each is necessary for a thorough assessment. Assessment should be done upon hospital admission and as initial screening performed in an outpatient setting.

Medical History and Clinical Exam

A medical history should include a review of social history, growth and development milestones, digestive abnormalities, any episodes of severe vomiting or diarrhea, trauma, and drug history. In the physical exam, actual physical manifestations of nutrient deficiencies are usually present only in children with severe deficiency states. Milder, more subclinical signs may be present in a child undergoing subtle forms of malnutrition, for example, pale conjunctivae as a manifestation of anemia. Most common findings in children are often on epithelial surfaces. Therefore, a thorough exam of the skin, hair, and nails is indicated, as is examination of mucosal surfaces, which readily reflect nutritional insults.

Because many signs are nonspecific and can be of nutritional or environmental etiology, laboratory assessment of the suspect nutrient is indicated when a physical sign is noted. Usually, abnormalities will be present if the physical sign is observed, unless the sign is indicative of a former nutritional insult that has since been corrected (e.g., depigmented bands in the hair). Since the presence of a physical sign is in the eye of the beholder, laboratory evaluation is essential to document objective data. Table 1 summarizes clinical signs that have been described in the malnourished child and adult (5–7). The suspect nutrient and supportive objective findings that can be identified in either the serum or urine and that indicate abnormalities are included (7,8). Those findings that involve bone may be supported by x-ray films.

Diet History and Evaluation

In pediatrics there are two parts to a diet history. The first is the feeding history, which is normally contained in the medical history, and the second is the documentation and evaluation of the child's present normal intake. Both are important to nutritional assessment; the feeding history describes past nutrition, and the intake history, present nutrition.

A thorough feeding history will document whether or not a child has experienced normal nutrient intake and if any foods have been eliminated. The feeding history should include the child's first food as an infant, either breast milk or type of formula, and the time and sequence of the introduction of foods, with any intolerances noted. Of particular interest is the age at which highly allergenic foods, such as cow's milk and eggs, were added to the diet and their tolerance. The feeding history should include any foods that were eliminated from the diet and the reason for the elimination. This documentation of elimination diets, noting the age of the child and the length of time for the elimination, may be important for later assessment. For children 2 to 5 years old it is advantageous to ask about aversions to foods and whether or not these foods have been completely eliminated from the diet. This is important, since the elimination of foods that normally contribute important nutrients to the diet may put the child at risk for nutritional deficiency.

The feeding history may also be accomplished using a questionnaire that is completed by the parent (Fig. 1). A brief questionnaire needs to be supplemented with further questioning; however, it provides some of the basic information needed for a diet history.

The second part is the food intake history, which includes documentation and evaluation of the present food intake pattern. There are many ways to conduct this; however, the most common method is to obtain a typical day's intake (24-hour recall) (9). The intake is then evaluated by comparing actual intake to recommended intake for age. This history should be taken by a dietitian who possesses the interviewing skills and knowledge of food composition and normal food patterns of specific age groups.

The day's intake should include everything the child normally eats and drinks for a 24-hour period. The foods are recorded in approximate amounts, since one cannot expect exactness in this kind of food history. This information is best obtained from the child's mother or the primary care-giver. It is worthwhile to divide the day into periods of time—early morning, midmorning, noon, afternoon, eve-

Table 1. Clinical Signs and Laboratory Findings in the Malnourished Child and Adult

Clinical Sign	Suspect Nutrient	Supportive Objective Findings
EPITHELIAL		
Skin		
Xerosis, dry scaling	Essential fatty acids	Triene/tetraene ratio > 0.4 (see Chapter 7)
Hyperkeratosis, plaques around hair follicles	Vitamin A	↓ Plasma retinol
Ecchymoses, petechiae	Vitamin K	Prolonged prothrombin time
	Vitamin C	↓ Serum ascorbic acid
Hair		
Easily plucked, dyspigmented, lackluster	Protein–calorie	↓ Total protein
		↓ Albumin
		↓ Transferrin
Nails		
Thin, spoon shaped	Iron	↓ Serum Fe
		↑ TIBC
MUCOSAL		
Mouth, lips, and tongue	B vitamins	
Angular stomatitis (inflammation at corners of mouth)	B_2 (riboflavin)	↓ RBC glutathione reductase
Cheilosis (reddened lips with fissures at angles)	B_2	See above
	B_6 (pyridoxine)	↓ Plasma Pyridoxal phosphate[a]
Glossitis (inflammation of tongue)	B_6	See above
	B_2	See above
	B_3 (niacin)	↓ Plasma tryptophan
		↓ Urinary N-methyl nicotinamide[a]
Magenta tongue	B_2	See above
Edema of tongue, tongue fissures	B_3	See above
Gums		
Spongy, bleeding	Vitamin C	↓ Plasma ascorbic acid
OCULAR		
Pale conjunctivae secondary to anemia	Iron	↓ Serum Fe, ↑ TIBC,
	Folic acid	↓ serum folic acid, or
		↓ RBC folic acid
	Vitamin B_{12}	↓ Serum B_{12}
	Copper	↓ Serum copper
Bitot's spots (grayish, yellow, or white foamy spots on the whites of the eye)	Vitamin A	↓ Plasma retinol
Conjunctival or corneal xerosis, keratomalacia (softening of part or all of cornea)	Vitamin A	↓ Plasma retinol
MUSCULOSKELETAL		
Craniotabes (thinning of the inner table of the skull); palpable enlargement of costochondral junctions ("rachitic rosary"); thickening of wrists and ankles	Vitamin D	↓ 25-OH-vit D
		↑ Alkaline phosphatase
		± ↓ Ca, ↓ PO_4
		Bone films

Table 1. (Continued)

Clinical Sign	Suspect Nutrient	Supportive Objective Findings
Scurvy (tenderness of extremities, hemorrhages under periosteum of long bones; enlargement of costochondral junction; cessation of osteogenesis of long bones)	Vitamin C	↓ Serum ascorbic acid Long bone films
Skeletal Lesions	Copper	↓ Serum copper X-ray film changes similar to scurvy since copper is also essential for normal collagen formation
Muscle wasting, prominence of body skeleton, poor muscle tone	Protein–calorie	↓ Serum proteins ↓ Arm muscle circumference
GENERAL Edema	Protein	↓ Serum proteins
Pallor 2° to anemia	Vitamin E (in premature infants)	↓ Serum Vitamin E ↑ Peroxide hemolysis Evidence of hemolysis on on blood smear
	Iron	↓ Serum Fe, ↑ TIBC
	Folic acid	↓ Serum folic acid Macrocytosis on RBC smear
	Vitamin B_{12}	↓ Serum B_{12} Macrocytosis on RBC smear
	Copper	↓ Serum copper
INTERNAL SYSTEMS Nervous Mental confusion	Protein	↓ Total protein, ↓ albumin, ↓ transferrin
	Vitamin B_1 (thiamine)	↓ RBC transketolase
Cardiovascular Beriberi (enlarged heart, congestive heart failure, tachycardia)	Vitamin B_1	Same as above
Tachycardia 2° to anemia	Iron Folic Acid B_{12} Copper Vitamin E (in premature infants)	See above
GASTROINTESTINAL Hepatomegaly	Protein–calorie	↓ Total protein, ↓ albumin, ↓ transferrin
GLANDULAR Thyroid enlargement	Iodine	↓ Total serum iodine: inorganic, PBI[a]

[a] Bio Science Laboratories, 7600 Tyrone Avenue, Van Nyes, Calif, 91405

Nutrition Questionnaire

1. Breast fed this child: Yes _____ No _____ How Long _____
2. Formula fed: Yes _____ No _____ What Brands _____
3. Solid foods started at what age? Fruits _____ Juices _____
   Cereals _____ Vegetables _____ Meats _____ Crackers _____
4. Directions: Please answer questions appropriate for the age of your child.

   A. *Infant*   Yes No
      If you are breast feeding, are you having any problems?   ___ ___
      If feeding formula, do you feed over 1 quart (32 oz) a day?   ___ ___
      Do you feed only breast or formula?   ___ ___
      Have you given your infant regular cow's milk on a regular basis?   ___ ___
      Please list the solid foods and amount you might feed in one day. _____
      _____
      _____

   B. *Over 1 year*   Yes No
      Does your child drink over 1 quart of milk per day?   ___ ___
      Does your child have a poor appetite at meal time?   ___ ___
      Do you think your child is underweight?   ___ ___
                                    overweight?   ___ ___
      Have you eliminated any foods from your child's diet?   ___ ___
      Do you have concerns about your child's diet?   ___ ___
      Please list your child's five favorite foods:
      _____ , _____ , _____ , _____ ,
      _____ , _____

Figure 1 Example of a feeding history questionaire to be completed by the parent.

ning, and bedtime. With children, intake normally begins in the morning. With infants, document feedings after midnight to the next midnight, in order to include night feedings.

Once the normal intake is recorded it is evaluated for key nutrient composition. Some dietitians have access to computer analysis for evaluation. With computer analysis, actual nutrients ingested are usually compared to recommended daily dietary allowances for age. When computer analysis is unavailable, another way to evaluate the diet is to use the food groups for classifying foods and then to compare the actual number of servings eaten to those recommended for age. Foods are classified into groups based on their nutrient composition. The use of food groups is particularly helpful in the evaluation of children's diets. If, for example, a food intake history reveals that the child does not ingest foods from the milk and milk products group, one would suspect a very low intake of calcium, vitamin D, riboflavin, and thiamine.

A useful way to check the accuracy of a 24-hour record is to do an approximation of the number of calories ingested. If it deviates greatly from what a normal caloric intake should be for a child the same age and weight, then one would question the accuracy of the information regarding amounts. The history should still be useful, however, for determining the quality of the diet. The form illustrated in Figure 2 is designed to facilitate the recording and evaluation of a typical day's intake. This form also contains a brief summary of the child's height and weight, along with an evaluation of the adequacy of calories ingested.

The interview should begin with questions such as "Was yesterday a typical day for your child?" or, if the child is hospitalized, "Can you describe a normal day's intake for your child?" Other questions that are important include "Are you with the child normally?" and "Does anyone else care for your child?" The interviewer goes on to say "I'd like for you to describe to me your child's intake for the day, including all food and beverages taken. Let's begin with the time your child woke up in the morning. What was the first thing eaten?" As the parent or care-giver describes the intake, a skilled interviewer will ask more probing questions to complete the history. For example, the interviewer may ask, "Does your child normally have a snack before bed?" After collecting the day's intake, the foods are classified into food groups and the number of servings from each group is summarized. The actual foods ingested are then compared with the recommended pattern for age (Table 2). For evaluation of calories, Table 3 contains recommended intake of calories per kilogram (11).

Anthropometric Measurements

Anthropometric measurements which are normally obtained in the routine examination of children include height, weight, and head circumference (until 3 years of age). These measurements are used to assess physical size and growth. The addition of upper arm circumference and skinfold thickness (most commonly triceps) allows for more accurate nutritional assessment, since these two measurements provide information regarding body composition. The skinfold thickness is a measurement of the subcutaneous fat layer, which is an indication of energy stores. The arm muscle area, which can be calculated from the upper arm circumference and skinfold measurement, is an indication of the status of skeletal muscle mass. These two measurements have gained acceptance and credibility in pediatrics because they are simple, noninvasive, and can be compared to established standards. Although these measurements may not be sensitive enough to reflect short-term changes, they may be used to document changes in body fat and somatic protein stores in response to long-term therapy (11,12).

The standards most commonly used for assessing physical growth for the United States population are the National Center for Health Statistics (NCHS) percentiles published in 1976. The NCHS percentiles are based on data collected from a large cross sectional and representative sample of infants, children, and adolescents in the United States (13,14). Smoother percentile curves were derived from the data for boys and girls from birth to 36 months for (1) head circumference for age, (2) recumbent length for age, (3) weight for age, (4) weight for length. For boys and girls from 2 to 18 years of age, percentile curves were derived for (1) stature for age and (2) body weight for age. A body weight for stature table is provided to assess weight for length of boys and girls up to middle childhood. All the curves described above are presented in Figure 3a–h. The curves for each growth chart contain seven percentiles: fifth, tenth, twenty-fifth, fiftieth, seventy-fifth, ninetieth, and ninety-fifth.

The use of these standards is accurate only when the measurement techniques are the same as those in the data collection. Infants should be weighed nude, and length should be measured in the recumbent position. The growth charts for birth

Diet History: Date_____ Name_____ Sex_____ Age_____ Ht_____ cm_____ % Wt_____ Kg_____ % Wt/Ht_____ %

Time/Place	Description of Food or Drink	Amount	Food Groups						Approximate Calories
			Milk and Milk Prod.	Protein	Grains	Fruits and Veg.	Fats	Other	
		Total Serv. Eaten							Total
Supplements:		# Sugg. for Age							# Sugg. /Kg
		Plus or Minus Diff.							Plus or Minus Difference

Figure 2 Example of a form used to record and evaluate daily intake.

Table 2. Recommended Food Patterns

Key Nutrients	Food Groups	Serving Size	Infants (mo) 0–4	4–8	8–12	Children (yr) 1–3	4–6	7–10	Adolescents (yr) 11–14	15–18
Protein, calcium, phosphorus, magnesium, vitamin A, D, B_{12} and riboflavin.	Milk and milk products Milk: nonfat, lowfat, whole	8 oz	Human milk or formula							
	Cheeses (brick and soft)	1.5 oz	18–36 oz		24–32 oz	2 serv	3 serv	3 serv	4 serv	4 or more serv
	Yogurt	8 oz								
Protein, phosphorus, iron, B_6, B_{12}, niacin riboflavin and thiamine	Protein foods Animal sources: meat, fish, poultry egg	3 oz 1 (2–3 ×/wk)		1/3 serv	1/2 serv	1 serv	1½ serv	2 serv	2 serv	2 or more serv
	Vegetable sources: dried beans, peas	3/4 cup				1/2 serv (veg pro)	1 serv (veg pro)	2 serv (veg pro)	2 serv (veg pro)	2 serv (veg pro)
	Peanut butter, nuts	1 oz								
	Soy products (tofu)	3 oz								
Iron, thiamine, riboflavin, niacin, and vitamin E.	Grains Cereals: cooked or dry	3/4 cup		1 serv	2 or more serv	3 or more serv	3 or more serv	4 or more serv	5 or more serv	6 or more serv
	Crackers and breads, whole grain or enriched	3–5 crackers or 1 slice bread								
	Starches: rice, noodles, grits	1/2 cup								
Vitamins C and A (carotene), riboflavin and folic acid.	Fruits and vegetables Vitamin C rich: orange, grapefruit, tomato, cantaloupe, berries	1/2 cup		1/2 serv	1/2 serv	1 serv	1 serv	1 serv	1 serv	1 serv
	Carotene rich: dark green (spinach, broccolli); greens or deep yellow (carrots, squash, sweet potato)	1/2 cup		1/2 serv	1/2 serv	1/2 serv	1 serv	1 serv	2 serv	2 serv
	Other fresh fruits and vegetables	1/2 cup			1/2 serv	1/2 serv	1 serv	1 serv	2 or more serv	2 or more serv
Vitamins A and E, and essential fatty acids	Fats Oils, butter, margarine	2 Tblsp			1/4 serv	1/2 serv	1 serv	1 serv	1 or more serv	1 or more serv
Energy	Other foods Contributors to energy: e.g., desserts, snack foods		— dependent upon caloric needs —							

Table 3. Suggested Calories per Kilogram

Age	Calories per kilogram
Infants	
0–0.5 yr	117
0.5–1.0 yr	105
Children	
1–3 yrs	100
4–6 yrs	85–90
7–10 yrs	80–85
11–14 yrs	boys: 60–64 girls: 48–55
15–18 yrs	boys: 43–49 girls: 38–40

SOURCE: Adapted from *Food and Nutrition Board, National Research Council Recommended Daily Dietary Allowances,* rev 9th ed and 10th ed. Washington, DC, National Academy of Sciences 1974, 1979.

to 36 months should only be used with recumbent length measurements. After 2 years of age children can be weighed in light garments and in the standing position for height in stocking feet. Children measured by this latter method should then be plotted on the growth charts for 2 to 18 years old. Accurate chronological age is essential when using growth charts for assessment. For more complete description of measurement techniques refer to the text by Fomon (15).

The growth charts have many uses in the clinical assessment of physical size and growth. A single plotting at the time of presentation may be used to assess how a child ranks in comparison to other children of the same age and sex in the United States. When a measurement is below the tenth percentile, it should first be checked for accuracy, and, if accurate, further evaluated. A useful parameter that may stimulate further evaluation is the weight for length for infants and children. If the child is fifth percentile or lower in weight for length, it may reflect a state of acute malnutrition. On the other hand, if the patient has decreased height for age, if may reflect chronic undernutrition (8). The normality of the growth rate can be assessed when there are interval measurements available for plotting. Under normal conditions the growth is channeled, and continues along channels during childhood, usually varying within two percentiles. Greater variation in the prepubescent child and the adolescent is common. However, if in childhood the plottings decrease progressively and a decrease of more than two percentiles is observed, the possibility of inadequate nutrition exists. The charts are helpful in differentiating the child who is small for age, but proportionately so, and the child who has disproportionate weight for length.

Roche and Himes (16) published incremental growth charts based on serial data from healthy white children in the United States. These charts are for 6 month intervals; they extend up to 18 years of age. The charts can be used to assess growth velocity, or increment divided by time measurements. These may be particularly useful when an infant or preadolescent child is identified as below the tenth percentile in size or when the growth channel has shifted dramatically. It may also be helpful to assess growth rate before and after therapy. The incremental growth charts are available for (1) weight: 6 months to 36 months; (2) recumbent length: 6 months to 36 months; (3) head circumference: 6 months to 36 months; (4) stature: 2 years to 18 years; (5) weight: 2 years to 18 years. There are separate charts for

NCHS percentiles for length and weight for age, boys, birth to 36 months.

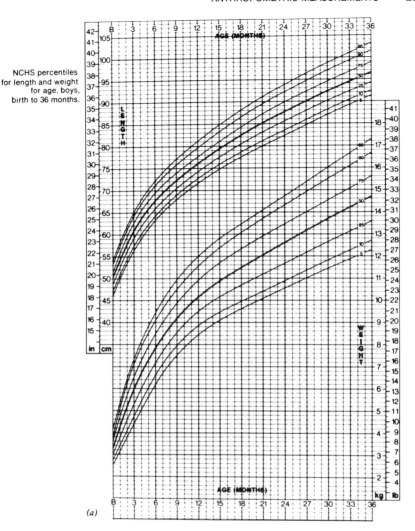

(a)

Figure 3a–h Adapted from Hamill PVV, Drizd TA, Johnson CL, Reed RB, Roche AF, Moore WM: Physical growth: National Center for Health Statistics percentiles. Courtesy of Ross Laboratories, Columbus, Ohio.

boys and girls, making a total of ten. We feel they can be used effectively with the NCHS growth charts (16).

The standards available for assessing skinfold thickness, mid-upper arm circumference, and arm muscle area in children come from the American and British literature. Standards for triceps and subscapular skinfold thickness developed by Tanner and Whitehouse appeared in the British literature in 1962 (17); revised standards were published in 1975 (18). Their percentile standards are based on measurements of the left side performed on boys and girls aged 1 month to 19 years. Although most clinicians use only a triceps skinfold measurement in nutri-

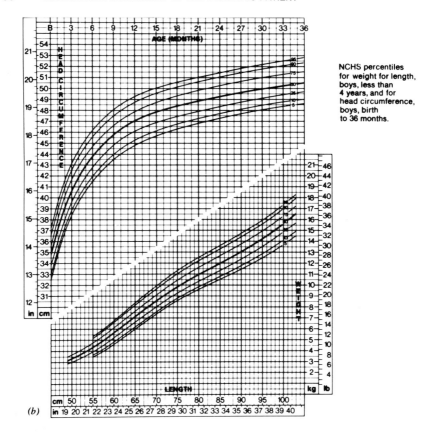

NCHS percentiles
for weight for length,
boys, less than
4 years, and for
head circumference,
boys, birth
to 36 months.

(b)

tional assessment, the subscapular measurement may also be useful. Tanner and Whitehouse recommend that two sites, one on the limbs and one on the trunk be measured. The subscapular measurement, particularly in young infants, is a simple measurement to perform. Tanner and Whitehouse standards are applicable only to measurements taken with the Harpenden and Holtain caliper. The authors emphasize that their standards represent actual percentiles observed and do not imply desirability of distribution of subcutaneous fat, although a child at third percentile should perhaps be considered undernourished. Tanner and Whitehouse's standards are presented in Figure 4.

In 1974 Frisancho developed norms for triceps skinfold and arm circumference, and arm muscle diameter, circumference, and area (19). The percentiles are for right arm measurements and were compiled from data collected from a sample of white males and females from birth to 44 years who participated in the Ten State Nutrition Survey of 1968–1970. Measurements were made with the Lange skinfold caliper. The percentiles for arm muscle diameter, arm muscle circumference and arm muscle area were derived from calculations for each individual. Frisancho advises that evaluations of arm muscle area are valuable in evaluations of nutritional status of children because they show greater changes with age than diameter

NCHS percentiles
length and weight
for age, girls,
birth to 36 months.

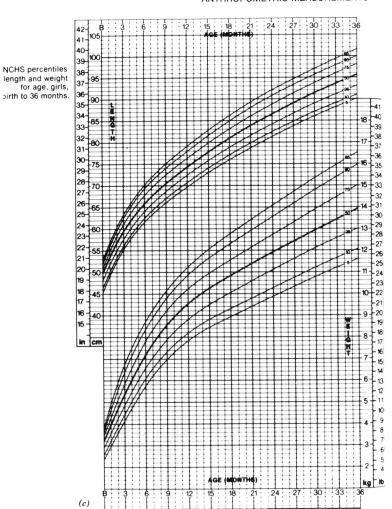

(c)

or circumference. Frisancho recently published new norms for triceps skinfold, arm circumference, arm muscle circumference, arm muscle area, and arm fat area (20). The norms differ from those previously published in that they are derived from data collected on white subjects participating in the Health and Nutrition Examination Survey I (Hanes I) during 1971–1974. Frisancho recommends that these more appropriate new norms replace those currently in use (20), and that they be used in conjunction with the NCHS weight for height percentiles for children. Because these two norms are based on the same population samples they provide a uniform reference.

In the Hanes survey, measurements of skinfold were made on the right side with the Lange skinfold caliper (21). Frisancho's percentiles for upper limb fat and muscle areas were derived from calculations for each subject. The equations for

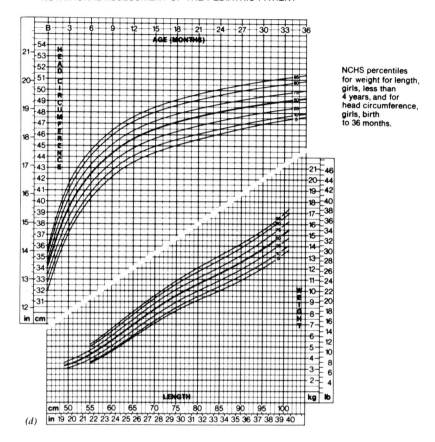

NCHS percentiles
for weight for length,
girls, less than
4 years, and for
head circumference,
girls, birth
to 36 months.

(d)

computation are contained in his article (20). For a simpler method of obtaining arm muscle area and arm muscle circumference, Gurney and Jelliffe devised an arm anthropometry nomogram for children (22). The nomogram can be used for rapid calculation of arm muscle circumference and arm muscle area for comparison with Frisancho's percentiles. Tables 4–6 contain Frisancho's new norms, and Figure 5 contains Gurney and Jelliffe's nomogram.

For very young infants, Oakley et al. reported in the British literature in 1977 standards for triceps and subscapular skinfolds (23). The data were collected on caucasian newborn infants 37–42 weeks after gestation, and at 0.25 kg birth weight intervals between 2.25 kg and 4.5 kg for males and females. These percentiles are particularly useful because one can use weight as well as age. Harpenden and Holtain calipers were used, and, as with Tanner and Whitehouse, the left side was measured. Their percentiles are presented in Figures 6–9.

For data on premature infants, a group of investigators headed by Vaucher at Tucson, Arizona measured caucasian infants from 24–42 weeks gestation (24). Their data is comprised of skinfold measurements taken at eight sites with bilateral measurements of the biceps, triceps, subscapular, and abdominal skinfolds using

NCHS percentiles
for stature and
weight for age, boys,
2 to 18 years.

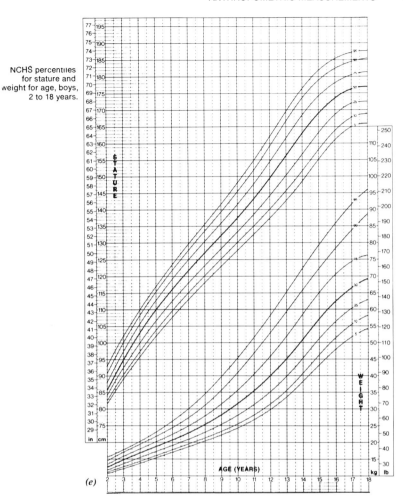

(e)

the Lange skinfold caliper. Their measurements also include arm circumference (a mean of the right and left)with calculated cross-sectional nonfat and fat area.

Methods for collection of anthropometric data with detailed description of the appropriate techniques required are contained in the articles we have cited above. Various texts also contain descriptions of techniques for measurements (6–8,15,25,26). Table 7 contains the methods developed for performing measurements for nutritional assessment of infants and children at Stanford University Hospital. It is most important that a standardized method be used and that a trained examiner perform the measurements.

When anthropometric data obtained from an infant or child indicate depleted lean body mass stores, laboratory confirmation should be obtained to complete the assessment. The status of lean body mass is evaluated by measurements of somatic and visceral proteins. This data is essential before a treatment plan is initiated. It

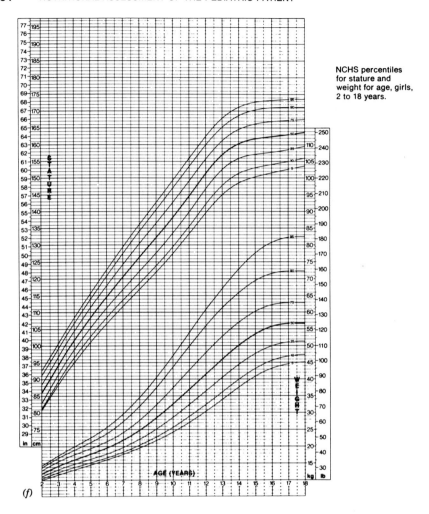

NCHS percentiles
for stature and
weight for age, girls,
2 to 18 years.

(f)

can also be used in conjunction with anthropometric measurements during treatment to assess recovery.

Laboratory Assessment

Laboratory tests are of particular value in nutritional assessment because they are objective and can be used to confirm subjective findings. Findings on clinical exam that can be supported by laboratory tests are discussed earlier and illustrated in Table 1. Further tests performed for the evaluation of nutritional status should provide information on somatic protein mass (skeletal muscle mass), visceral protein mass (interior organ protein), and the cellular immune system.

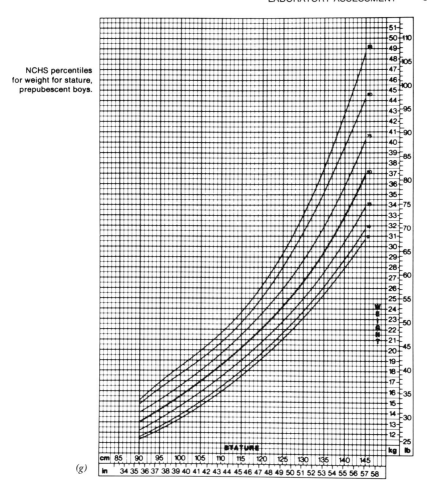

NCHS percentiles for weight for stature, prepubescent boys.

(g)

The somatic protein mass is assessed by the measurement of creatinine excretion. Creatinine (creatinine anhydride) is derived from creatine, a nitrogenous compound synthesized in the body. Because the conversion of creatine to creatinine occurs only in muscle, its excretion in the urine is a reflection of muscle mass (27,28). In protein–calorie malnutrition (PCM) there is loss of body protein. Children with severe PCM have reduced creatinine excretion, which increases as the child recovers (29). Viteri and Alvarado demonstrated the use of their creatinine height index (CHI) to evaluate the magnitude of protein deficiency in children with PCM and during recovery and protein repletion (29). They define the CHI as a ratio consisting of the creatinine excretion of a child per unit of time (24 hours) divided by the normal excretion value for a child of the same height, regardless of age. The CHI has been devised for estimating the relative muscle mass of children. The child's height rather than weight is used, since height is more indicative of lean body mass, whereas weight reflects fat tissue as well. Viteri and Alvarado found a

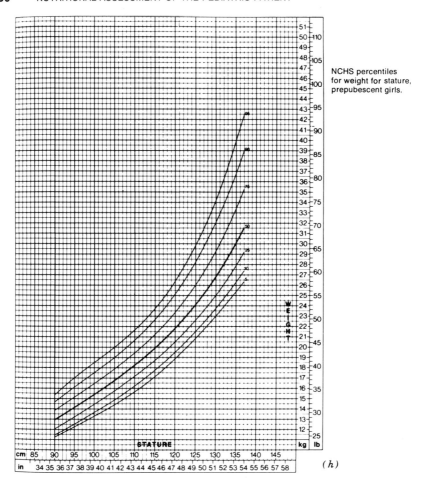

NCHS percentiles for weight for stature, prepubescent girls.

(h)

negative correlation between CHI and nitrogen retention, indicating the physiological significance of the CHI in estimating protein nutrition (29).

Bistrian and Blackburn then suggested a role for this technique in the nutritional assessment of surgical patients (30). In their study, they found the CHI to be more sensitive than other measures of nutritional status such as nitrogen balance and serum albumin. The CHI has now been incorporated into nutritional assessment and has gained acceptance as a sensitive indicator of somatic protein status. Many prefer to use the CHI calculation times 100, which is a calculation of percentage of standard. With children the main limitation to this test is that the data base available for ideal values of urinary creatinine is limited. Viteri and Alvarado's publication contains expected creatinine excretion of children ranging in height from 50–132 cm (29). Cheek contains tables for normal male infants and for females and males with heights to 175 cm (31). Merritt has combined the two sources into one table for easier reference (8). The test also requires an accurate 24-hour urine collection

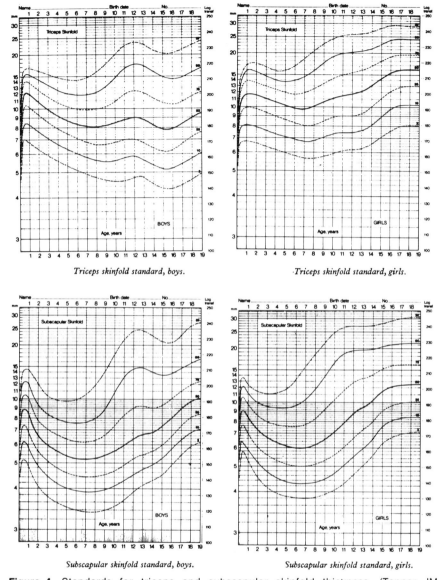

Triceps skinfold standard, boys.

·Triceps skinfold standard, girls.

Subscapular skinfold standard, boys.

Subscapular skinfold standard, girls.

Figure 4 Standards for triceps and subscapular skinfold thickness. (Tanner JM, Whitehouse RH: Revised standards for triceps and subscapular skinfolds in British children. *Arch Dis Child* 50:142, 1975. Reprinted with permission.)

Table 4. Percentiles for Triceps Skinfold for Whites of the United States Health and Nutrition Examination Survey I of 1971 to 1974

Age group	Males								Females							
	n	5	10	25	50	75	90	95	n	5	10	25	50	75	90	95
1–1.9	228	6	7	8	10	12	14	16	204	6	7	8	10	12	14	16
2–2.9	223	6	7	8	10	12	14	15	208	6	8	9	10	12	15	16
3–3.9	220	6	7	8	10	11	14	15	208	7	8	9	11	12	14	15
4–4.9	230	6	6	8	9	11	12	14	208	7	8	8	10	12	14	16
5–5.9	214	6	6	8	9	11	14	15	219	6	7	8	10	12	15	18
6–6.9	117	5	6	7	8	10	13	16	118	6	6	8	10	12	14	16
7–7.9	122	5	6	7	9	12	15	17	126	6	7	9	11	13	16	18
8–8.9	117	5	6	7	8	10	13	16	118	6	8	9	12	15	18	24
9–9.9	121	6	6	7	10	13	17	18	125	8	8	10	13	16	20	22
10–10.9	146	6	6	8	10	14	18	21	152	7	8	10	12	17	23	27
11–11.9	122	6	6	8	11	16	20	24	117	7	8	10	13	18	24	28
12–12.9	153	6	6	8	11	14	22	28	129	8	9	11	14	18	23	27
13–13.9	134	5	5	7	10	14	22	26	151	8	8	12	15	21	26	30
14–14.9	131	4	5	7	9	14	21	24	141	9	10	13	16	21	26	28
15–15.9	128	4	5	6	8	11	18	24	117	8	10	12	17	21	25	32
16–16.9	131	4	5	6	8	12	16	22	142	10	12	15	18	22	26	31
17–17.9	133	5	5	6	8	12	16	19	114	10	12	13	19	24	30	37
18–18.9	91	4	5	6	9	13	20	24	109	10	12	15	18	22	26	30
19–24.9	531	4	5	7	10	15	20	22	1060	10	11	14	18	24	30	34
25–34.9	971	5	6	8	12	16	20	24	1987	10	12	16	21	27	34	37
35–44.9	806	5	6	8	12	16	20	23	1614	12	14	18	23	29	35	38
45–54.9	898	6	6	8	12	15	20	25	1047	12	16	20	25	30	36	40
55–64.9	734	5	6	8	11	14	19	22	809	12	16	20	25	31	36	38
65–74.9	1503	4	6	8	11	15	19	22	1670	12	14	18	24	29	34	36

Triceps Skinfold Percentiles (mm²)

SOURCE: Frisancho AR: New norms of upper limb fat and muscle areas for assessment of nutritional status. *Am J Clin Nutr* 34:2540–2545, 1981. Reprinted with permission.

(which is often difficult to obtain), and the urine output and renal function must be normal. The presence of infection has been reported to cause elevation of creatinine excretion (32,33).

Nitrogen balance determinations can also be performed in the hospital setting; this test also requires a 24-hour urine collection. The balance study is a measure of the net effect of protein anabolism and catabolism. The nitrogen intake is calculated from food nitrogen ingested and requires a strict recording of the child's intake. The excretion of nitrogen is measured by urinary urea, (as urea makes up about 90% of total urinary nitrogen) with factors added to account for stool, skin, and nonurinary nitrogen loss. For a more detailed discussion refer to Grant (6), Foman (34), and Cheek (35). A negative nitrogen balance, with a greater amount of nitrogen being excreted than ingested, may be indicative of catabolism and may occur in malnutrition or starvation. Positive nitrogen balance, with more nitrogen being ingested than excreted, reflects net protein anabolism. One may observe this in a malnourished patient during recovery. Nitrogen balance studies are difficult to perform in children because nitrogen intake is often overestimated and nitrogen output underestimated. Therefore, tests results must be viewed with a scrutinizing eye. Some clinicians use nitrogen balance determinations during the recovery period as a measure of repletion of muscle mass (36). Hendry reports nitrogen balance studies to be of value to predict nitrogen requirements of small premature infants (37). Reichman et al. report its use in premature infants who demonstrated deposition rates of protein comparable to the fetus and rates of fat deposition three times that of the fetus (38).

Another biochemical measure under study for use in estimating somatic protein mass is urinary 3-methylhistidine (3MH) (39,40). This amino acid is contained in muscle protein, is released when muscle protein is degraded, and is not recycled, but is quantitatively excreted in the urine. It is, therefore, indicative of muscle turnover (muscle protein catabolism). Kim et al. in their study of primarily adult patients, found it to be a good index of both the status of protein nutrition and the fluctuation of muscle protein catabolism (40). Seashore et al. suggest that a 3MH/creatinine ratio can be useful clinically as a sensitive indicator of metabolic status, particularly in infants receiving parenteral nutrition (PN) (41). Most conclude that this method can be used to measure total body muscle mass only if a reliable 24-hour urine collection can be accomplished and if no increased rate of muscle turnover is present. This assay requires an amino acid analyzer.

We feel that a routine assessment of the somatic protein compartment can be simply and accurately accomplished by a determination of CHI, a measurement of arm circumference and triceps skinfold with a calculation of arm muscle area. Table 8 includes a brief description of indicators, including the calculation of arm muscle circumference.

The visceral (interior organ) protein mass is evaluated by a measure of the serum concentrations of liver secretory transport proteins. Their acceptance as useful parameters in initial nutritional screening and during treatment and recovery is based on publications that demonstrate their value for assessing visceral protein status in the pediatric population (42–44,46–50). The decision as to which proteins to assess should be based on the knowledge of what each measurement can contribute to your assessment. A serum albumin is useful in assessing PCM. In the pediatric literature, PCM is recognized as presenting in two forms, kwashiorkor and marasmus. The finding of edema on the physical exam, and severe hypop-

Table 5. Percentiles of Upper Arm Circumference (mm) and Estimated Upper Arm Muscle Circumference (mm) for Whites of the United States Health and Nutrition Examination Survey I of 1971 to 1974

Age Group	Arm Circumference (mm)							Arm Muscle Circumference (mm)						
	5	10	25	50	75	90	95	5	10	25	50	75	90	95
Males														
1–1.9	142	146	150	159	170	176	183	110	113	119	127	135	144	147
2–2.9	141	145	153	162	170	178	185	111	114	122	130	140	146	150
3–3.9	150	153	160	167	175	184	190	117	123	131	137	143	148	153
4–4.9	149	154	162	171	180	186	192	123	126	133	141	148	156	159
5–5.9	153	160	167	175	185	195	204	128	133	140	147	154	162	169
6–6.9	155	159	167	179	188	209	228	131	135	142	151	161	170	177
7–7.9	162	167	177	187	201	223	230	137	139	151	160	168	177	190
8–8.9	162	170	177	190	202	220	245	140	145	154	162	170	182	187
9–9.9	175	178	187	200	217	249	257	151	154	161	170	183	196	202
10–10.9	181	184	196	210	231	262	274	156	160	166	180	191	209	221
11–11.9	186	190	202	223	244	261	280	159	165	173	183	195	205	230
12–12.9	193	200	214	232	254	282	303	167	171	182	195	210	223	241
13–13.9	194	211	228	247	263	286	301	172	179	196	211	226	238	245
14–14.9	220	226	237	253	283	303	322	189	199	212	223	240	260	264
15–15.9	222	229	244	264	284	311	320	199	204	218	237	254	266	272
16–16.9	244	248	262	278	303	324	343	213	225	234	249	269	287	296
17–17.9	246	253	267	285	308	336	347	224	231	245	258	273	294	312
18–18.9	245	260	276	297	321	353	379	226	237	252	264	283	298	324
19–24.9	262	272	288	308	331	355	372	238	245	257	273	289	309	321
25–34.9	271	282	300	319	342	362	375	243	250	264	279	298	314	326
35–44.9	278	287	305	326	345	363	374	247	255	269	286	302	318	327
45–54.9	267	281	301	322	342	362	376	239	249	265	281	300	315	326
55–64.9	258	273	296	317	336	355	369	236	245	260	278	295	310	320
65–74.9	248	263	285	307	325	344	355	223	235	251	268	284	298	306

Females

Age (years)														
1–1.9	138	142	148	156	164	172	177	105	111	117	124	132	139	143
2–2.9	142	145	152	160	167	176	184	111	114	119	126	133	142	147
3–3.9	143	150	158	167	175	183	189	113	119	124	132	140	146	152
4–4.9	149	154	160	169	177	184	191	115	121	128	136	144	152	157
5–5.9	153	157	165	175	185	203	211	125	128	134	142	151	159	165
6–6.9	156	162	170	176	187	204	211	130	133	138	145	154	166	171
7–7.9	164	167	174	183	199	216	231	129	135	142	151	160	171	176
8–8.9	168	172	183	195	214	247	261	138	140	151	160	171	183	194
9–9.9	178	182	194	211	224	251	260	147	150	158	167	180	194	198
10–10.9	174	182	193	210	228	251	265	148	150	159	170	180	190	197
11–11.9	185	194	208	224	248	276	303	150	158	171	181	196	217	223
12–12.9	194	203	216	237	256	282	294	162	166	180	191	201	214	220
13–13.9	202	211	223	243	271	301	338	169	175	183	198	211	226	240
14–14.9	214	223	237	252	272	304	322	174	179	190	201	216	232	247
15–15.9	208	221	239	254	279	300	322	175	178	189	202	215	228	244
16–16.9	218	224	241	258	283	318	334	170	180	190	202	216	234	249
17–17.9	220	227	241	264	295	324	350	175	183	194	205	221	239	257
18–18.9	222	227	241	258	281	312	325	174	179	191	202	215	237	245
19–24.9	221	230	247	265	290	319	345	179	185	195	207	221	236	249
25–34.9	233	240	256	277	304	342	368	183	188	199	212	228	246	264
35–44.9	241	251	267	290	317	356	378	186	192	205	218	236	257	272
45–54.9	242	256	274	299	328	362	384	187	193	206	220	238	260	274
55–64.9	243	257	280	303	335	367	385	187	196	209	225	244	266	280
65–74.9	240	252	274	299	326	356	373	185	195	208	225	244	264	279

SOURCE: Frisancho AR: New norms of upper limb fat and muscle areas for assessment of nutritional status. Am J Clin Nutr 34:2540–2545, 1981. Reprinted with permission.

Table 6. Percentiles for Estimates of Upper Arm Fat Area (mm²) and Upper Arm Muscle Area (mm²) for Whites of the United States Health Examination Survey I of 1971 to 1974

Males

Age group	Arm Muscle Area Percentiles (mm²)							Arm Fat Area Percentiles (mm²)						
	5	10	25	50	75	90	95	5	10	25	50	75	90	95
1–1.9	956	1014	1133	1278	1447	1644	1720	452	486	590	741	895	1036	1176
2–2.9	973	1040	1190	1345	1557	1690	1787	434	504	578	737	871	1044	1148
3–3.9	1095	1201	1357	1484	1618	1750	1853	464	519	590	736	868	1071	1151
4–4.9	1207	1264	1408	1579	1747	1926	2008	428	494	598	722	859	989	1085
5–5.9	1298	1411	1550	1720	1884	2089	2285	446	488	582	713	914	1176	1299
6–6.9	1360	1447	1605	1815	2056	2297	2493	371	446	539	678	896	1115	1519
7–7.9	1497	1548	1808	2027	2246	2494	2886	423	473	574	758	1011	1393	1511
8–8.9	1550	1664	1895	2089	2296	2628	2788	410	460	588	725	1003	1248	1558
9–9.9	1811	1884	2067	2288	2657	3053	3257	485	527	635	859	1252	1864	2081
10–10.9	1930	2027	2182	2575	2903	3486	3882	523	543	738	982	1376	1906	2609
11–11.9	2016	2156	2382	2670	3022	3359	4226	536	595	754	1148	1710	2348	2574
12–12.9	2216	2339	2649	3022	3496	3968	4640	554	650	874	1172	1558	2536	3580
13–13.9	2363	2546	3044	3553	4081	4502	4794	475	570	812	1096	1702	2744	3322
14–14.9	2830	3147	3586	3963	4575	5368	5530	453	563	786	1082	1608	2746	3508
15–15.9	3138	3317	3788	4481	5134	5631	5900	521	595	690	931	1423	2434	3100
16–16.9	3625	4044	4352	4951	5753	6576	6980	542	593	844	1078	1746	2280	3041
17–17.9	3998	4252	4777	5286	5950	6886	7726	598	698	827	1096	1636	2407	2888
18–18.9	4070	4481	5066	5552	6374	7067	8355	560	665	860	1264	1947	3302	3928
19–24.9	4508	4777	5274	5913	6660	7606	8200	594	743	963	1406	2231	3098	3652
25–34.9	4694	4963	5541	6214	7067	7847	8436	675	831	1174	1752	2459	3246	3786
35–44.9	4844	5181	5740	6490	7265	8034	8488	703	851	1310	1792	2463	3098	3624
45–54.9	4546	4946	5589	6297	7142	7918	8458	749	922	1254	1741	2359	3245	3928
55–64.9	4422	4783	5381	6144	6919	7670	8149	658	839	1166	1645	2236	2976	3466
65–74.9	3973	4411	5031	5716	6432	7074	7453	573	753	1122	1621	2199	2876	3327

Females

Age														
1–1.9	885	973	1084	1221	1378	1535	1621	401	466	578	706	847	1022	1140
2–2.9	973	1029	1119	1269	1405	1595	1727	469	526	642	747	894	1061	1173
3–3.9	1014	1133	1227	1396	1563	1690	1846	473	529	656	822	967	1106	1158
4–4.9	1058	1171	1313	1475	1644	1832	1958	490	541	654	766	907	1109	1236
5–5.9	1238	1301	1432	1598	1825	2012	2159	470	529	647	812	991	1330	1536
6–6.9	1354	1414	1513	1683	1877	2182	2323	464	508	638	827	1009	1263	1436
7–7.9	1330	1441	1602	1815	2045	2332	2469	491	560	706	920	1135	1407	1644
8–8.9	1513	1566	1808	2034	2327	2657	2996	527	634	769	1042	1383	1872	2482
9–9.9	1723	1788	1976	2227	2571	2987	3112	642	690	933	1219	1584	2171	2524
10–10.9	1740	1784	2019	2296	2583	2873	3093	616	702	842	1141	1608	2500	3005
11–11.9	1784	1987	2316	2612	3071	3739	3953	707	802	1015	1301	1942	2730	3690
12–12.9	2092	2182	2579	2904	3225	3655	3847	782	854	1090	1511	2056	2666	3369
13–13.9	2269	2426	2657	3130	3529	4081	4568	726	838	1219	1625	2374	3272	4150
14–14.9	2418	2562	2874	3220	3704	4294	4850	981	1043	1423	1818	2403	3250	3765
15–15.9	2426	2518	2847	3248	3689	4123	4756	839	1126	1396	1886	2544	3093	4195
16–16.9	2308	2567	2865	3248	3718	4353	4946	1126	1351	1663	2006	2598	3374	4236
17–17.9	2442	2674	2996	3336	3883	4552	5251	1042	1267	1463	2104	2977	3864	5159
18–18.9	2398	2538	2917	3243	3694	4461	4767	1003	1230	1616	2104	2617	3508	3733
19–24.9	2538	2728	3026	3406	3877	4439	4940	1046	1198	1596	2166	2959	4050	4896
25–34.9	2661	2826	3148	3573	4138	4806	5541	1173	1399	1841	2548	3512	4690	5560
35–44.9	2750	2948	3359	3783	4428	5240	5877	1336	1619	2158	2898	3932	5093	5847
45–54.9	2784	2956	3378	3858	4520	5375	5964	1459	1803	2447	3244	4229	5416	6140
55–64.9	2784	3063	3477	4045	4750	5632	6247	1345	1879	2520	3369	4360	5276	6152
65–74.9	2737	3018	3444	4019	4739	5566	6214	1363	1681	2266	3063	3943	4914	5530

SOURCE: Friancho AR: New norms of upper limb fat and muscle areas for assessment of nutritional status. *Am J Clin Nutr* 34:2540–2545, 1981. Reprinted with permission.

43

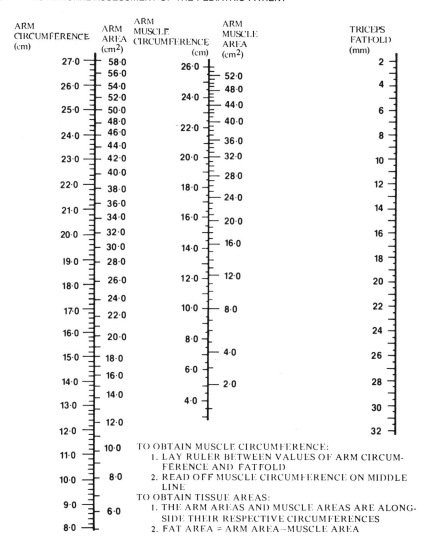

Figure 5 Arm anthropometry nomogram for children. (Gurney JM, Jelliffe DB: Arm anthropometry in nutritional assessment: Nomogram for rapid calculation of muscle circumference and cross-sectional muscle and fat areas. *Am J Clin Nutr* 26:912, 1973. Copyright© 1973, American Society for Clinical Nutrition. Reprinted with permission.)

roteinemia and hypoalbuminemia on the laboratory exam are the distinguishing characteristics of kwashiorkor. In marasmus plasma protein and albumin concentrations can be relatively normal (44). The difference, as demonstrated in this parameter, is thought to be secondary to well-preserved metabolic processes in the marasmic child contrasted to a more severe pathologic condition in kwashiorkor (43).

Bistrian reports this same observation in adults. He considers PCM as occurring in a spectrum ranging from marasmus, with depletion of skeletal protein and fat

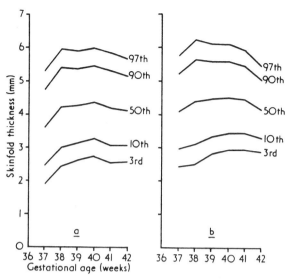

Figure 6 Variations of triceps skinfold thickness with gestational age for (a) males and (b) females. (Oakley JR, Parsons RJ, Whitelaw AGL: Standards for skinfold thickness in British newborn infants. *Arch Dis Child* 52:287, 1977. Reprinted with permission.)

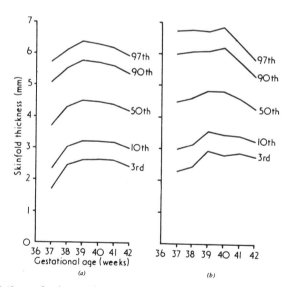

Figure 7 Variations of subscapular skinfold thickness with gestational age for (a) males and (b) females. (Oakley Jr, Parsons RJ, Whitelaw AGL: Standards for skinfold thickness in British newborn infants. *Arch Dis Child* 52:287, 1977. Reprinted with permission.)

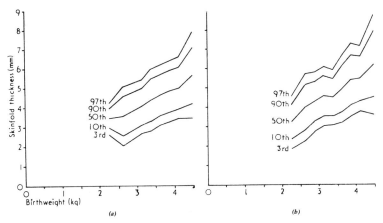

Figure 8 Variations of subscapular skinfold thickness with birthweight for (a) males and (b) females. (Oakley JR, Parsons RJ, Whitelaw AGL: Standards for skinfold thickness in British newborn infants. *Arch Dis Child* 52:287, 1977. Reprinted with permission.)

but preservation of serum albumin, to adult kwashiorkor, or visceral attrition, in which serum albumin is severely affected (2,45). The biochemical measure of albumin can be used to distinguish the two types of PCM. However, because there is a large body pool of albumin with a long serum half-life, its concentration in the serum diminishes slowly and is a late manifestation of visceral protein wasting.

Serum transferrin is a more sensitive indicator than albumin. Transferrin has a shorter half-life and is reported to be a more sensitive indicator of nutritional status in children, particularly during the recovery phase, and reflects early response to total parenteral nutrition (TPN) therapy (46). Transferrin can be measured directly in some laboratories or it can be estimated from the measurement of total iron binding capacity. Transferrin levels are elevated in the anemic; therefore, it is not a

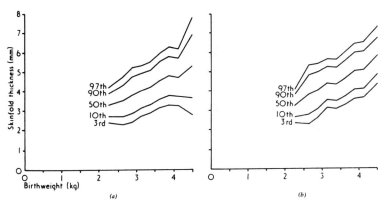

Figure 9 Variations of triceps skinfold thickness with birthweight for (a) males and (b) females. (Oakley JR, Parsons RJ, Whitelaw AGL: Standards for skinfold thickness in British newborn infants. *Arch Dis Child* 52:287, 1977. Reprinted with permission.)

Table 7. Methods for Collecting Anthropometric Data

Method for Mid-Arm Circumference in Infants and Children
Instrument: Narrow fiberglass tape
1. With infant being held up (neonates may need to lie on side), or child standing, flex the arm to 90°. The midpoint of the upper arm is halfway between the tip of the acromion process and the tip of the olecranon (elbow). Palpate the tip of the acromion process and place the end of the tape there. Pull straight back and down, measuring the distance to the tip of the elbow. Place a mark on the arm midway between the two points.
2. With the arm hanging freely measure the circumference of the arm at the midpoint. For the neonate, the arm rests on the body. The tape, kept in a horizontal plane, should rest on the arm without causing indentations. Record duplicate measures to the nearest millimeter.

Method for Triceps Skinfold Measurement in Infants and Children
Instrument: Lange caliper
            Narrow fiberglass tape
Triceps
1. With infant being held up (neonates may need to lie on side) or child standing, expose the entire arm. The triceps skinfold is measured at the midpoint of the upper arm. The midpoint is midway between the acromion and olecranon on the posterior aspect of arm.
2. With the arm flexed 90°, palpate the tips of the acromion process and the olecranon, place the tape between these two points, and locate midpoint, making a mark with felt pen at midpoint.
3. With the thumb and forefinger of the left hand placed approximately 2 cm apart, pick up the skinfold just above midpoint marking. Fold is parallel to the arm. Arm should now be in relaxed position. The pinch should include two thicknesses of skin and subcutaneous fat with no muscle.
4. With the right hand, apply calipers on the midline mark at a depth equal to the thickness of the fold. The right hand should relax entirely to allow the jaws of the caliper to exert full pressure. The left hand maintains its pinch.
5. The measurement is read to the nearest millimeter as soon as the needle is steady (approximately 2–3 seconds).
6. Duplicate measurements are recorded with regrasping of the skinfold for each measurement.

Method for Subscapular Skinfold Measurement in Infants and Children
Instrument: Lange Caliper
1. The subscapular skinfold is measured just below the inferior angle of the scapula.
2. With infant being held up (neonates lying on stomach) or child standing, the examiner, with the left hand, follows the line of the scapula, picking up the skinfold with a vertical pinch. Thumb and forefinger are approximately 2 cm apart. Skinfold held should include 2 thicknesses of skin and subcutaneous fat.
3. With calipers in the right hand, apply jaws of calipers just under the pinch point. As the left hand maintains the pinch, the right hand should relax entirely, so that the jaws of the calipers can exert full pressure.
4. Measurement is read to the nearest millimeter as soon as the needle becomes steady (2–3 seconds).
5. Duplicate measurements are recorded with complete regrasping of the skinfold.

Table 8. Assessment of Somatic Protein Compartment (Muscle Mass)

Indicator	Measurement	Interpretation
Creatine: The skeletal muscle pool of creatine is reflected in creatinine excretion.	Measure creatinine excreted in 24° urine. Compare to expected standard excretion for height and sex. % standard calculated. $$\frac{24° \text{ creatinine excreted}}{\text{Normal value for child of same height and sex}} \times 100 = CHI^a$$	Indirect measure of muscle mass <80% of standard = moderate depletion of active skeletal mass, <60% = severe depletion Limitation: Small data base for children. Must have normal renal function and urine output.
Arm muscle circumference	Calculated from measurements of mid arm circumference (MAC) and triceps skinfold thickness (TSF) Arm muscle circumference in cm (AMC) can be calculated: AMC = MAC in cm − (0.314 × TSF in mm)	Only an estimate of muscle mass reserve.
Arm muscle area	Compare to standards and calculate deficit. M = arm muscle area in square cm. $$M = \frac{(Ca - \pi S)^2}{4\pi}$$ Ca = MAC in cm S = TSF in cm π = 3.14 Can be compared to tables of standards to determine degree of deficit.	Especially useful in children where arm muscle area changes more with age than does arm muscle circumference.

^a Creatine height index.

valid indicator of visceral protein status if the child has iron deficiency anemia. It is also not a useful measurement when hormones or medications that decrease protein synthesis are being used (8). Because of these influences on transferrin synthesis, one may select to use the measurements of other hepatic proteins.

The measurement of the thyroxine-binding prealbumin/retinol-binding protein complex is suggested by Ingenbleek and co-workers as having the highest sensitivity to an alteration in nutritional status (47). In 1972, they reported the measurement of thyroxine-binding prealbumin (TBPA) as a sensitive indicator of protein deficiency and its improvement with nutritional treatment. They felt it allowed the detection of prekwashiorkor and the differential diagnosis of various forms of PCM. The sensitivity of this protein was related to three factors: (1) biosynthesis of TBPA by the liver, which reacts promptly to protein deficiency; (2) the richness of TBPA in tryptophan; and (3) the rapid turnover of this protein (48). Later, this same group of investigators reported on the role of retinol-binding protein (RBP) in PCM. In their study of 39 children aged 18–30 months with severe malnutrition the RBP doubled its plasma level after one week and tripled after two weeks of appropriate refeeding. The return to normal of RBP ran in close parallel with prealbumin (PA), implying that both components remain bound by 1 : 1 molar ratio in the PA-RBP complex (49).

Smith et al. demonstrated that children with varying degrees of PCM showed significant increases in the serum concentrations of vitamin A, RBP, and PA by the end of the second week and further progressive increases by the fourth week with appropriate refeeding; the serum concentrations were highly correlated with each other (50). Because these two proteins parallel one another, prealbumin measurements have been recommended for routine use. However, measuring both PA and RBP may be helpful in detecting early malnutrition and, as demonstrated in the references cited, serve as highly sensitive indicators of the response to refeeding. These proteins, with normal values for interpretation of results, are included in Table 9.

A function of the visceral protein mass is cellular immunity. This function is evaluated by total lymphocyte count and cutaneous hypersensitivity to common antigens to determine immune competence. The total lymphocyte count (TLC) is derived from the routine complete blood count (CBC) with differential count. The TLC is equal to the percentage of lymphocytes in the peripheral smear multiplied by the white cell count (WBC). Decreased lymphocyte count can be secondary to a vast number of acute or chronic states, including malnutrition (2,4,45). The TLC is used as a screening indicator of immune status. The response of a patient's lymphocyte count to nutritional support can be used as a favorable prognostic sign during nutritional repletion. Table 9 provides normal values for evaluating the lymphocyte count.

Several investigators have reported anergy in the malnourished child (51,57). Anergy is a decrease or actual loss of the body's ability to mount an immune response to foreign antigens. This loss or inability, known as impaired cell-mediated immunity or immunoincompetence, may result in serious clinical complications since the body's ability to fight infection is reduced. Immune competence can be assessed with delayed hypersensitivity skin testing. This is unlike immediate hypersensitivity skin testing which involves an antibody response to intradermally injected antigens with the development of a reaction within minutes. Delayed hypersensitivity reactions require the local attraction from the blood stream of specific

Table 9. Assessment of Visceral Protein Compartment

Serum Protein	Origin/Turn Over Rate (half-life)	Function	Normal Value	Comment
Albumin	Hepatic, 14–20 days	Carrier protein: makes up 50–60% of serum proteins; contributes to intravascular oncotic pressure	Normal >6 mo: 3.5–5 mg/dl. <3.4 warrents further evaluation. <2.5 = severe depletion.	Commonly used on initial screening. Not a good measure for short term response to nutritional therapy due to longer half-life. Dehydration causes falsely elevated values.
Transferrin	Hepatic, 8–10.5 days	Carrier protein for iron	Normal >6 mo: 180–260 mg/dl. 100–200 warrants further evaluation; 100 mg/dl = severe depletion. can be estimated by using Fe binding capacity (TIBC): Serum transferrin (mg/100 ml) = (TIBC × 0.8)–43 Depressed serum transferrin suspected if TIBC <250 µg%.	More sensitive measure of protein deficiency due to shorter half-life. Not to be used as indicator of protein status in presence of Fe deficiency states, as serum transferrin will be elevated. Decreased by hormones and medications that limit protein synthesis.
Prealbumin	Hepatic, 2–3 days	Carrier protein for thyroxin: thyroxinbinding prealbumin (TBPA). Carrier protein for retinol binding protein.	Normal 20–50 mg/dl; <10 mg/dl = severe depletion	Can be used for monitoring of nutritional therapy as it is more responsive to therapy than transferrin and albumin. Recommended for routine clinical use since PA + RBP strictly parallel each other in behavior and the serum concentration of PA is 4–5× higher than RBP.

| | | | 37.2 ± 7.3 mcg/ml
 <3 mcg/dl = severe depletion | Sensitive indicator of protein and energy deprivation even of short term duration. Can be used to monitor response to parenteral or enteral therapy. Primarily used in research. |

| Retinol-binding protein | Hepatic, 12 hours; is released from liver complexed with Vitamin A (retinol). | Carrier protein for Vitamin A; RBP binds to prealbumin in 1:1 ratio for transport. | | |

Assessment of Immunocompetence (The Most Important Function of the Visceral Protein Compartment)

Measurement	Calculation	Function	Normal Value	Comment
1. Total lymphocyte count (TLC)/mm³	TLC = WBC × % lymphocytes	75% of lymphocytes are T cells—important in cell mediated immunity; 25% are B cells—important in humoral immunity	>2500 in first 3 mo of life, otherwise normal is >1800	Provides a general guide to patient's ability to respond to infection. <2500 in first 3 mo of life may be abnormal. Values <1500 represent deficiency at any age. Values <1000 represent severe lymphopenia (associated with severe impairment).
2. Use of intradermal skin test antigens (to assess cell mediated immunity)—see text				

lymphocytes previously sensitized to the injected antigen. Because the accumulation of sufficient lymphocytes at the injection site requires time, delayed hypersensitivity is measured at 24, 48 and 72 hours after the injection. The evaluation of the immune response is accomplished through the skin testing to antigens to which the person is thought to have been sensitized previously. There are two such antigens: (1) ubiquitous, for example *Candida* (responsible for yeast infection) and *Trichophyton* (responsible for athlete's foot) and (2) previously injected antigens, for example, mumps vaccine. A number of challenge antigens is usually necessary to determine a positive delayed hypersensitivity response. Various antigens have been used for skin testing in children (54, 59). Some of these have not been approved by the FDA for this purpose. Table 10 contains antigens that have been used in skin testing; however, there are no clear cut guidelines to use for skin testing in pediatrics. Where possible, references are provided for further reading. If skin testing is used, a review of the current literature would be helpful before deciding which antigens to use, as well as for determining dilution, dosage, and interpretation of the results. As a general rule, young infants are usually not tested. A positive result is dependent upon previous exposure, and the percentage of positive responses increases with age.

In skin testing, three antigens are normally administered. (Table 10 will help you decide which three antigens are appropriate.) The following procedures are recommended by two members of our nutritional support team in order to provide uniform and reproducible results (52):

1. Give 0.1 ml intradermally with a 25-gauge needle. With needle bevel up, lift the first layer of skin only, raising a wheal (subcutaneous administration will result in a false negative reaction; do not allow fluid to leak onto skin).

2. Administer on the volar flexor surface of the forearm with sufficient distance between antigens to prevent positive reactions from overlapping one another.

3. Circle the site of administration with a pen. Administer in alphabetical order (e.g., *Candida*, mumps, *Trichophyton*).

4. Document administration (on the skin test sheet record date, time, locations, and antigens used).

5. Read at 24 and 48 hours. Reactions peak at 48 hours—occasionally a first time reactor may not have a response until 72 hours have elapsed. Note both erythema and induration.

6. The margin of induration should be marked using the ball point pen technique. Lightly move the pen toward the injection site from four sides; slight resistance is noted when the pen reaches the margin of induration. Diameter of induration is measured with a millimeter ruler. Five or more millimeters of induration is generally accepted as a positive response; however, erythema alone may signify a positive reaction to mumps (52).

A positive response is induration greater than 5 mm to any of the tests administered. Anergy is the inability to demonstrate a reaction to at least one test. A negative response may correlate with biochemical findings of protein malnutrition, e.g., decreased levels of transferrin and albumin. However, a negative skin test result must be interpreted with caution. When a child demonstrates a negative response, it may indicate either anergy or that there has been no previous exposure to the antigen. Table 11 lists factors that have been shown to decrease reactivity to

Table 10. Antigens

1. Candida (Dermatophyton "0")[52,53]
     (1 : 10, 1 : 100, 1 : 500 dilution)
2. Diphtheria–tetanus[58]
     (1 : 100 dilution)
     Given to immunized children
3. Mumps (20 CFU/ml)[51,52]
     Administered to infants over 1 year
     Because this antigen is cultivated in chick embryo, if the child is sensitive to egg, he
     or she may react in 2–4 hr.
4. PPD (Purified protein derivative)[57]
     (1 TU, 5 TU, 250 TU)
5. Tetanus toxoid[51,54,59]
     (10 Lf/ml; prior to skin testing, dilute the solution 1 : 5 with sterile saline—final
     concentration of toxoid = 2 Lf/ml)
     Given to immunized children who have had 3 or more immunizations.
6. Tricophyton[51]
     (1 : 30, 1 : 100, 1 : 500 dilution)
     This skin test is a good alternative to streptokinase/streptodornase which is no
     longer available.

skin test antigens (52,53,56,58). Most clinicians feel that if true anergy is demonstrated, the result identifies the child to be at high risk for infection, and precautions should be taken to protect the child. A recent article has cautioned that anergy should not be used as the sole indication for delay of operative treatment or for initiation of parenteral nutrition (55). Rather, the skin test results must be interpreted in light of all other indicators of nutritional assessment.

A final consideration in nutritional assessment is the functional status of the intestinal tract. Gastrointestinal dysfunction can be caused by malnutrition alone, secondary to multiple disease entities (e.g., congenital heart disease, malignancy, renal insufficiency, central nervous system disease), or by primary pathology within the gastrointestinal tract (e.g., short bowel syndrome, celiac disease, soy or milk protein intolerance, inflammatory bowel disease, cystic fibrosis, biliary atresia, neonatal hepatitis).

Table 11. Factors that may be Associated with Decreased Reactivity to Skin Testing

Lack of exposure to the antigen; common in infants
Corticosteroids: levels increase secondary to trauma or after surgery
Elevation in BUN
Fever
Simultaneous administration of skin tests, with a weaker reaction suppressed by a
    strong reaction
Elevated WBC
Cancer
Iron Deficiency
Radiation
Immunosuppressive drugs
Immunologic deficiency

Table 12. Functional Status of Gastrointestinal Tract

Test	Dosage	Interpretation
Upper small bowel mucosa integrity		
D-xylose: A pentose absorbed by passive diffusion. The amount absorbed depends upon intactness of mucosal surface. (If acute diarrhea is present results may be misleading; a low value may also occur if the patient has delayed gastric emptying).	Give orally 0.5 g/kg body wt (or 14.5 g/m^2) in a 10% solution p̄ a 4–6 hr fast (max. dose = 25 g); measure xylose in serum fasting, and at 60 min.	A 25 mg % rise above the fasting level occurs with normal mucosal function. The 1 hr D-xylose is a sensitive indicator of severe intestinal damage. An intestinal biopsy should be considered in all patients with a D-xylose <20 mg/dl. With borderline results (20–25 mg/dl), clinical decisions must be individualized.
Carbohydrate Absorption		
Disaccharide absorption: Normally disaccharides are hydrolyzed to monosaccharides by specific disaccharidases of upper small bowel mucosa. Tests evaluate damage to the mucosa and/or enzyme deficiencies. (False values may occur in patients with delayed gastric emptying.)		
Lactose tolerance Lactose → glucose + galactose	Give orally 2 g/kg (max. dose 50 g) as a 10% solution (p̄ a 4–6 hr fast); measure plasma levels of glucose at fasting 30, 60, 90, and 120 min.	In the normal child, the serum glucose level rises more than 30 mg/dl over the test period. With lactose intolerance the rise is usually <20 mg/dl.
Sucrose tolerance Sucrose → glucose + fructose	Give orally 2 g/kg in a 10% solution (p̄ a 4–6 hr fast); measure plasma levels of glucose at fasting 30, 60, 90, and 120 min.	>30 mg% rise should occur at any time from fasting. A rise of <20 mg/dl should be interpreted as sucrose intolerance.
Maltose Tolerance Maltose → glucose + glucose	Give orally 1 g/kg in a 10% solution (p̄ a 4–6 hr fast); measure plasma levels of glucose at fasting 30, 60, 90, and 120 min.	>30 mg% rise should occur at any time from fasting. A rise of <20 mg/dl should be interpreted as maltose intolerance.
Clinitest tablet For reducing substances in stool for the presence of lactose or maltose.[a]		0.25% or less = negative 0.25%–0.5% = suspect 0.5% = abnormal [a]Sucrose is not a reducing sugar and the test requires the use of HCl instead of H$_2$O + boiling briefly.

Stool pH
Unabsorbed disaccharides pass into the distal ileum and colon where intestinal bacteria ferment them to short chain volatile acids in quantities sufficient to lower the stool pH to 5.5 or less.

Fecal pH of <5.5 is abnormal.

Breath hydrogen
Give a challenge dose of a disaccharide, either lactose or sucrose. Unabsorbable carbohydrate will be metabolized by bacteria and hydrogen will be released and then excreted in breath.

Dosages + times for measurement are identical to challenges above (may need to obtain 2½ hr + 3 hr samples in some patients with delayed gastric emptying or poor motility).

>20 ppm breath hydrogen above baseline indicates carbohydrate malabsorption.

Fat absorption
Dietary fat absorption

Fecal fat
Actual fat intake is documented. Parent keeps a 72 hr. diet history and a dietitian then calculates daily fat intake. All stool specimens are collected for that 72 hr. period in a pre-weighed paint can (and kept on ice or in refrigerator).

Child is fed:
<12 mos: 25–30 g fat/day;
1–3 yr: 35 g fat/day;
>3 yr: 40 g fat/day;
adolescent: 75–100 g fat/day for three days.

$$\frac{\text{Dietary fat} - \text{fecal fat}}{\text{dietary fat}} \times 100 = \text{coefficient of absorption}$$

Coefficient of absorption normals: premie 60–75%; newborn 80–85%; 10 mo–3 yr 85–95%; >3 yr 95%.

Fat soluble vitamin absorption:
(carotene screens for vitamin A absorption; protime screens for vitamin K absorption)

Serum carotene
Child must have eaten foods containing carotene (e.g. carrots, squash, sweet potatoes, pumpkin)

<50 µg/dl = steatorrhea
50–100 µg/dl = probably ok
>100 µg/dl = normal

Carotene challenge
Give infant 4.5 oz of carrots (small jar of baby food) each day for one week. Obtain baseline carotene + carotene after 1 week of the challenge

carotene change >30 above baseline = no steatorrhea.

Prothrombin time

>60% is normal (newborn infants have ↓ levels)

Malnutrition alone is not an indication for parenteral nutrition. When possible, enteral feeding should be utilized since nutrients are metabolized far more efficiently by this route. Therefore, the feasibility of oral, nasogastric, nasojejunal, gastrostomy, or needle–catheter jejunostomy should be determined before deciding to bypass the gastrointestinal tract and institute parenteral support. The patient's appetite, mucosal and intraluminal digestive function, and food transit time are important when considering an enteral regimen (60).

If severe gastrointestinal dysfunction is present, the only alternative will be parenteral nutrition. If there are selective areas of dysfunction, the treatment of choice may be enteral feedings with either defined formula diets or specific nutritional supplements (see chapter on Transition from Parenteral to Enteral Feedings for tables depicting the products available). If the intestinal tract is determined to be intact, adding appropriate nutritional supplements to the existing dietary regimen may be sufficient. Table 12 summarizes the tests used to assess gastrointestinal function with guidelines for their interpretation (61–63).

Application of Nutritional Assessment

A complete nutritional assessment requires (1) a medical history and clinical exam, (2) a diet history and evaluation, (3) anthropometric measurements, and (4) laboratory assessment. It is not practical to perform full nutritional assessment on all hospitalized patients. According to Merritt and Blackburn (8) the presence of recent weight loss of greater than 5% (excluding dehydration), a weight to height ratio below the fifth percentile, a serum albumin of less than 3.5 g/dl, or a specific diagnosis associated with the development of protein–calorie malnutrition would warrant complete nutritional assessment.

Nutritional assessment can separate patients into three groups: (1) those for whom nutritional therapy is imperative, (2) those for whom it is advisable, and (3) those who do not require further intervention (8). Merritt and Blackburn would assign a patient to:

Group 1 if serum albumin is <2.5 g/dl, transferrin level is <100 µg/dl (after 6 months), and the lymphocyte count is <1000/mm^3 (except in patients on chemotherapy or radiation therapy); or if the patient is anergic (beyond infancy and in patients not on steroids) in the presence of weight:height >2 SD below normal or <80% of standard, arm muscle area <5th percentile, or CHI <60% of standard; or if the patient has marginal skeletal or visceral protein status and is markedly stressed. Group 1 definitely requires *repletion* therapy (8).

Group 2 if serum albumin is <3 g/dl or the transferrin is <150 µg/dl, if the lymphocyte count is <1500/mm^3, if the weight:height is >2 SD below normal or <80% of standard, if the arm muscle area is <5th percentile, or if the CHI is <80% of standard. This group requires close monitoring for evidence of further nutritional depletion and at least *maintenance* nutritional support if full repletion is not feasible. If these patients also have sepsis secondary to surgery or major injury, they should be placed in Group 1 (8).

Group 3 if no nutritional deficits are documented, if the patient has no chronic disease, and if the patient will not encounter markedly stressful situations in the hospital. Normal patients who develop an infection, undergo starvation, or undergo major surgery require repeat assessment in 1–2 weeks (8).

The data collected during nutritional assessment provide a baseline for evaluating effects of future therapy. In a malnourished patient success of nutritional therapy can be documented by improvement of biochemical parameters, anthropometric measurements, and nitrogen balance studies from baseline determinations. Baseline data, even if initially normal, are helpful if subsequent treatment (e.g., chemotherapy, surgery, radiation therapy) results in nutritional deficits. Cooper and co-workers (64) recently demonstrated that acute protein calorie malnutrition is far more prevalent among hospitalized pediatric patients than is generally appreciated and that *comprehensive nutritional assessment* is essential to identify the "at risk," nutritionally deprived pediatric surgical patient.

Monitoring patients at risk for developing nutritional deficits routinely includes daily weights, weekly serum albumin and transferrin measurement and lymphocyte count, anthropometric measurements every two weeks, and weekly CHI determinations. The use of other parameters depends on the clinical course of the patient and the length of hospitalization. Clearly the effects of hospitalization on the nutritional status of a child require further study (65).

The patient's underlying condition must be taken into account when interpreting data from laboratory, clinical, dietetic, and anthropometric investigations. Ultimately, there is still a great deal of reliance on clinical impressions and judgement (66).

Part of the decision in determining the mode of nutritional support is based on whether the child requires maintenance or repletion therapy. If growth has been compromised, repletion therapy will be necessary for catch-up growth (8,67). A hypermetabolic child requires maintenance nutritional therapy plus additional allowances for stress factors (8). Although parenteral nutrition is used to replete the malnourished child, it may also be used prophylactically when prolonged starvation is expected (68).

Based upon the assessment of the gastrointestinal tract, a decision will be made of how to provide maintenance or repletion therapy. Indications for PN are described in Chapter 1; PN requirements are described in Chapters 3–10. Peripheral PN is usually adequate to provide maintenance therapy. If repletion therapy is indicated, central vein PN is required. Enteral requirements are discussed in Chapter 20.

References

1. Butterworth CE: The skeleton in the hospital closet. *Nutrition Today* 9:4, 1974.

2. Bistrian BR, Blackburn GL, Vitale J, et al: Prevalence of malnutrition in general medical patients. *JAMA* 235:1567, 1976.

3. Blackburn GL, Bistrian BR, Baltej SM, et al: Nutritional and metabolic assessment of the hospitalized patient. *JPEN* 1:11, 1977.

4. Merritt RJ, Suskind RM: Nutritional survey of hospitalized pediatric patients. *Am J Clin Nutr* 32:1320, 1979.

5. McLaren DS: Nutritional Assessment, in McLaren DS, Burman D (eds): *Textbook of Paediatric Nutrition.* Edinburgh, Churchill Livingstone, 1976, p. 91.

6. Grant A: *Nutritional Assessment Guidelines,* ed 2. Berkeley, Calif, Cutter Medical, 1979.

7. Ekvall S: Assessment of nutritional status, in Palmer S, Edvall S (eds): *Pediatric Nutrition in Development Disorders.* Charles C Thomas, Springfield, Ill, 1978, p 502.

8. Merritt RJ, Blackburn GL: Nutritional assessment and metabolic response to illness of the hospitalized child, in Suskind RM (ed): *Textbook of Pediatric Nutrition.* New York, Raven Press, 1981, p 285.

9. Zerfas AJ, Shorr IJ, Neumann CG: Office assessment of nutritional status. *Pediatr Clin North Am,* 24:253, 1977.

10. *Recommended Daily Dietary Allowances* ed 10. Washington DC, National Academy of Sciences, National Research Council, Food and Nutrition Board, Washington, DC, 1979.

11. Kerner JA, Hattner JA, Sunshine P: The use of skinfold thickness and mid upper arm circumferences in the nutritional assessment of low birth weight infants. *Pediatr Res* 13:401, 1979.

12. Brans YW, Summers JE, Dweck HS, et al: A noninvasive approach to body composition in the neonate: Dynamic skinfold measurements. *Pediatr Res* 8:215, 1974.

13. National Center for Health Statistics growth charts, 1976. *Monthly Vital Statistics Report* 25 (Suppl) No. (HRA) 76-1120. Rockville, Md, Health Resources Administratin, 1976.

14. Hamill PV, Drizd TA, Johnson CL, et al: Physical growth: National Center for Health Statistics percentiles. *Am J Clin Nutr* 32:607, 1979.

15. Fomon SJ: *Nutritional Disorders of Children. Prevention, Screening, and Follow-up.* U.S. Dept of Health, Education, and Welfare publication No. (HSA) 76-5612. Rockville, Md, Public Health Service, 1976, p 14.

16. Roche AF, Himes JH: Incremental growth charts. *Am J Clin Nutr* 33:2041, 1980.

17. Tanner JM, Whitehouse RH: Standards for subcutaneous fat in British children. Percentiles of thickness of skinfolds over triceps and below scapula. *Br Med J* 1:446, 1962.

18. Tanner JM, Whitehouse RH: Revised standards for triceps and subscapular skinfolds in British children. *Arch Dis Child* 50:142, 1975.

19. Frisancho AR: Triceps skinfold and upper arm muscle size norms for assessment of nutritional status. *Am J Clin Nutr* 27:1052, 1974.

20. Frisancho AR: New norms of upper limb fat and muscle areas for assessment of nutritional status. *Am J Clin Nutr* 34:2540. 1981.

21. *Anthropometric and Clinical Findings. Preliminary Findings of the First Health and Examination Survey. U.S. 1971–72.* U.S. Dept of Health, Education, and Welfare (HRA) 75-1229. Rockville, Md, National Center for Health Statistics 1975.

22. Gurney JM, Jelliffe DB: Arm anthropometry in nutritional assessment: Nomogram for rapid calculation of muscle circumference and cross-sectional muscle and fat areas. *Am J Clin Nutr* 26:912, 1973.

23. Oakley JR, Parsons RJ, Whitelaw AG: Standards for skinfold thickness in British newborn infants. *Arch Dis Child* 52:287, 1977.

24. Vaucher YE, Harrison GG, Udall JN, et al: Estimation of fat deposition in utero: Multiple skinfold thickness measurements in preterm and term neonates. *Clin Res* 28:127A, 1980.

25. Weiner JS, Lourie JA (ed): *Human Biology: A Guide to Field Methods.* International Biological Programme Handbook No. 9, Oxford, England, Blackwell Scientific Publications, 1969, p 7.

26. Benke A, Wilmore J: *Evaluation and Regulation of Body Build and Composition.* Englewood Cliffs, NJ, Prentice Hall, 1974, p 38.

27. Cheek DB: A new look at growth, in Cheek DB (ed): *Human Growth.* Philadelphia, Lea & Febiger, 1968, p 3.

28. Graystone JE: Creatinine excretion during growth, in Cheek DB (ed): *Human Growth.* Philadelphia, Lea & Febiger, 1968, p 182.

29. Viteri FE, Alvarado J: The creatinine height index: Its use in the estimation of the degree of protein depletion and repletion in protein calorie malnourished children. *Pediatrics* 46:696, 1970.

30. Bistrian BR, Blackburn GL, Sherman M, et al: Therapeutic index of nutritional depletion in hospitalized patients. *Surg Gynecol Obstet* 141:512, 1975.

31. Cheek DB (ed): *Human Growth.* Philadelphia, Lea & Febiger, 1968, p 745.

32. Beisel WR: Magnitude of the host nutritional responses to infection. *Am J Clin Nutr* 30:1236, 1977.

33. Reindorp S, Whitehead RG: Changes in serum creatine kinase and other biological measurements associated with musculature in children recovering from kwashiorkor. *Br J Nutr* 25:273, 1971.

34. Fomon SJ: Collection of urine and feces and metabolic balance studies, in Fomon SJ (ed): *Infant Nutrition* ed 2. Philadelphia, WB Saunders Co, 1974, p 549.

35. Graystone JE, Ortgies AM: Methods for studying body composition. Part VI, in Cheek DB (ed): *Human Growth.* Philadelphia, Lea & Febiger, 1968, p 661.

36. Golden M, Waterlow JC, Picou D: The relationship between dietary intake, weight change, nitrogen balance, and protein turnover in man. *Am J Clin Nutr* 30:1345, 1977.

37. Hendry PG, James BE, MacMahon RA: Nitrogen balance studies during oral and complete intravenous feeding of small premature infants. *Aust Paediatr J* 14:6, 1978.

38. Reichman B, Chessex P, Putet G, et al: Diet, fat accretion, and growth in premature infants. *N Engl J Med* 305:1495, 1981.

39. Long CL, Schiller WR, Blakemore WS, et al: Muscle protein catabolism in the septic patient as measured by 3-methylhistidine excretion. *Am J Clin Nutr* 30:1349, 1977.

40. Kim CW, Okada A, Itakura T, et al: Urinary excretion of 3-methylhistidine in patients receiving parenteral nutrition. *JPEN* 3:255, 1979.

41. Seashore JH, Huszar GB, Davis EM: Urinary 3-methylhistidine excretion and nitrogen balance in healthy and stressed premature infants. *J Pediatr Surg* 15:400, 1980.

42. Owen G, Lippman G: Nutritional status of infants and young children: U.S.A. *Pediatr Clin North Am* 24:211, 1977.

43. Human protein deficiency—Biochemical changes and functional implications. *Nutr Reviews* 35:294, 1977.

44. Coward WA, Whitehead RG, Lunn PG: Reasons why hypoalbuminemia may or may not appear in protein–energy malnutriton. *Br J Nutr* 38:115, 1977.

45. Bistrian BR: Interaction of nutrition and infection in the hospital setting. *Am J Clin Nutr* 30:1228, 1977.

46. Rickard KA, Matchett N, Ballantine TV, et al: Serum transferrin: An early indicator of nutritional status in children with advanced cancer. *Surg Forum* 30:78, 1979.

47. Ingenbleek Y, Van Den Schrieck HG, De Nayer P, et al: Albumin transferrin and thyroxine-binding prealbumin/retinol-binding protein (TABA-RBP) complex in assessment of malnutrition. *Clin Chim Acta* 63:61, 1975.

48. Ingenbleek Y, De Visscher M, De Nayer P: Measurement of prealbumin as index of protein–calorie malnutrition. *Lancet* 2:106, 1972.

49. Ingenbleek V, Van Den Schrieck HG, De Nayer P, et al: The role of retinol-binding protein–calorie malnutrition. *Metabolism* 24:633, 1975.

50. Smith FR, Goodman DS, Zaklama M, et al: Serum vitamin A, retinol binding protein, and prealbumin concentrations in protein–calorie malnutriton. 1. A functional decrease in hepatic retinol release. *Am J Clin Nutr* 26:973, 1973.

51. Chandra RK, Scrimshaw NS: Immunocompetence in nutritional assessment. *Am J Clin Nutr* 33:2694, 1980.

52. Rupp C, Andolina A: Skin testing for anergy. *Drug Information Service Newsletter* (Stanford University Hospital) 3:2, 1981.

53. Strauss RG: Iron deficiency, infections, and immune function: A reassessment. *Am J Clin Nutr* 31:660, 1978.

54. Borut TC, Ank BJ, Gard SE, et al: Tetanus toxoid skin test in children: Correlation with in vitro lymphoctye stimulation and monocyte chemotaxis. *J Pediatr* 97:567, 1980.

55. Simonowitz D, Oreskovich M, Dellinger E, et al: Value of nutritional support in anergic patients. *Nutr Support Serv* 1:29, 1981.

56. Martin DJ: Skin test antigens. *Nutritional Support Services* 1:49, 1981.

57. McMurray DN, Loomis SA, Casazza LJ, et al: Development of impaired cell-mediated immunity in mild and moderate malnutrition. *Am J Clin Nutr* 34:68, 1981.

58. Kaufman DB, de Mendonea WC, Newton J: Diptheria–tetanus skin testing. *Am J Dis Child* 134:479, 1980.

59. Steele RW, Suttle DE, Le Master PC, et al: Screening for cell-mediated immunity in children. *Am J Dis Child* 130:1218, 1976.

60. Sutphen JL: Nutritional support of the pediatric patient. *Clinical Consultations in Nutritional Support* 1:1, 1981.

61. Kraut JR, Lloyd-Still JD: The 1-hr blood xylose test in the evaluation of malabsorption in infants and children. *Am J Clin Nutr* 33:2328, 1980.

62. Tests of carbohydrate digestion and absorption, in Roy CC, Silverman A, Cozzetto FJ (eds): *Pediatric Clinical Gastroenterology*, ed 2. St Louis, CV Mosby Co, 1975, p 684.

63. Tests of fat absorption and metabolism, in Roy CC, Silverman A, Cozzetto FJ (eds): *Pediatric Clinical Gastroenterology*, ed 2. St Louis, CV Mosby Co, 1975. p 692.

64. Cooper A, Jakobowski D, Spiker J, et al: Nutritional assessment: An integral part of the preoperative pediatric surgical evaluation. *J Pediatr Surg* 16(4) (Suppl 1):554, 1981.

65. Parsons HG, Francoeur TE, Howland P, et al: The nutritional status of hospitalized children. *Am J Clin Nutr* 33:1140, 1980.

66. Grant JP, Custer PB, Thurlow J: Current techniques of nutritional assessment. Symposium on surgical nutrition. *Surg Clin North Am* 61:437, 1981.

67. Picou DM: Evaluation and treatment of the malnourished child, in Suskind RM (ed): *Textbook of Pediatric Nutrition*. New York, Raven Press, 1981, p 217.

68. Filler RM: Parenteral support of the surgically ill child, in Suskind RM (ed): *Textbook of Pediatric Nutrition*. New York, Raven Press, 1981, p 341.

Part II
Specific Requirements

3
Caloric Requirements

John A. Kerner, Jr.

Premature Infants

The number of calories that the preterm infant requires in order to gain weight optimally has been calculated to be approximately 85–130 cal/kg/day (Table 1). These requirements are based on the needs of an infant who is receiving feedings enterally and also take into consideration the fat malabsorption known to occur in premature infants. Approximately 75 cal/kg/day is the usual estimate for resting energy expenditure; resting energy requirements include maintenance of the basal metabolic rate (approximately 50 cal/kg/day) plus requirements for activity and response to cold stress. Modern nursery management has decreased resting caloric expenditure. With careful control of the environmental temperature, energy expenditure in response to cold stress can be reduced considerably (1). Oxygen consumption studies of relatively inactive infants maintained in a strictly thermoneutral environment suggest that daily resting caloric expenditure is closer to 50 cal/kg/day than 75 cal/kg/day (2).

Obviously, the infant who receives all his nutrients intravenously requires fewer calories. Adequate growth in neonates has been demonstrated with parenteral intakes of 88–90 cal/kg/day (3,4).

A controlled trial (5) of 14 appropriate for gestational age (AGA) premature infants evaluated two isocaloric intravenous feeding regimens, each providing *60 cal/kg/day*—one providing glucose alone, the other providing *glucose plus 2.5 g/kg/day of crystalline amino acids*. Infants on the regimen containing glucose alone had a negative mean nitrogen balance, whereas those fed glucose plus amino acids had a positive balance. There was no significant weight gain in either group.

Recently, in a study of premature infants of 25–33 weeks gestation who were being fed exclusively with peripheral parenteral nutrition (PN), nonprotein energy intakes averaging 80 cal/kg/day, as compared to 50 cal/kg/day, resulted in higher daily nitrogen retention and weight gain. At energy intakes greater than 70 cal/kg/day, further increases in energy intake had only minimal effect on nitrogen retention, suggesting that the basal metabolic needs of the infant were being met at 70 cal/kg/day (6). Intravenous infusion of energy intakes providing greater than *70 cal/kg/day* and nitrogen intakes of 430–560 mg/kg/day (*2.7–3.5g protein/kg/day*) resulted in nitrogen accretion and growth rates similar to in utero values (6).

Table 1. Enteral Caloric Requirements for the Preterm Infant (cal/kg/day)

Basal requirements	40– 50
Activity	5– 15
Cold stress	0– 10
Fecal losses	10– 15
Specific dynamic action	10
Growth	20– 30
Total	85–130

SOURCE: Kerner JA Jr, Sunshine P: *Seminars in Perinatology* 3:420, 1979. Reproduced with permission.

Rubecz and co-workers have pointed out that an individual approach to the estimation of caloric need is necessary for each infant (7) because the components of total heat production (basal metabolic rate, specific dynamic action, activity, thermoregulatory heat production) may vary a great deal depending on maturity, postnatal age, feeding, and thermal conditions. They also cautioned that intravenous calories be high enough to cover maintenance energy expenditure and low enough to avoid undesirable metabolic complications. When they infused a balanced solution containing approximately *70 cal/kg/day* (7.18 g/kg/day glucose, 1.54 g/kg/day amino acids, 3.16 g/kg/day of intravenous fat) to low birth weight infants, the plasma metabolic profile was normal (7).

It is often difficult, if not impossible, initially to provide the very low birth weight infant with even 30 or 40 cal/kg/day, especially if the infant has respiratory distress and/or is receiving assisted ventilation. Glucose intolerance may occur with the infusion of a 10% solution of dextrose, and attempts to provide even 120 ml/kg/day may result in fluid overload. It may require as long as 2–3 weeks to be able to infuse 60–70 cal/kg/day in some infants (8).

Infants and Older Children

Caloric requirements for pediatric patients on total parenteral nutrition (TPN) are summarized in Table 2 (9). Special circumstances that increase caloric needs are shown in Table 3 (9). General guidelines for oral caloric requirements are depicted in the Recommended Dietary Allowance (RDA) tables in Appendix I.

The tables mentioned should be used merely as guidelines. Each patient will have special circumstances that determine overall caloric needs. Rutten et al. (10) have proposed that the basal energy expenditure (BEE) equation when multiplied by a factor of 1.75 can assess a patient's caloric needs (10). A recent study (11) shows that indirect calorimetry (measuring oxygen consumption and respiratory quotient) consistently predicted higher caloric expenditure than did the equation of Rutten et al. Indirect calorimetry is easily performed in adults and older children and may prove to be a sensitive way to predict a patient's caloric needs.

A recent study by Merritt et al. (12) estimated caloric and protein requirements in six pediatric patients with acute non-lymphocytic leukemia. Mean total caloric requirement for weight maintenance was 136% of estimated basal metabolic rate,

Table 2. Caloric Requirements on TPN

Age (yr)	cal/kg/day
0– 1	90–120
1– 7	75– 90
7–12	60– 75
12–18	30– 60

SOURCE: Modified from Wesley R, Saran PA, Khalidi N, et al (eds): *Parenteral and Enteral Nutrition Manual of the University of Michigan Medical Center.* Chicago, Abbott Laboratories, 1980.

which is much lower than the RDA for healthy children. The mean protein requirement was 108% of the RDA. The difference between the caloric requirements of these children compared to normal requirements was probably due to limitation of their activity imposed by illness and their confinement to a laminar air flow unit. Many more such studies involving the whole spectrum of pediatric illnesses, both acute and chronic, are needed to help further define necessary caloric requirements.

Ziegler et al. (13) have suggested that the critical issue in selecting the route of intravenous nutrition (peripheral vs. central) is the estimated caloric requirements of the patient in question (see detailed discussion of peripheral vs. central PN in Chapter 1). It is clear that central vein PN allows delivery of sufficient nutrients to permit "normal" growth.

Levy and co-workers (14) point out that peripheral PN (limited to glucose concentrations of 10%) cannot be expected to produce "normal" growth unless unusually large volumes or large doses of fat emulsions are infused. To provide only 100 cal/kg/day requires 200 ml/kg/day if lipid intake is restricted to 3 g/kg/day (30 ml/kg/day of a 10% fat emulsion). If fluids are restricted to 150 ml/kg/day, lipid must be supplied at 6 g/kg/day, which may be excessive (see Chapter 7) to provide 100 cal/

Table 3. Circumstances That Increase Caloric Requirements

Fever	12% for each degree above 37°C
Cardiac failure	15–25%
Major surgery	20–30%
Burns	up to 100%
Severe sepsis	40–50%
Long-term growth failure	50–100%
Protein–calorie malnutrition (PCM)[a]	

SOURCE: Modified from Wesley R, Saran PA, Khalidi N, et al (eds): *Parenteral and Enteral Nutrition Manual of the University of Michigan Medical Center.* Chicago, Abbott Laboratories, 1980.

[a]A normal neonate needs approximately 80 cal/kg/day for basal needs and 110–120 cal/kg/day for growth. An infant with PCM needs 120 cal/kg/day for basal needs and 150–175 cal/kg/day for growth. An older child with PCM needs > 2× the basal energy requirement for growth to occur. (Suskind RM: Nutritional support of the secondarily malnourished child. *ASPEN Postgraduate Course.* 6th Clinical Congress, San Francisco, February, 1982.)

In PCM patients, approximately 6 cal are required for each gram of weight gain, at least during infancy. Thus, given the basal requirements for infants with PCM above, one can calculate the initial rate of weight gain during recovery from malnutrition (Kerr D, Ashworth A, Picou D, et al: Accelerated recovery from infant malnutrition with high calorie feeding, in Gardner LI, Amacher P (eds): *Endocrine Aspects of Malnutrition.* Santa Ynez, Calif, Kroc Foundation, 1973, p 467.)

kg/day. Utilizing reasonable restrictions of both fluids (150 ml/kg/day) and fat (3 g/kg/day) will provide approximately 80 cal/kg/day—only slightly more than an infant's resting requirements. Thus, peripheral PN seems more appropriate for a patient under minimal stress with a limited course on intravenous nutrition for whom full growth and development is not the therapeutic goal (14).

Practical Guidelines

PRETERM INFANTS

1. An intravenous regimen providing *60 cal/kg/day* (which includes 2.5 g/kg/day of amino acids) will result in positive nitrogen balance.
2. Intravenous intakes of approximately *70–90 cal/kg day* will result in weight gain.
   a. Intakes of > 70 cal/kg/day (including 2.7–3.5 g/kg/day protein) results in nitrogen accretion and growth rates similar to in utero values.
   b. Ideally, the caloric intake should be "balanced"—providing glucose, protein, and fat.
3. Fluid restrictions secondary to severe respiratory, cardiac, or renal disease may prevent the delivery of adequate calories (even if given by central TPN)—see Chapter 4.

OLDER INFANTS AND CHILDREN

1. Follow the guidelines in Table 2 for baseline caloric needs.
2. Follow the recommendations in Table 3 to estimate reasons for increased caloric needs.

GENERAL COMMENTS

1. Peripheral PN will provide approximately 80 cal/kg/day.
2. Peripheral PN seems best suited for minimally stressed patients undergoing a limited course on intravenous nutrition for whom full growth and development is not the therapeutic goal.
3. Central PN is indicated when full growth and development is essential.

References

1. Heird WC, Anderson TL: Nutritional requirements and methods of feeding low birth weight infants, in Gluck L (ed): *Current Problems in Pediatrics.* Chicago, Year Book Medical Publishers, 1977, vol 7, p 6.
2. Mestyan J, Jarai I, Fekete M: The total energy expenditure and its components in premature infants maintained under different nursing and environmental conditions. *Pediatr Res* 2:161, 1968.

3. Coran AG: The long-term total intravenous feeding of infants using peripheral veins. *J. Pediatr Surg* 8:801, 1973.

4. Cashore WJ, Sedaghatian MR, Usher RH: Nutritional supplements with intravenously administered lipid, protein hydrolysate, and glucose in small premature infants. *Pediatrics* 56:88, 1975.

5. Anderson TL, Muttart CR, Bieber MA, et al: A controlled trial of glucose versus glucose and amino acids in premature infants. *J. Pediatr* 94:947, 1979.

6. Zlotkin SH, Bryan MH, Anderson CH: Intravenous nitrogen and energy intakes required to duplicate in utero nitrogen accretion in prematurely born human infants. *J Pediatr* 99:115, 1981.

7. Rubecz I, Mestyan J, Varga P, et al: Metabolic and hormonal responses to low birth weight infants to intravenously infused calories not exceeding the maintenance energy expenditure. *Arch Dis Child* 54:499, 1979.

8. Heird WC, Driscoll JM Jr, Winters RW: Total parenteral nutrition in infants of very low birth weight, in Elliot K, Knight, J (eds): *Size at Birth.* Ciba Foundation Symposium 27 (New Series). Amsterdam, Associated Scientific Publishers, 1974, p 329.

9. Wesley JR, Saran PA, Khalidi N, et al (eds): *Parenteral and Enteral Nutrition Manual of the University of Michigan Medical Center.* Chicago, Abbott Laboratories, 1980, p 17.

10. Rutten P, Blackburn GL, Flatt JP, et al: Determination of optimal hyperalimentation infusion rate. *J Surg Res* 18:477, 1975.

11. Gazzaniga AB, Polachek JR, Wilson AF, et al: Indirect calorimetry as a guide to caloric replacement during total parenteral nutrition. *Am J Surg* 136:128, 1978.

12. Merritt RJ, Ashley JM, Siegel SE, et al: Calorie and protein requirements of pediatric patients with acute nonlymphocytic leukemia. *JPEN* 4:20, 1981.

13. Ziegler M, Jakobowski D, Hoelzer D: Route of pediatric parenteral nutrition: Proposed criteria revision. *J Pediatr Surg* 15:472, 1980.

14. Levy JS, Winters RW, Heird WC: Total parenteral nutrition in pediatric patients. *Pediatr in Review* 2:99, 1980.

4
Fluid Requirements

John A. Kerner, Jr.

The determination of fluid requirements for parenteral nutrition (PN) in pediatrics necessitates knowledge of several important aspects of "maintenance" fluid requirements.

1. There is a standard approach to calculating the maintenance fluid requirements of full term infants and older children.
2. Preterm infants have their own unique requirements.
3. Maintenance fluid regimens are calorically inadequate and will not promote growth. Such regimens are suitable for short periods of time only.
4. To provide the necessary calories for PN (hyperalimentation), discussed in Chapter 3, fluid volumes must be administered *in excess* of maintenance amounts.

A number of excellent review articles have been written describing fluid requirements of preterm infants, older infants, and children (1–4).

Maintenance Therapy

Maintenance intravenous fluid therapy in pediatrics replaces ongoing normal losses of fluids and electrolytes. Such therapy is required in any patient unable to tolerate a normal oral intake. The purpose of this treatment is to maintain the patient's normal fluid balance and to prevent deficits from occurring.

Any infant or child deprived of a normal oral intake will continue to lose basal amounts of fluids and electrolytes in urine, feces, and sweat and will also have additional evaporative (insensible) losses from the lungs and skin. Normal maintenance water requirements are depicted in Table 1. Note that maintenance water requirements normally average 100 ml/100 cal/day (1 ml/1 cal used). Hence, any physiological process that increases the caloric requirements of a child will increase the fluid requirements as well (see Table 3 in Chapter 3).

Table 1. Normal Maintenance Water Requirements

		Quantity (ml/100 cal/day)	
	Source of Water	Range	Average
Output	Insensible		
	pulmonary	10–20	15
	skin	25–35	30
	Urine	50–70	60
	Stool	5–10	7
	Sweat	0–20	0
	Total Output		112
Intake	Water of oxidation	10–15	12
	Average Maintenance Requirement		100

SOURCE: Gruskin AB: Fluid therapy in children. *Urol Clin North Am* 3:279, 1976. Reproduced with permission.

Deficit Therapy and Ongoing Losses

Losses of fluids and electrolytes that occurred before the initiation of medical support are replaced by "deficit" therapy. Such deficits may have resulted either from inadequate oral intake, excessive losses (e.g., diarrhea or diabetic ketoacidosis), or a combination of both. The goal of deficit therapy is to correct the deficit, and the fluids required to do so must be *added* to the calculated maintenance requirements.

In addition to the provision of maintenance fluids and fluids required to replete a determined deficit, fluids may also be needed to replace *ongoing losses*. For example, diarrhea or nasogastric suction will result in losses not provided for by maintenance requirements. These ongoing losses must be appropriately replaced.

Fluid Requirements

Fluid requirements can be altered by numerous clinical situations. For example, fever will increase ventilation (increasing insensible loss from the lungs) and increase sweating (increasing loss of water from the skin). Hyperventilation increases insensible losses by 5–20 ml/100 cal/day (2). Visible sweating increases sweat losses by 5–25 ml/100 cal/day (2). Renal disease may result in either oliguria or polyuria. Therapy, such as the use of a mist tent, will reduce insensible losses by 5–30 ml/100 cal/day (2).

Maintenance fluid requirements for pediatric patients, with the exception of the low birth weight infant, can be simply calculated using the recommendations in Table 2.

Unique Requirements of the Preterm Infant

Total body water (TBW) content of the fetus is high and decreases with increasing gestational age. It is estimated that TBW constitutes 94% of the fetal weight during

Table 2. Daily Maintenance Fluids in Pediatrics

By Body Surface:	1500–1800 ml/m^2/day
By Weight:	
Body weight	*Fluids required per day*
1–10 kg	100 ml/kg
11–20 kg	1000 ml plus 50 ml/kg for each kg above 10 kg
Above 20 kg	1500 ml plus 20 ml/kg for each kg above 20 kg

the third month of gestation, and decreases to approximately 80% by 32 weeks of gestation and to about 78% at term (5). In addition, as maturation proceeds intracellular water (ICW) forms a greater percentage of TBW while extracellular water (ECW) decreases. ECW decreases from about 60% body weight in the fifth month of gestation to about 45% at term; ICW increases from 25% of body weight during the fifth month to 33% at term (6).

The major source of water loss following birth is insensible water loss (IWL), that water lost through the skin by evaporation and from the respiratory tract, the latter accounting for 10–30% of the total IWL. Measurements of IWL using direct weighing techniques show that IWL varies from 17–64 ml/kg/24 hr, depending on the baby's birth weight. Very low birth weight infants often lose up to 10–15% of their body weight during the first week of life (5). These infants may have had very high water losses, up to 80–100 ml/kg/day, and there is an inverse correlation between birth weight and IWL.

Mechanisms that account for this excess water loss in low birth weight infants include

Their very large surface area relative to body weight

The minimal amount of subcutaneous fat present

The very thin epidermis which is very permeable

The large TBW and ECW content of these infants

The maintenance water requirements in low birth weight infants is the sum of the IWL, renal water excretion, and stool loss. In addition, water is required for the formation of new tissue mass during growth (1,7).

Although the infant born at term can adapt somewhat to fluid deprivation or fluid excesses, the preterm infant adapts poorly because of the inability of the renal system to conserve water and the mechanisms accounting for excess water loss previously described. Obviously if the patient is not given adequate fluids, hyperosmolarity, hypernatremia, and dehydration may ensue. If too much fluid is given intravenously, edema and congestive heart failure will also develop, especially if the infant is receiving warm, humidified gases with assisted ventilation or is cared for in a warm, humidified environment. Factors increasing or decreasing fluid requirements in preterm infants are shown in Table 3.

Wu and Hodgman demonstrated that infants cared for under radiant warmers had a significantly increased IWL as compared to those cared for in conventional incubators. The loss was greater under the infrared radiant warmer than under either the IMI (Industrial Medical Instruments) radiant warmer or the nichrome wire radiant warmer (8). Interestingly, they demonstrated that the percentage increase in water loss under radiant warmers as compared to loss in conventional incubators was greater in infants weighing more than 1500 g than those weighing

Table 3. Water Requirements in Premature Infants

Factors Increasing Requirements
Radiant warmers[8]
Conventional single walled incubators[8,10]
Phototherapy[a]
An ambient temperature above the neutral thermal range
Respiratory distress
Any hypermetabolic problem
Elevated body temperature
Furosemide treatment
Diarrhea
Glycosuria (with associated osmotic diuresis)
Intravenous alimentation[24]
Factors Decreasing Requirements
Heat shields[10]
Thermal blankets[15]
Double walled incubators[b]
Placing the infant in relatively high humidity
Use of warm humidified air via endotracheal tube
Renal oliguria

---

[a] Oh W, Karechi H: Phototherapy and insensible water loss in the newborn infant. *Am J Dis Child* 124:230, 1972.

[b] Yeh TF, Voora S, Lilien J: Oxygen consumption and insensible water loss in premature infants in single versus double-walled incubators. *J Pediatr* 97:967, 1980.

less than 1500 g. Our clinical experience is somewhat at variance with the data of Wu and Hodgman in that the IWL in infants cared for under radiant warmers is often more than tripled, especially if the infant weighs less than 1000 g (9).

Wu and Hodgman have also demonstrated that infants who weighed more than 1500 g had a greater percentage of IWL when placed under phototherapy as compared to those infants who weighed less than 1500 g (8). Again, this is somewhat contrary to our clinical experience with the use of phototherapy, in which there appears to be a greater percentage of fluid loss in the more immature infant (9).

Fanaroff and co-workers demonstrated that IWL could be markedly decreased with the use of a heat shield inside of a conventional incubator, especially in those infants who were less than 1250 g and less than 10 days of age (10). Because there is a direct relationship between insensible or evaporative water loss and basal metabolic rate, the data implied that there were markedly elevated metabolic rates in these extremely frail infants. This seemed extremely unlikely because, if true, the infants would have rapidly depleted their limited caloric reserves. Darnall and Ariagno demonstrated that minimal rates of oxygen consumption could be achieved under radiant warmers—where insensible water losses have been demonstrated to be increased—and theorized that large increases in insensible water loss could occur without a concomitant rise in metabolic rate (11). This concept of dissociation between insensible water loss and metabolic rate has been confirmed by simultaneous measurement of oxygen consumption and insensible water loss by Bell and co-workers (12). Okken and co-workers found that evaporative heat loss made up about 23% of the total loss by the large preterm infant, but could account for as much as 60% of heat loss by small, preterm infants nursed in single-wall

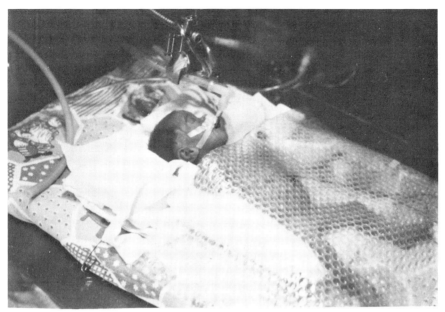

Figure 1 Infant cared for under a radiant warmer with a "thermal blanket" in place. (Kerner JA Jr, Sunshine P: Parenteral alimentation. *Semin Perinatol* 3:419, 1979.) Reproduced with permission.

incubators (13). A heat shield has also been proven to decrease insensible water loss in infants under a radiant warmer (14).

Marks and co-workers convincingly demonstrated that the use of a thermal blanket markedly decreased the insensible fluid loss of babies cared for in conventional incubators (15), and although not well documented, it is probable that this also occurs in infants cared for under radiant warmers. Again, despite the fact that the insensible water loss was decreased, Darnall and Ariagno showed that the oxygen consumption was identical whether or not the baby was covered with a thermal blanket as long as the infant was in a neutral thermal environment (16).

Because of the many variables encountered, we have recommended that the intravenous infusion of fluid be initiated at the rate of 40–60 ml/kg/day in the low birth weight infant and that this be increased slowly over the first week of life to 100–200 ml/kg/day. These are the rates that are used if the infant is cared for in a servo-controlled incubator; increased rates of fluid infusion may be necessary if the infant is cared for under a radiant warmer. With the use of a thermal blanket (Fig. 1), we have been able to decrease fluid loss significantly and avoid both overhydration and underhydration.

Usually by the end of the second week of life the infant can tolerate up to 130–140 ml/kg/day. If infants cared for in conventional incubators receive more than 150 ml/kg/day, they may develop evidence of congestive heart failure with opening of the ductus arteriosus. The signs of fluid overload are often not recognized readily, since cardiomegaly, hepatic enlargement, and pulmonary edema are not conspicuous particularly if the infant has respiratory distress and is receiving assisted ventilation. Often, the only sign of failure is a gradual elevation of the infant's $PaCO_2$ or inappropriately rapid weight gain.

Complications of Overhydration in the High Risk Infant

PATENT DUCTUS ARTERIOSUS

Persistent patent ductus arteriosus (PDA) is a common clinical problem in intensive care nurseries. Functional closure usually occurs in the first 24 hours of life and anatomical closure occurs within weeks in the term infant. Closure is normally delayed in preterm infants. Hypoxia and other factors associated with respiratory distress syndrome (RDS) may keep the ductus patent. The incidence of PDA is inversely related to gestational age and is highest in sickest infants—reportedly as high as 80% in infants less than or equal to 30 weeks gestation (17).

Functional closure of the ductus arteriosus depends on many factors, including fluid administration. Excessive water administration to preterm infants in the first days of life results in a higher incidence of clinically evident PDA (18). In a retrospective study, Brown and co-workers demonstrated that the incidence of patent ductus arteriosus associated with congestive heart failure as well as the development of bronchopulmonary dysplasia (BPD) was most closely correlated with increased rates of fluid infusions in infants with hyaline membrane disease (118 ± 8 ml/kg/day vs. 150 ± 11 ml/kg/day) (19).

BRONCHOPULMONARY DYSPLASIA

BPD is a chronic lung disease of preterm infants that follows RDS and is usually seen after prolonged intubation and oxygen exposure. Lung oxygen toxicity is associated with increased pulmonary microvascular permeability and increased pulmonary water. Retrospective reviews suggest that BPD is related to increased fluid administration in the first 5 days of life (19) and to PDA (20).

NECROTIZING ENTEROCOLITIS

Necrotizing enterocolitis (NEC) is characterized by abdominal distention, intolerance to feedings, apnea, temperature instability, and guaiac-positive stools. The primary abnormality is intestinal musocal injury. Classic NEC also requires the presence of invasive gas-producing organisms and an appropriate substrate for bacterial growth. Infants who develop NEC are usually premature and stressed by hypoxia, acidosis, and hypotension.

Many factors may lead to the mucosal injury, and fluid overload appears to be related to this injury. In enteral feeding regimens, NEC may be related to the use of large volumes or rapid increases in volume (21). Bell et al. (22) studied 170 premature infants (birthweights 751–2000 g) in a randomized sequential trial comparing "high" and "low" volumes of fluid intake. The low-volume group received only enough water to supply average estimated requirements, and the high-volume group received an excess of at least 20 ml/kg/day (mean excess was 47 ml/kg/day). More cases of necrotizing enterocolitis occurred in the high-volume group (22).

INTRAVENTRICULAR HEMORRHAGE IN THE PRETERM INFANT

The incidence of periventricular and intraventricular hemorrhage (IVH) is inversely correlated with gestational age. Severe IVH has an extremely poor prognosis, and thus prevention is extremely important. A retrospective review of infants less than 1400 g showed that those with IVH had received excessive volume expansion in the first hours of life (23).

Individualized Fluid Management

It is apparent from the data presented that the water losses in low birth weight infants vary tremendously according to birth weight and many other environmental factors. It must be emphasized that *no* measurements of IWL have been made in *sick* infants (e.g., those on ventilators), and these studies need to be performed to allow us to make more intelligent decisions about fluid management of such babies. Previously suggested intakes of fluids have been based on data obtained on *well* infants and *may be excessive* for the tiny, sick babies that neonatal intensive care nurseries are now treating.

After the initial fluid administration of 40–60 ml/kg/day, many centers base all subsequent fluid requirements on the infant's needs, rather than using "cookbook" guidelines. The needs are defined by clinical examination of the patient, the peripheral perfusion, the presence or absence of edema, central venous pressure readings, urine output and osmolality (or specific gravity), and measurements of hematocrit, blood urea nitrogen, and electrolytes. The infant's body weight must be evaluated at least daily and as often as every 8 hours if his or her condition is unstable. In determining fluid needs the type of incubator that is being used and the techniques employed to curtail fluid losses must also be considered. In addition, the above fluid restrictions prohibit the provision of adequate calories. Adequate caloric intake cannot be attained until the infant has entered the recovery phase of the disease. At this point administration of much larger fluid volumes, to achieve adequate caloric intake, positive nitrogen balance, and growth is more feasible.

Parenteral Nutrition

As depicted in Table 3, PN solutions with intravenous fat emulsion are still another potential cause of increased insensible water loss as a result of increased metabolic rate and thermogenesis (24). Weight gain and positive nitrogen balance have been demonstrated in many patients supported solely by intravenous nutrition. In the past there has been debate about whether the weight gain observed is due to an increase in lean body mass or simply due to water retention secondary to the large volume of fluids infused. Using the deuterium oxide dilution technique, the total body water changes of five infants maintained on TPN have been determined (25,26). The results support tissue accretion rather than water retention as the mechanism of weight gain in the long-term, large-volume, TPN of these infants (25,26).

Table 4. Fluid Recommendations for Parenteral Nutrition

Initial volume for patients free of cardiovascular or renal disease:

<10 kg = 100 ml/kg/day

10–30 kg = 2000 ml/m²/day

30–50 kg = 100 ml/hr (2.4 liters/day)

>50 kg = 125 ml/hr (3 liters/day)

Volume may be increased by

10 ml/kg/day in infants until the desired caloric intake is achieved (to a maximum of 200 ml/kg/day, *if tolerated*).

>10 kg: by 10% of initial volume/day until desired caloric intake is achieved (to a maximum of 4000 ml/m²/day, *if tolerated*).

Practical Guidelines for Fluid Requirements in Parenteral Nutrition

1. For low birth weight infants, follow the recommendations for fluid use described in the sections on "Unique Requirements of the Preterm Infant" and "Individualized Fluid Management" in this chapter. Complications of overhydration in the high risk infant limit the degree that fluids can be advanced to increase calories (fluid volume is the rate limiting step; thus clinical problems such as PDA, CHF, and BPD may require restriction of fluids to the extent that adequate calories cannot be provided, even with PN).

2. For older infants and children, follow the recommendations in Table 4.

References

1. Bell EF, Oh W: Fluid and electrolyte balance in very low birth weight infants. *Clin Perinatol* 6:139, 1979.

2. Gruskin AB: Fluid therapy in children. *Urol Clin North Am* 3:277, 1976.

3. Oh W: Disorders of fluid and electrolytes in newborn infants. *Pediatr Clin North Am* 23:601, 1976.

4. Dreszer M: Fluid and electrolyte requirements in the newborn infant. *Pediatr Clin North Am* 24:537, 1977.

5. Friis-Hansen B: Changes in body water compartments during growth. *Acta Paediatr Scand* (Suppl 110) 46:1, 1957.

6. Oh W: Fluid and electrolyte management, in Avery GB (ed): *Neonatology: Pathophysiology and Management of the Newborn.* Philadelphia, JB Lippincott Co, 1975, p 471.

7. Heird WC, Anderson TL: Nutritional requirements and methods of feeding low birth weight infants. *Curr Probl Pediatr* 7:15, 1977.

8. Wu PYK, Hodgman JE: Insensible water loss in premature infants: Changes with postnatal development and nonionizing radiant energy. *Pediatrics* 54:704, 1974.

9. Kerner JA Jr, Sunshine P: Parenteral alimentation. *Semin Perinatol* 3:417, 1979.

10. Fanaroff M, Wald M, Gruber HS, et al: Insensible water loss in low birth weight infants. *Pediatrics* 50:236, 1972.

11. Darnall RA Jr, Ariagno RL: Minimal oxygen consumption in infants cared for under overhead radiant warmers compared with conventional incubators. *J Pediatr* 93:283, 1976.

12. Bell EF, Weinstein MR, Oh W: Heat balance in premature infants: Comparative effects of convectively heated incubator and radiant warmer, with and without plastic shield. *J Pediatr* 96:460, 1980.

13. Okken A, Jonxis JHP, Respene P, et al: Insensible water loss and metabolic rate in low birth-weight newborn infants. *Pediatr Res* 13:1072, 1979.

14. Yeh TF, Amma P, Lilien LO, et al: Reduction of insensible water loss in premature infants under the radiant warmer. *J Pediatr* 94:651, 1979.

15. Marks KH, Friedman Z, Maisels MJ: A simple device for reducing insensible water loss in low birth weight infants. *Pediatrics* 60:223, 1977.

16. Darnall RA Jr, Ariagno RL: Resting oxygen consumption of premature infants covered with a thermal blanket. *Pediatrics* 63:547, 1979.

17. Emmanouilides GC: Persistent patency of the ductus arteriosus in premature infants: Incidence, perinatal factors and natural history, in Heymann MA, Rudolph AM, (eds): *The Ductus Arteriosus Report of the Seventy-Fifth Ross Conference on Pediatric Research.* Columbus, Ohio, Ross Laboratories, 1978, p 63.

18. Stevenson JG: Fluid administration in the association of patent ductus arteriosus complicating respiratory distress syndrome. *J Pediatr* 90:257, 1977.

19. Brown ER, Stark A, Sosenko I, et al: Bronchopulmonary dysplasia: Possible relationship to pulmonary edema. *J Pediatr* 92:982, 1978.

20. Brown ER: Increased risk of bronchopulmonary dysplasia in infants with patent ductus arteriosus. *J Pediatr* 95:865, 1979.

21. Goldman HI: Feeding and necrotizing enterocolitis. *Am J Dis Child* 134:553, 1980.

22. Bell EF, Warburton D, Stonestreet BS, et al: Effects of fluid administration on the development of symptomatic patent ductus arteriosus and congestive heart failure in premature infants. *N Engl J Med* 302:598, 1980.

23. Goldberg RN, Chung D, Goldman SL, et al: The association of rapid volume expansion and intraventricular hemorrhage in the preterm infant. *J Pediatr* 96:1060, 1980.

24. Marks KH, Farrell TP, Friedman Z, et al: Intravenous alimentation and insensible water loss in low-birth-weight infants. *Pediatrics* 63:543, 1979.

25. Rhodin AG, Coran AG, Weintraub WH, et al: Total body water changes during high volume peripheral hyperalimentation. *Surg Gynecol Obstet* 148:196, 1979.

26. Polley TZ Jr, Benner JW, Rhodin A, et al: Changes in total body water in infants receiving total intravenous nutrition. *J Surg Res* 26:555, 1979.

5
Carbohydrate Requirements

John A. Kerner, Jr.

Metabolism of both the central nervous system and the hematopoietic tissue is dependent to a large extent on glucose, but it is not essential that these glucose requirements be supplied exogenously (either from the diet or intravenously). Glucose can be produced from exogenously administered protein or endogenous protein stores (gluconeogenesis). Thus, unlike the amino acid and essential fatty acid requirements discussed in the next two chapters, no absolute requirement for carbohydrate has been demonstrated (1). The pathways of gluconeogenesis in the low birth weight infant are not completely understood, and the high incidence of hypoglycemia in these infants has been attributed to immaturity of hepatic gluconeogenesis mechanisms (2). In *all* infants during the first 2 days of life there is decreased, but not absent, gluconeogenic pathway activity. Low carbohydrate diets tend to produce ketosis, especially if the protein content is also low. Newborn infants and low birth weight infants do not appear to develop ketosis, unlike older patients (1). For these reasons, carbohydrates should provide approximately 40–45% of the total caloric content of most dietary regimens, including those specifically designed for low birth weight infants.

The Use of Intravenous Glucose

GLUCOSE INTOLERANCE IN PREMATURE INFANTS

Currently, glucose is the main source of calories in patients receiving parenteral nutrition (PN). The ability to metabolize glucose is limited in neonates compared with that in older infants and children. In premature infants it may be limited even more.

The infusion of glucose (dextrose) in term and older infants can be initiated at a rate of 7–8 mg/kg/min (420–480 mg/kg/hr), and rapidly increased to 12–14 mg/kg/min without difficulty. However, a large number of the very low birth weight infants develop significant hyperglycemia if the glucose infusion rate is in excess of 400 mg/kg/hr (9.6 g/kg/day), the equivalent of 10% dextrose at 100 ml/kg/day (3). The hyperglycemia occurs within the first 24–48 hours after the infusion has been initiated and is encountered most frequently in the very immature infant (4). Interestingly, even in very immature infants, hyperglycemia does not occur as readily in those infants who are also receiving intravenous infusion of amino acids along with the dextrose (5). These data suggested that the amino acids may have been stimulating the release of greater amounts of insulin, although concentrations of insulin in plasma had not been measured.

In a study by Cowett and co-workers, low birth weight infants who were appropriate for gestational age were infused with varying amounts of glucose ranging from 8.1–14 mg/kg/min over 3 hours (6). At the lower rates of infusion (8.1 mg/kg/min) the infants had insignificant changes in the concentration of plasma glucose or insulin. When 11.2 mg/kg/min of glucose was given, half of the infants became hyperglycemic. These infants had lower insulin responses at 2 hours after starting the infusion than those who did not become hyperglycemic. The authors speculated that the infants "who had fewer clinical complications during the neonatal period may have had more active pancreatic beta-cell response to plasma glucose concentrations resulting in lower risk for hyperglycemia (and glucosuria) when exogenous glucose was provided" (6). All the infants in the study developed hyperglycemia when given 14 mg/kg/min, demonstrating that the tolerance to glucose of these infants had been exceeded (6).

The reasons for the limited glucose tolerance in neonates is not clear. Possible causes include: (1) decreased insulin production, (2) insulin resistance, (3) increased hepatic glucose production, (4) immature hepatic enzyme systems, (5) insulin receptors being abnormal in number or function.

1. *Decreased insulin production.* Premature infants show a less consistent rise in plasma insulin after glucose loading during the first 24 hours than later (7). Even a term infant's insulin response to carbohydrate is sluggish (8).

2. *Insulin resistance.* Goldman and Hirata (9) attempted to avoid hyperglycemia by providing exogenous insulin with parenteral alimentation to four very low birth weight infants. However, the exogenous insulin did not affect glucose tolerance as expected. With seemingly appropriate preinfusion and extraordinarily high insulin levels during infusion, glucose intolerance remained. Thus, insulin resistance and not insulin deficiency may be at fault (9).

3. *Increased hepatic glucose production.* Sherwood and co-workers (10) reported that in some premature rhesus monkeys, hyperglycemia and endogenous insulin did not suppress hepatic glucose output. It is not known whether the glucose output is secondary to gluconeogenesis or glycogenolysis. There is evidence that the phenomenon described by Sherwood and co-workers may also occur in human infants. Pollack et al. (11) demonstrated that some very low birth weight infants infused with glucose become hyperglycemic despite an increase in endogenous insulin secretion.

4. Hepatic enzyme systems responsible for glycogenesis, which would decrease peripheral glucose values, may be deficient (9).

5. The infant's insulin receptors may be abnormal in number or function (9). No data exist for premature infants, but it has been demonstrated in rats that insulin receptors increase in number as gestational age increases (12).

Finally, other hormonal systems may play a role in the glucose metabolism of the neonate. Stressed very low birth weight infants are afflicted with more hyperglycemia than their unstressed peers, despite higher serum levels of insulin and lower levels of cortisol (13).

Further studies, in both human infants and appropriate animal models, will have to be performed to further elucidate the mechanisms of glucose intolerance in very low birth weight infants.

Attempts to modulate the adverse effects of intravenous dextrose with the use of insulin have been extremely difficult because of the variable response of the infants to the hormone. While in the study of Goldman and Hirata (9) a continuous infusion of insulin had little to no effect, others have found that even miniscule amounts of insulin may cause the concentration of glucose in blood to plummet from hyperglycemic to hypoglycemic levels in very short periods of time (14).

Another technique used to avoid severe hyperglycemic responses is to infuse other carbohydrates such as galactose along with the glucose. Using this technique, Avery was able to demonstrate a more normoglycemic response of the infant and thus avoid hyperglycemic reactions (15). Even small, ill infants who became hyperglycemic when given infusions of 10% dextrose became normoglycemic when an infusion combination of 5% dextrose plus 5% galactose was used. Avery noted no toxicity due to the galactose and observed that neither galactosuria nor hypergalactosemia resulted.

Hyperglycemia, per se, cannot only cause an osmotic diuresis with concomitant loss of electrolytes but can actually increase serum osmolality to such a degree that the infant may develop hyperosmolar coma and even intracranial hemorrhage. Thus, careful monitoring of the serum glucose during infusion, especially during the first 24–48 hours in the very low birth weight infant is mandatory in order to avoid the complications of severe hyperglycemia. On the whole, infants weighing less than 1000 g at birth should initially receive no more than 6 mg glucose/kg/min and those weighing between 1000 g and 1500 g should not receive more than 8 mg/kg/min. Even with these low rates of glucose infusion, hyperglycemia could conceivably occur. After the infant has stabilized and is able to tolerate the glucose infusion, the concentrations can be increased slowly with careful monitoring. When the infant is able to tolerate the infusion of approximately 100 ml/kg/day of 10% dextrose (7mg/kg/min), then amino acids can be added to the infusion. As the infant demonstrates tolerance to increasing concentrations of dextrose, the rate of infusion can be increased appropriately. Any infant who suddenly demonstrates glucosuria at a concentration of dextrose infusion that had previously been tolerated is suspect for sepsis. This is often the initial finding in an infected infant. Hypoglycemia has not been a major problem in infants receiving parenteral nutrition and the only time it is of concern is when the infusion of glucose is stopped abruptly. This complication can also occur in any infant who is receiving parenteral nutrition and the infusion has to be discontinued because of complications or infiltration of the peripheral intravenous site. In such cases, glucose infusions should be restarted immediately to avoid rebound hypoglycemia.

Use of Intravenous Glucose in Older Infants and Children

The very large glucose loads delivered with central PN might be expected to cause glucose intolerance in many patients, but in fact this complication is relatively uncommon. Das and Filler (16) performed glucose balance studies in infants given total parenteral nutrition (TPN) with 20% dextrose. Plasma insulin concentration increased significantly and appropriately during infusion of hypertonic dextrose (16). Most individuals are relatively glucose intolerant for a few days following major trauma or surgery due to high circulating levels of cortisol and glucagon (17). TPN is, therefore, not given during the immediate post-traumatic period since there is considerable evidence that nutrients cannot be used effectively in the presence of these counter-regulatory hormones. Sepsis, as mentioned in the section on low birth weight infants, is another important cause of glucose intolerance in older infants and children. The sudden onset of glucosuria in a patient receiving PN, at a dose of glucose previously tolerated, may be an early sign of bacteremia. Steroids administered to a pediatric patient may also cause hyperglycemia.

The syndrome of hyperglycemic nonketotic dehydration has been reviewed extensively by Kaminski (18) who reported six cases among 200 adults who were receiving TPN with hypertonic dextrose. Most of the patients had a family history of diabetes and either sepsis or other metabolic stress. The fully developed syndrome with coma and a significant mortality rate (16%) can be prevented by frequent monitoring of blood and urine glucose.

In pediatrics, hyperglycemic nonketotic dehydration occurs almost exclusively in small premature infants. Hyperglycemia (blood glucose > 200 mg/dl) and persistent glucosuria (3 + or more on successive determinations) were observed by one center in six patients, five of whom weighed less than 2000 g (17).

Plasma insulin concentration increases in response to infusion of hypertonic dextrose. Abrupt cessation of the infusion may lead to profound hypoglycemia with secondary seizures and coma. If the central catheter becomes clotted or dislodged, a peripheral intravenous infusion of 10% dextrose must be started promptly. Patients should be tapered slowly from hypertonic dextrose solutions when PN is being electively discontinued.

Experience with cyclic TPN in outpatients has shown that hypoglycemia rarely develops in well-nourished individuals who have adequate glycogen stores; therefore, they can be weaned over several hours (17). Premature infants and malnourished or stressed patients, however, are at greater risk and should be weaned over 12–36 hours.

When patients require severe fluid restriction, some authors recommend increasing the dextrose concentration to 30% or 35% so that the same number of calories can be infused in a smaller volume of fluid (17). There is concern about the increased risk of thrombosis with such hypertonic solutions (see Table 1 for osmolarity of dextrose solutions), especially in premature infants. Since the catheter is approximately the same diameter as the vessel cannulated, the chance of adequate dilution of the hypertonic solution is less than in larger patients (S. Shochat, personal communication, April, 1982).

Use of Other Carbohydrates

GALACTOSE

Using galactose along with glucose in premature infants Avery (15) was able to avoid hyperglycemic reactions that occurred when giving dextrose alone (see sec-

Table 1. Caloric Density and Osmolarity of Dextrose Solutions

Dextrose Solution	Cal/ml	Calculated Osmolarity (mOsm/L)
D5W	0.17	252
D7.5W	0.25	378
D10W	0.34	505
D15W	0.51	758
D20W	0.68	1010
D25W	0.85	1263
D30W	1.02	1515

tion on glucose intolerance in premature infants). No toxicity from the galactose was noted (15).

Pribylova and Kozlova (19) have also found no undesirable effects of galactose administration to full term neonates. Their study demonstrated that galactose is quickly metabolized by the newborn and provides minimal stimulation of insulin secretion (19). More studies need to be completed before recommendations can be made for the routine use of galactose.

FRUCTOSE

Numerous complications have been reported during fructose infusion: increased levels of blood lactate, hepatomegaly, and decreased levels of hepatic inorganic phosphate and ATP (20–23). In low birth weight infants less than 7 days old, serum lactate levels rise considerably (24), four to five times more than after an equivalent load of galactose (25). Fructose, therefore, is contraindicated for use as an intravenous nutrient in children.

ALCOHOL

Intravenous infusion of alcohol has been recommended in order to provide additional caloric supplementation for infants of low birth weight (26). The concentrations have varied between 0.5% and 1%, and as each gram of alcohol is metabolized, 7 cal are generated, while contributing little to the volume and osmolality of the infusate. More current information suggests, however, that alcohol is poorly metabolized by neonates.

The activity of alcohol dehydrogenase, the rate-limiting oxidizing enzyme in the metabolism of alcohol, is 10–15% that of the adult when measured in the liver of term infants; adult levels of activity are not achieved until the child has reached 5 years of age (27). The vast majority of infants who have been given small quantities of alcohol in parenteral nutrition infusions have demonstrated few adverse reactions to alcohol and showed few, if any, signs of ethanol intoxication even at serum levels greater than 100 mg/dl (28).

We cared for an infant who had received intravenous alcohol as part of the nutritional supplementation, and only when the alcohol level exceeded 250 mg/dl did the infant demonstrate lethargy and apnea. Considering that the level of intoxication in adults is approximately 100 mg/dl, and that even 50 mg/dl decreases reaction time, the effects of increased alcohol levels on the developing central nervous system of a preterm infant should be of concern. It is obvious that with the use of lipid emulsions and dextrose plus amino acid substrates for intravenous infusions, the use of alcohol in preterm infants is not indicated. The long-term follow-up on infants who have been given intravenous alcohol is currently being studied, and preliminary data suggest that these small amounts of alcohol have had no adverse effect on the infants (SG Babson, personal communication to Dr. Philip Sunshine, February, 1979).

MALTOSE

Preliminary studies in adults suggest that maltose could be an acceptable source of calories for parenteral alimentation. In equimolar concentrations, maltose provides twice as many calories per unit of volume as glucose, but only half the osmolar load. It elicits metabolic effects similar to those of glucose, except for the absence of hyperglycemia (29). A rise in total serum-reducing substances in the presence of normoglycemia suggests that maltose enters the cells intact and is metabolized. Unfortunately no data are available yet on maltose tolerance in neonates, so recommendations for use cannot be made.

The Need for "Balanced" TPN Including Carbohydrate and Fat

A balanced TPN solution, including both carbohydrate and fat (as nonnitrogen calories) may avoid (1) fatty infiltration of the liver, (2) water retention, and (3) worsening already severe respiratory compromise.

1. Fatty Infiltration of the Liver. An excessive load of carbohydrate can cause fatty infiltration of the liver; the incidence of this complication can be reduced by replacing some of the carbohydrate calories with intravenous fat calories (30–34). In a study of TPN in rats, after 4 weeks of protein depletion the animals were nutritionally repleted with one of four isonitrogenous, isovolemic intravenous diets of varying caloric content and composition (35). After 6 days massive hepatomegaly and fatty deposition were noted in animals repleted with regimens supplying all nonnitrogenous calories as fat or carbohydrate. Hepatic "steatosis" was avoided when a "balanced" regimen of 75% carbohydrate and 25% fat was used (see the discussion of hepatic dysfunction in Chapter 13).

2. Water Retention. (See the discussion on nitrogen retention in Chapter 7.)

3. Worsening of Already Severe Respiratory Compromise. In adults it has been shown that high glucose loads may be detrimental to the hypermetabolic patient with decreased pulmonary reserve (31). Glucose metabolism increases carbon dioxide production and minute ventilation, which may aggravate ventilator weaning or precipitate pulmonary failure (30, 31). Metabolism of each potential energy substrate (e.g., protein, carbohydrate, fat) has a respiratory quotient (RQ) defined as the ratio of carbon dioxide produced to oxygen consumed. Metabolism of carbohydrate yields an RQ of 1.0; protein yields 0.8; and fat produces 0.7 (30, 36). RQs near 1.0 tend to reduce respiratory reserve capacity and may be detrimental in the acutely ill patient with pulmonary insufficiency (31, 37).

Changes in CO_2 production and O_2 consumption induced by TPN using either glucose as the entire source of nonprotein calories (the glucose system) or fat emulsions as 50% of the nonprotein calories (the lipid system) have been analyzed in patients with chronic nutritional depletion or who are acutely ill secondary to injury and infection (38). In patients with chronic nutritional depletion, shifting from the lipid to the glucose system caused a 20% increase in CO_2 production, which resulted in a 26% increase in minute ventilation. In the acutely ill patients receiving the glucose system, CO_2 production was significantly higher than in those receiving the lipid system. Fat emulsions can serve as a source of nonprotein calories and are associated with less CO_2 production than isocaloric amounts of glucose (38).

Practical Guidelines

1. Glucose (dextrose) provides 3.4 cal/g when given in the monohydrate form.
2. Maximum dextrose concentrations allowable in infants and children are
   a. 10% by peripheral vein. Concentrations above 10% are associated with an increased incidence of phlebitis, secondary to increased solution osmolarity, and thus a decreased "lifespan" of peripheral lines (39).
   b 20% by central vein.
   c. 25% by central vein in severely malnourished patients.
3. Carbohydrates are initiated in a slow, stepwise fashion to allow an appropriate response of endogenous insulin and thus prevent glucosuria (and subsequent osmotic diuresis).
4. For very low birth weight premature infants it is critical that the carbohydrate intake be calculated in terms of g/kg/day (or per hour or minute) rather

Table 2. Required Glucose Concentration by Rate of Glucose Infusion and Rate of Water Infusion

Glucose Infusion Rate		Fluid Infusion Rate			
		ml/kg/24 hr	96	144	192
mg/kg/min	g/kg/24 hr	ml/kg/hr	4	6	8
5.0	7.2		7.5%	5.0%	3.8%
7.5	10.8		11.3%	7.5%	5.6%
10.0	14.4		15.0%	10.0%	7.5%
12.5	18.0		18.8%	12.5%	9.4%

SOURCE: Yu VYH, James BE, Hendry PG, et al: Glucose tolerance in very low birth weight infants. *Aust Paediatr J* 15:150, 1979. Reproduced with permission.

Table 3. Recommendations for Dextrose Use

Premature and Newborn Infants		Older Infants and Children	Teenagers and Adults
Day 1	D 5	D 5	D 5
2	D 5	D 7.5	D10[a]
3	D 7.5	D10[a]	D15
4	D 7.5	D12.5	D20
5	D10[a]	D15	
6	D10[a]	D17.5	
7	D12.5	D20	
8	D12.5		
9	D15		
10	D15		
11	D17.5		
12	D17.5		
13	D20		
14	D20		

[a]Maximum allowable by peripheral vein.

than as arbitrary concentrations of dextrose given at rates to meet fluid requirements. Table 2 provides the necessary calculations.

   a. Careful monitoring of dextrose infusions, especially during the first 24–48 hours in the very low birth weight infant is crucial to avoid the complications of severe hyperglycemia (for specifics of monitoring see Chapter 15).

   b. Infants < 1000 g at birth should start at no more than 6 mg glucose/kg/min; those weighing between 1000–1500 g should not receive more than 8 mg/kg/min initially. Even at these low rates of infusion, hyperglycemia may still occur.

   c. After the infant has stabilized and is able to tolerate the dextrose infusions, the concentrations can be increased slowly, but the infant must be monitored carefully.

   d. Insulin should not be used in premature infants on PN because of highly variable responses.

5. Any infant or child who suddenly demonstrates glucosuria at a concentration of dextrose that had previously been tolerated is suspect for sepsis.

6. If the central catheter becomes clotted or dislodged, a peripheral IV infusion of 10% dextrose must be started promptly to avoid hypoglycemia.

7. Parenteral nutrition should ideally be discontinued only for a patient on adequate enteral nutrition, and should be gradually tapered over 1–2 days. Close observation for rebound hypoglycemia after abrupt termination of parenteral nutrition is essential.

8. Advances in carbohydrate load in very low birth weight infants are described in 4b and 4c with the help of Table 2.

9. In more mature premature infants, term infants, and older infants and children, advance the dextrose concentrations as recommended in Table 3.

References

1. Heird WC, Anderson TL: Nutritional requirements and methods of feeding low birth weight infants. *Curr Probl Pediatr* 7(8):13, 1977.

2. Gutberlet RB, Cornblath M: Neonatal hypoglycemia revisted, 1975. *Pediatrics* 58:10, 1976.

3. Dweck HS, Cassady G: Glucose intolerance in infants of very low birth weight. I. Incidence of hyperglycemia in infants of birth weight 1100 grams or less. *Pediatrics* 53:189, 1974.

4. Miranda LEV, Dweck HS: Perinatal glucose homeostasis: The unique character of hyperglycemia and hypoglycemia in infants of very low birth weight. *Clin Perinatol* 4:351, 1977.

5. Chance GW: Results in very low birth weight infants (< 1300 gm birth weight), in Winters RW, Hasselmeyer EG (eds): *Intravenous Nutrition in the High Risk Infant.* New York, John Wiley & Sons, 1975, p. 39.

6. Cowett RM, Oh W, Pollack A, et al: Glucose disposal of low birth weight infants. Steady state hyperglycemia produced by constant intravenous glucose infusion. *Pediatrics* 63:389, 1979.

7. Salle B, Ruitton-Ugliengo A: Glucose disappearance rate, insulin response and growth hormone response in the small for gestational age and premature infant of very low birth weight. *Biol Neonate* 29:1, 1976.

8. Tobin JD, Roux JF, Soeldner JS: Human fetal insulin response after acute maternal glucose administration during labor. *Pediatrics* 44:668, 1969.

9. Goldman SL, Hirata T: Attenuated response to insulin in very low birth weight infants. *Pediatr Res* 14:50, 1980.

10. Sherwood WG, Hill DE, Chance GW: Glucose homeostasis in preterm rhesus monkey neonates. *Pediatr Res* 11:874, 1977.

11. Pollak A, Cowett RM, Schwartz R, et al: Glucose disposal in low birth weight infants during steady state hyperglycemia: Effects of exogenous insulin administration. *Pediatrics* 61:546, 1978.

12. Blazquez E, Rubaclava B, Montesano R, et al: Development of insulin and glucagon binding and the adenylate cyclase response in liver membranes of the prenatal, postnatal, and adult rat: Evidence of glucagon "resistance." *Endocrinology* 98:1014, 1976.

13. Lilien LD, Rosenfeld RL, Baccaro MM, et al: Hyperglycemia in stressed small premature neonates. *J Pediatr* 94:454, 1979.

14. Brans YW: Parenteral nutrition of the very low birth weight neonate: A critical review. *Clin Perinatol* 4:367, 1977.

15. Avery GB: Galactose: Its potential use in the glucose-intolerant premature infant, in Stein L, Oh W, Friis-Hansen B (eds): *Intensive Care in the Newborn* ed 2. New York, Masson, 1978, p 261.

16. Das JB, Filler RM, Rubin VG, et al: Intravenous dextrose amino-acid feeding: The metabolic response in the surgical neonate. *J Pediatr Surg* 5:127, 1970.

17. Seashore JH: Metabolic complications of parenteral nutrition in infants and children. *Surg Clin North Am* 60:1239, 1980.

18. Kaminski MV: A review of hyperosmolar, hyperglycemic nonketotic dehydration (HHND): Etiology, pathophysiology, and prevention during intravenous hyperalimentation. *JPEN* 2:690, 1978.

19. Pribylova J, Kozlova J: Glucose and galactose infusions in newborns of diabetic and healthy mothers. *Biol Neonate* 36:193, 1979.

20. Förster H, Haslbeck M, Mehnert H: Zur Bedeutung der Kohlenhydrate in der parenteralen Ernährung. *Infusionstherapie* 1:199, 1973/74.

21. Bässler K-H, Reimold WV: Lactatbildung aus Zuckern und Zuckeralkoholen in Erythrozyten. *Klin Wochenschr* 43:169, 1965.

22. Bode JCh, Zelder O, Rumpelt HJ, et al: Depletion of liver adenosine phosphates and metabolic effects of intravenous infusion of fructose or sorbitol in man and in the rat. *Eur J Clin Invest* 3:436, 1973.

23. Bode JCh: Stoffwechselstörungen durch intravenöse Gabe von Fructose oder Sorbit. *Internist* 14:334, 1973.

24. Schwartz R, Gamsu H, Mulligan PB, et al: Transient intolerance to exogenous fructose in the newborn. *J Clin Invest* 43:333, 1964.

25. Cornblath M, Wybregt SH, Baens GS: Studies of carbohydrate metabolism in the newborn infant. VII. Tests of carbohydrate tolerance in premature infants. *Pediatrics* 32:1007, 1963.

26. Benda GI, Babson SG: Peripheral intravenous alimentation of the small premature infant. *J Pediatr* 79:494, 1971.

27. Pikkarainen PH, Räihä NCR: Development of alcohol dehydrogenase activity in human liver. *Pediatr Res* 1:165, 1967.

28. Peden VH, Sammon TJ, Downey DA: Intravenously induced infantile intoxication with ethanol. *J Pediatr* 83:490, 1973.

29. Young JM, Wesser E: The metabolism of circulating maltose in man. *J Clin Invest* 50:986, 1971.

30. Wilmore DW, Curreri PW, Spitzer KW, et al: Supranormal dietary intake in thermally injured hypermetabolic patients. *Surg Gynecol Obstet* 133:881, 1971.

31. Askanazi J, Rosenbaum SH, Hyman E, et al: Effect of total parenteral nutrition on gas exchange and breathing patterns. *Crit Care Med* 7:125, 1979.

32. Sheldon GF, Baker C: Complication of nutritional support. *Crit Care* 8:35, 1980.

33. Benotti PN, Bothe A, Miller JDB, et al: Cyclic hyperalimentation. *Compr Ther* 2(8):27, 1976.

34. Maini B, Blackburn GL, Bistrian BR, et al: Cyclic hyperalimentation: An optimal technique for preservation of visceral protein. *J Surg Res* 20:515, 1976.

35. Buzby GP, Mullen JL, Stein TP, et al: Manipulation of TPN caloric substrate and fatty infiltration of the liver. *J Surg Res* 31:46, 1981.

36. Elwyn DH: Nutritional requirements in adult surgical patients. *Crit Care Med* 8:9, 1980.

37. Duke JH, Kinney JM, Broell JR, et al: Metabolic evaluation of high calorie alimentation in surgical patients. *Surg Forum* 27:74, 1976.

38. Askanazi J, Nordenstrom J, Rosenbaum SH, et al: Nutrition for the patient with respiratory failure: Glucose vs. fat. *Anesthesiology* 54:373, 1981.

39. Sinatra F: Unpublished data.

6
Protein Requirements

John A. Kerner, Jr.

Available Solutions

Two general types of nitrogen sources are available for parenteral nutrition (PN)—hydrolysates of fibrin or casein and various mixtures of crystalline amino acids. Both types provide most of the essential as well as nonessential amino acids (1). Hydrolysates are protein solutions in which 55% of the protein source has been hydrolyzed to component amino acids. The remaining 45% is largely in the form of dipeptides and tripeptides that are not fully utilized by the body (2).

Both hydrolysates and crystalline L-amino acids have demonstrated effectiveness in clinical use; however, metabolic studies comparing the two generally show better nitrogen utilization of L-amino acids (3). The L-amino acids permit a more rigidly controlled intake of protein precursors than do the hydrolysates (4). Because of the differences stated above, protein hydrolysates (the first protein solutions available for intravenous use) are being replaced by crystalline L-amino acids in many institutions (3). Both Stanford University Hospital and Children's Hospital at Stanford use crystalline L-amino acids exclusively.

Protein Requirements in Premature Infants

Protein requirements for premature infants have been the subject of a great deal of debate over the past 40 years. Even when preterm infants are fed enterally, the recommended amounts of protein for "optimal" growth have ranged from 2–9 g/kg/day. Davidson and co-workers demonstrated that in infants weighing less than 1500 g at birth, especially in those who weighed less than 1000 g, the minimal amount of protein required for optimal growth was approximately 3 g/kg/day. This protein was supplied by a cow's milk casein formula, and the study results demonstrated that the more immature the infant, the greater were the protein requirements for optimal growth (5). Studies by Kagan and co-workers demonstrated that the greater weight gain experienced in preterm infants fed cow's milk formulas, as compared to those fed human milk, was due to greater retention of extracellular water and not necessarily to increased dry weight (6). More recently, Räihä and co-workers suggested that the protein content of human milk would allow the immature infant to grow at an appropriate rate, even though not quite as rapidly as he would grow either on a casein or whey-based milk preparation which provided greater concentrations of protein (7,8). The debate regarding optimal amount of protein intake as well as the proper type of ingested protein may continue for many years, although many investigators now agree that more than 3 g/kg/day is not necessary. Controlled studies evaluating protein requirements, when supplements of other nutrients are concurrently provided, are extremely arduous and time consuming to perform.

Since there is lack of agreement concerning the optimal amount of protein that should be given enterally to very low birth weight infants, the amount to be given parenterally certainly has not been elucidated. Initially, when infants were given intravenous nutrition the protein content of the infusion was often similar to that given to adults; therefore, the infants received 4–5 g/kg/day of protein. Unfortunately, the infants and children could not tolerate the large quantity of protein being infused, and they readily developed azotemia, hyperaminoaciduria, hyperaminoacidemia, and even hyperammonemia (9). However, most infants tolerated 2–3 g/kg/day of protein. The small preterm infants also tolerated the lesser amount of protein or amino acids, and there were few, if any, indications for infusing greater amounts of protein. Often, amounts of protein to be given were determined arbitrarily; then the infant was monitored carefully in order to avoid the complications that could ensue from either excessive or inadequate amounts of amino acids.

Since the quantities and types of amino acids that are required by different patients may vary greatly, the use of a single amino acid preparation for all age groups and disease states has not been feasible or wise. For example, the formulation that is appropriate for an adult recovering from gastrointestinal surgery would not necessarily be appropriate for the preterm infant.

The minimum requirement of amino acids for preterm infants has been formulated by studies of Holt and Synderman (10) and Fomon and Filer (11), and were based on the studies of oral feeding of these compounds. The amount required intravenously might be quite different from the amount required orally, and the formulations of the ideal amino acid mixture that should be given to preterm infants may vary from one investigator to the next.

Both Snyderman (12) and Ghadimi (13) have proposed "ideal" amino acid mixtures for preterm infants. Table 1 consists of the recommendations of both Snyderman and Ghadimi (GF-1). Their recommendations are compared to the currently available mixtures of amino acids if diluted and prepared as 2% solutions.

It is apparent that the products available for use in preterm infants (shown in Table 1) have more nonessential amino acids than are theoretically required, and little, if any, cysteine, tyrosine, or taurine. Although cysteine and tyrosine are not essential amino acids for term infants, they probably are "essential" for preterm infants. In the balance studies of Snyderman (14) the removal of either cysteine or tyrosine from the premature infant's diet resulted in impaired growth and nitrogen retention, and a depressed level of that particular amino acid in plasma. Based on studies by Sturman, Gaull, and Räihä, cysteine must be considered an essential amino acid for preterm infants since their hepatic cystathionase activity is greatly decreased and they cannot convert methionine to cysteine as rapidly as do term infants (15).

Table 1. Concentrations of Amino Acids Adjusted to 2% Solutions and Compared to Recommendations of Amino Acid Requirements

			Solution			
Amino Acid	Snyderman[12] (mg/kg/day)	GF-1[13] (mg/kg/day)	Travasol (mg/100 ml)	Freamine II (mg/100 ml)	Aminosyn (mg/100 ml)	Freamine III (mg/100 ml)
L-leucine	240	400	124	181	188	181
L-phenylalanine	144	100	124	113	88	113
L-methionine	72	15	116	106	80	106
L-lysine	168	120	116	205	144	205
L-isoleucine	180	200	96	139	144	139
L-valine	168	200	92	132	160	132
L-histidine	58	50	88	56	60	56
L-threonine	144	60	84	80	104	80
L-tryptophan	36	30	36	31	32	31
L-alanine	444	100	415	141	256	141
L-arginine	122	250	207	73	196	191[a]
L-proline	192	50	84	224	171	224
L-tyrosine	144	12.5	8	—	18	—
L-cysteine	72	85	—	<5	—	<5
L-taurine	—	—	—	—	—	—
L-serine	166	100	—	118	84	118
L-glycine	396	100	415	400	256	280[a]
L-glutamate	48	12.5	—	—	—	—

[a]Note the two changes in Freamine III compared to Freamine II.

CYSTEINE

Currently, the lack of cysteine in crystalline amino acid solutions or protein hydrolysates available in the United States is primarily due to the poor solubility of cystine, the oxidized form of cysteine (16). In other countries cysteine *is* present in products in significant quantity, for example, Vamin (Pharmacia, Montreal, Quebec) (16) and Amino acid solution 4200 (17).

Intravenous amino acid solutions may be supplemented before infusion to provide 100 mg of L-cysteine HCl (77 mg base)/kg/day (provided by Abbott Laboratories). Recently, such supplementation (77 mg/kg/day of cysteine) was studied by Zlotkin and co-workers (16). Their purpose was to examine the hypothesis that cysteine is an essential amino acid for the intravenously fed newborn. Group and pair-matched comparisons showed that nitrogen retention, weight change, and growth in length and head circumference were *not* affected by this supplementation. Cysteine supplemented infants exhibited a small increase in 3-methylhistidine excretion compared to pair-matched controls, suggesting that either an increase in muscle catabolism or an increase in muscle mass may have occurred (16). No definitive conclusions were made by the authors, and further studies are necessary to assess the need for supplemental cysteine.

TAURINE

Gaull and co-workers noted that taurine must also be considered an essential amino acid in preterm infants since it is synthesized from cysteine (18). They note that taurine is an important component of the developing retina, central nervous system, and cardiac muscle in laboratory animals and possibly in humans as well; theoretically, its omission may result in metabolic complications.

TYROSINE

In one recent study only two out of 11 crystalline amino acid solutions (Vamin 7% and Amino acid solution 4200) had detectable levels of cysteine and tyrosine (17). Despite the fact that many infants have received long-term PN with amino acid preparations that have been deficient in cysteine, tyrosine, and taurine, no recognizable complications of these deficiencies have yet been reported.

ELEVATED CONCENTRATIONS OF AMINO ACIDS

Another problem that had been noted previously when infants were given increased quantities of amino acids (4–5 g/kg/day) was the increased serum concentrations of tyrosine and phenylalanine. This problem was also noted by Rassin and co-workers in infants fed 3% cow's milk formulae (19). When the amino acid preparations are infused at the rate of 2–3 g/kg/day, these complications tend to be mitigated.

Considering all available data, we have not been able to document any superiority of one of the available amino acid mixtures over another. We currently recommend that an infant be given 0.5% amino acids initially with the dextrose infusion and that the amino acid concentration be increased gradually until the infant is receiving 2–2.5 g/kg/day.

Table 2. Protein Requirements for Parenteral
Nutrition (g/kg/day)

Premature and term infants	2.0–2.5
Older infants	2.5–3.0
Older children	1.5–2.5
Adults	1.0–1.5

Our recommendation for protein requirements is shown in Table 2. Recent studies have shown that higher protein requirements than those shown in Table 2 are required for optimal nitrogen retention in premature neonates. Zlotkin and coworkers showed that when energy intake was greater than 70 cal/kg/day the infusion of nitrogen providing 430–560 mg/kg/day (*2.7–3.5* g of protein/kg/day) duplicated intrauterine nitrogen accretion rates (20). Although this amount of amino acids may result in "ideal" nitrogen accretion rates, it may induce metabolic complications in premature neonates who are unable to tolerate these increased levels of protein intake (21). Hyperammonemia is more common in patients whose protein intake is high. Cholestatic liver disease (discussed in Chapter 13) occurs frequently in premature infants on parenteral nutrition, and epidemiologic studies suggest that increased amounts of amino acids predisposed preterm infants to this complication (22).

Protein Requirements in Older Infants and Children

Daily amino acid intakes of approximately 2–3 g/kg of body weight for infants and approximately 1.0–1.5 g/kg of body weight for adults, when provided along with adequate nonnitrogen calories, are generally sufficient to satisfy protein needs and promote positive nitrogen balance in such patients. Increased amounts may be required in patients with severely catabolic states. Such higher intakes, especially in infants, must be accompanied by frequent laboratory evaluation, including blood urea nitrogen and blood ammonia, when possible. The general "pediatric" recommendation for protein requirements while on PN is 1.7–2.5 g/kg/day (23). Our recommendations for protein intake for patients of various ages on PN are shown in Table 2.

An inadequate protein intake has short-termed repercussions, including poor weight gain and low serum albumin with associated edema, and potential long-term repercussions such as decreased DNA content in the brain (24).

Complications of Protein Administration

Complications associated with intravenous protein use are shown in Table 3. Most protein hydrolysates, containing large proportions of chloride salts, have been replaced with synthetic amino acid solutions containing acetate salts; therefore, it is unusual for an infant to develop metabolic acidosis as a complication of parenteral nutrition. On the other hand, premature infants and patients with kidney or liver

Table 3. Complications of Excess Protein Administration

Short-Term Complications	Long-Term Complications
Hyperchloremic metabolic acidosis (with protein hydrolysates)	Abnormal plasma aminograms
	Cholestatic jaundice
Azotemia	Hepatic dysfunction
Hyperammonemia	

disease *are* at an increased risk of developing acidosis while receiving PN. Thus, frequent monitoring of serum electrolytes and blood pH are indicated (23). Excessive nitrogen intake may result in azotemia which can be detected with frequent monitoring of blood urea nitrogen.

HYPERAMMONEMIA

Elevated blood ammonia levels during PN have been observed in full-term and premature infants as well as in adults, although it appears more frequently in premature infants. Johnson et al. (25) observed hyperammonemia in infants receiving TPN containing either fibrin or casein hydrolysates as the nitrogen source. Since the free ammonia content of these hydrolysate preparations is quite high, it was assumed that infusion of preformed ammonia might be responsible, at least in part, for the observed hyperammonemia. Hyperammonemia during PN was also reported by Ghadimi (26). Heird et al. (27) subsequently described hyperammonemia in infants receiving a negligible amount of ammonia, using a crystalline amino acid solution. They found that supplementing the amino acid solution with 0.5–1.0 mmol/kg/day of arginine hydrochloride mitigated elevated blood ammonias (27). The newer amino acid solutions (Aminosyn, Travasol, Freamine III) contain significantly more arginine than the protein hydrolysates or the earlier amino acid preparations (e.g., Freamine and Freamine II). This fact and the general practice of reducing protein administration (see Table 2) have definitely decreased, but not eliminated, the incidence of hyperammonemia. In a recent review Seashore and co-workers found that 75% of their infants and children had one or more elevated blood ammonia concentrations greater than 150μg/dl (88.2 μmol/liter) (28).

Clinical manifestations of hyperammonemia are lethargy and decreased responsiveness, proceeding to twitching and grand mal seizures. Cessation of PN is usually followed by a decrease of blood ammonia levels and reversal of clinical symptoms (27).

Hyperammonemia may be caused by deranged hepatic function due to hepatocellular damage, as documented by elevations of serum bilirubin, transaminases, and abnormal hepatic histology. It may also be caused by injury to subcellular organelles (e.g., mitochondria) in which even short periods of hypoxia can inhibit oxidative phosphorylation and affect mitochondrial function (29).

Hyperammonemia is not unique to patients receiving PN. Goldberg et al. (30) described hyperammonemia (305–960 μg/dl) in eight infants who had suffered perinatal asphyxia, and who had not received any intravenous amino acids. In the four survivors hyperammonemia was associated with hepatic dysfunction and central nervous system irritability, convulsions, hyperthermia, exaggerated sinus arrhythmia, and wide neonatal heart rate oscillations (30). As in infants with PN-associated hepatic dysfunction, their clinical improvement coincided with falling blood ammonia levels (29,30).

Transient hyperammonemia in preterm infants, a problem of unknown etiology, has also been described (31,32). Ellison and Cowger (32) described two preterm infants with blood ammonia levels of 2400–2800 μg/dl associated with profound neurologic depression, persistent seizures, and coma. They were treated effectively with exchange transfusion and peritoneal dialysis (32). Therefore, serum ammonia should be included in the laboratory work-up of any premature infant with repeated seizures.

Septic infants appear to be at particular risk for hyperammonemia as compared to nonseptic subjects (33). Additional studies are needed to confirm this latter association.

It is probable that most, if not all, of the blood ammonia in infants receiving PN results from decreased ammonia detoxification and metabolism and inefficient synthesis of urea (29). In adults 50% of arterial ammonia is metablized in skeletal muscle. In premature infants and malnourished children decreased muscle mass may be contributing to the hyperammonemia (29).

Normal levels for blood ammonia are shown in Table 4. Capillary samples are less reliable because it is difficult to avoid contamination and levels may be falsely elevated (34). Care is needed to avoid gross hemolysis since red cell damage will also result in misleadingly high results (35). Details for ideal collection of blood samples for blood ammonia are described by Beddis et al (35).

There are no agreed upon guidelines for when to adjust intravenous protein intake based on blood ammonia. Seashore reduces protein intake if the ammonia exceeds 147 μmol/liter (250 μg/100 ml) (28). Based upon our experience, this seems to be a reasonable cut-off point. We have performed 261 blood ammonia determinations on sick infants who required PN in our intensive care nursery, using a kit available from Sigma and scaling it down so that only microliter amounts of blood were needed. Values ranged from 9–182 μmol/liter, mean 65 ± 28 ($\pm$ SD) μmol/liter. Our values correlate well with those of previous investigators (see Table 4) (36). None of our monitored infants exhibited any clinical symptoms of hyperammonemia.

ABNORMAL PLASMA AMINOGRAMS

Plasma amino acid concentrations reflect the amino acid distribution in the protein source (37–39). None of the currently available amino acid mixtures results in a "normal" plasma amino acid pattern when administered to children (37,40,41). Blood levels of branched-chain amino acids and lysine during PN are usually far below the postprandial levels of formula-fed infants (42), and often below those of infants fed human milk (43). As mentioned before, plasma concentrations of cysteine and tyrosine, both thought to be essential amino acids for the infant, are extremely low (15,44). No available amino acid solution in the United States contains appreciable amounts of these amino acids. Elevated plasma concentrations of many amino acids are of equal concern. Some amino acid mixtures, for example, result in plasma glycine levels approximately four times postprandial values (45). High plasma glutamate levels have been shown to damage the central nervous

Table 4. Normal Levels of Blood NH_3

Age Group	μmol/liter	μg/100 ml	Comments
Adults			
(Stanford Hospital)	11–35		
Children and Adults[35]	4–35		
Full-term infants	27.5		
AGA[36]	(mean)		
Low birth weight infants, AGA and SGA[36]	37–76		↑ Blood NH_3 occurred in almost all low birth weight infants (compared to adult or full-term infant values) and persisted for 2 mo postnatally.
Neonates[35]			
740–3880 g	32–255	44.8–357	
(mean weight 1823 g)	(mean 94.5)	(mean 132.3)	
ICU neonates[33]	52.9 (mean)	90 (mean)	"Normal" was up to 150 μg/100 ml (88.2 μmol/liter) = 2 S.D. above the mean.
Infants and children			75% had 1 or more elevations above 150 μg/100 ml (88.2 μmol/liter). Seashore accepts blood NH_3 up to 250 μg/100 ml (147 μmol/liter) before decreasing protein intake.[28]
ICU neonates at Stanford	9–182 (mean 65)		

system of growing mice and monkeys (46). Inborn errors of metabolism, which lead to elevations of phenylalanine, glycine, and other amino acids, have profoundly harmful effects on human growth and development (28).

Imbalance of plasma amino acids or, perhaps, toxicity of one or more amino acids may be responsible for hepatic dysfunction and cholestasis (discussed in detail in the section on hepatic dysfunction in Chapter 13). Since plasma amino acid determinations are expensive, difficult to obtain, and not of immediate clinical value, monitoring of plasma amino acids is not mandatory (1). However, if a center can provide aminograms, their data could be used to develop more appropriate amino acid solutions.

Extensive research is underway to develop amino acid mixtures appropriate for children. Bürger and co-workers have developed a mixture based on the transfer rates of individual amino acids that apparently results in normal amino acid blood levels. They compared their solution to a "mother's milk-adapted" solution now available in Europe (47). Both solutions were clinically well tolerated and resulted in positive nitrogen balance. However, in situations of increased stress, the transfer rate-based amino acid solution resulted in a more advantageous nitrogen balance. The "mother's milk-adapted" solution resulted in clearcut imbalances for methionine, and the authors concluded that this latter mixture was not appropriate for long-term PN in premature infants (47). Clearly, further research is required to develop optimal amino acid solutions tailored to the individual needs of all pediatric patients.

Monitoring

Careful monitoring of the urea nitrogen and ammonia in blood will help the clinician recognize when too much protein is being given to the infant or child. Usually, but not always, azotemia precedes hyperammonemia. Measurement of ammonia using small quantities of blood is not an easy task, and techniques using 0.1–0.2 ml of blood are not always accurate. In caring for an infant with congenital absence of hepatic ornithine transcarbamylase, Goldstein et al. found that an increased excretion of orotic acid, an intermediary in the pyrimidine biosynthetic pathway, was noted before the infant developed hyperammonemia (48). We have demonstrated that increased excretion of orotic acid expressed as μg/mg creatinine often heralds the appearance of hyperammonemia. Although extensive data are lacking, this technique may prove to be valuable in assessing the infant's ability to metabolize the infusion of amino acids appropriately.

Practical Guidelines

1. Protein requirements for pediatric patients of all ages are shown in Table 2.
2. In general, the *amino acid concentration* in *peripheral veins should not exceed 2%* (because of the increased osmolality of more concentrated solutions, which is associated with increased incidence of thrombophlebitis). Amino acid solutions through *central lines* usually *need not exceed 3%*.
3. We recommend gradual progression of amino acid concentrations as shown in Table 5.

Table 5. Advancement of Amino Acid Concentration (%) in Parenteral Nutrition in Children

Day	Neonates	Older Infants and Children
1	0.5	1.0
2	0.5	1.5
3	1.0	2.0[a]
4	1.0	2.5 ⎱ for central line
5	1.5	3.0 ⎰ use only
6	1.5	
7	2.0[a]	
8	2.0	
9	2.5 ⎱	
10	2.5 ⎟ for central	
11	3.0 ⎟ line use only	
12	3.0 ⎰	

[a]Maximum concentration of amino acids that is well tolerated by peripheral vein administration.

Table 6. Total Parenteral Nutrition Solutions Available From Pharmacy

TPN Solution	Nonprotein Calories/ Gram Nitrogen	Nonprotein Calories/ 100 ml	Nitrogen (Grams/100 ml)
D5% AA 0.5%[a]	216:1	17	0.08
D7.5% AA 1.0%	162:1	26	0.16
D10% AA 1.0%	216:1	34	0.16
D12.5% AA 1.5%	182:1	43	0.24
D15% AA 2.0%	162:1	51	0.31
D17.5% AA 2.0%	191:1	60	0.31
D20% AA 2.0%	216:1	68	0.31
D25% AA 2.5%	216:1	85	0.39
D25% AA 3.5%	155:1	85	0.55
D35% AA 4.25%	178:1	119	0.67

[a]Dextrose provides 3.4 calories/gram when given parenterally in monohydrate form.
AA = amino acids.

4. Ideally, with each increase in amino acid concentration a BUN should be obtained to be sure the increase in protein is tolerated.

5. If possible, blood NH_3 determinations should be performed one to two times weekly, to monitor for protein tolerance and perhaps for early evidence of sepsis (33).

6. Please note in newborns receiving 140 ml/kg/day of fluids: if that solution contains 1.5% amino acids, the patient is receiving 2.1 g/kg/day of protein. At the same rate, 2% amino acids provides 2.8 g/kg/day of protein which *may* be in excess of the tolerance of many infants.

7. To promote efficient net protein utilization (i.e., not to use the protein source exclusively as an energy source) approximately 150–200 nonprotein calories are required per gram of nitrogen.

   a. Nitrogen content (grams) $= \dfrac{\text{protein (grams)}}{6.25}$

   b. 1 g protein $\xrightarrow{\text{contains}}$ 0.16 g nitrogen

   c. Therefore, 24–32 nonnitrogen calories must be supplied per gram of protein infused to yield a proper ratio of 150–200 : 1

   (1) $\dfrac{\text{Nonnitrogen calories}}{N(g)} = \dfrac{24}{0.16} = \dfrac{150}{1}; \dfrac{32}{0.16} = \dfrac{200}{1}$

   (2) If 2 g/kg/day of protein as amino acids is supplied, then 48–64 cal/kg/day of nonnitrogen calories must be supplied to insure adequate protein utilization.

   (3) If 2.5 g/kg/day of protein is supplied, then 60–70 cal/kg/day of nonnitrogen calories must be supplied.

8. See Table 6 for nonprotein calorie per gram of nitrogen ratios for various dextrose amino acid solutions. These solutions do not contain intravenous fat. If intravenous fat is used, it will contribute to nonprotein calories.

References

1. Levy JS, Winters RW, Heird WC: Total parenteral nutrition in pediatric patients. *Pediatrics in Review* 2:99, 1981.

2. Fischer JE: Parenteral and enteral nutrition. *Disease-a-Month* 24:23, 1981.

3. Hooley RA: Parenteral nutrition—General concepts. Part II. *Nutritional Support Services* 1:41, 1981.

4. Heird WC: Total parenteral nutrition, in Lebenthal E (ed): *Textbook of Gastroenterology and Nutrition in Infancy.* New York, Raven Press, 1981, p 633.

5. Davidson M, Levine SZ, Bauer CH, et al: Feeding studies in low-birth weight infants. I. Relationships of dietary protein, fat and electrolytes to rates of weight gain, clinical courses and serum chemical concentrations. *J Pediatr* 70:695, 1967.

6. Kagan BM, Stainincova V, Felix NS, et al: Body composition of premature infants: Relation to nutrition. *Am J Clin Nutr* 25:1153, 1972.

7. Räihä NCR, Heinonen K, Rassin DK, et al: Milk protein quantity and quality in low birth weight infants. I. Metabolic responses and effects on growth. *Pediatrics* 57:659, 1976.

8. Rassin DK, Gaull GE, Heinonen K, et al: Milk protein quantity and quality in low birth weight infants. II. Effects on selected aliphatic amino acids in plasma and urine. *Pediatrics* 59:407, 1977.

9. Johnson JD, Albritton WL, Sunshine P: Hyperammonemia accompanying parenteral nutrition in newborn infants. *J Pediatr* 81:154, 1972.

10. Holt LE, Jr, Snyderman SE: The amino acid requirements of children, in Nyhan WL (ed): *Amino Acid Metabolism and Genetic Variation.* New York, McGraw-Hill, 1967, p 381.

11. Fomon SJ, Filer LJ, Jr: Amino acid requirements for normal growth, in Nyhan WL (ed): *Amino Acid Metabolism and Genetic Variation.* New York, McGraw-Hill, 1967, p 391.

12. Snyderman SE: Recommendations for parenteral amino acid requirements, in Winters RW, Hasselmeyer EG (eds): *Intravenous Nutrition in the High Risk Infant.* New York, John Wiley & Sons, 1975, p 422.

13. Ghadimi H: Newly devised amino acid solutions for intravenous administration, in Ghadimi H (ed): *Total Parenteral Nutrition: Premises and Promises.* New York, John Wiley & Sons, 1975, p 393.

14. Snyderman SE: The protein and amino acid requirements of the premature infant, in Jonxis JHP, Visser HKA, Troelstra JA (eds) *Metabolic Processes in the Fetus and Newborn Infant.* Baltimore, Williams & Wilkins, 1971, p 128.

15. Sturman JA, Gaull G, Räihä NCR: Absence of cystathionase in human fetal liver: Is cystine essential? *Science* 169:74, 1970.

16. Zlotkin SH, Bryan MH, Anderson GH: Cysteine supplementation to cysteine-free intravenous feeding regimens in newborn infants. *Am J Clin Nutr* 34:914, 1981.

17. Knuiman JT, Monnens L, Trijbels F, et al: Amino acid solutions: Composition and suitability for intravenous feeding in infants. *Infusionsther Klin Ernaehr* 8:4, 1981.

18. Gaull GE, Rassin DK, Räihä NCR, et al: Milk protein quantity and quality in low birth weight infants. III. Effects on sulfur amino acids in plasma and urine. *J Pediatr* 90:348, 1977.

19. Rassin DK, Gaull GE, Räihä NCR: Milk protein quantity and quality in low birth weight infants. IV. Effects on tyrosine and phenylalanine in plasma and urine. *J Pediatr* 90:356, 1977.

20. Zlotkin SH, Bryan MH, Anderson GH: Intravenous nitrogen and energy intakes required to duplicate in utero nitrogen accretion in prematurely born human infants. *J Pediatr* 99:115, 1981.

21. Merritt RJ: Neonatal nutritional support. *Clinical Consultations in Nutritional Support* 1:5, 1981.

22. Vileisis RA, Inwod RJ, Hunt CE: Prospective controlled study of parenteral nutrition—Associated cholestatic jaundice: Effect of protein intake. *J Pediatr* 96:893, 1980.

23. Wesley JR, Saran PA, Khalidi N, et al: *Parenteral and Enternal Nutrition Manual* of the University of Michigan Medical Center. Chicago, Abbott Laboratories, 1980, p 43.

24. Denson SE, Palma PA, Adcock EW: TPN for the neonate, Part l: Macronutrients. *Nutritional Support Services* 1(8): 24, 1981.

25. Johnson JD, Albritton WL, Sunshine P: Hyperammonemia accompanying parenteral nutrition in newborn infants. *J Pediatr* 81:154, 1972.

26. Ghadimi H, Abaci F, Kumar S, et al: Biochemical aspects of intravenous alimentation. *Pediatrics* 48:955, 1971.

27. Heird WC, Nicholson JF, Driscoll JM, et al: Hyperammonemia resulting from intravenous alimentation using a mixture of synthetic L-amino acids: A preliminary report. *J Pediatr* 81:162, 1972.

28. Seashore JH: Metablic complications of parenteral nutrition in infants and children. *Surg Clin North Am* 60:1239, 1980.

29. Poley JR: Liver and nutrition: Hepatic complications of total parenteral nutrition, in Lebenthal E (ed): *Textbook of Gastroenterology and Nutrition in Infancy.* New York, Raven Press, 1981, p 747.

30. Goldberg RN, Cabal LA, Sinatra FR, et al: Hyperammonemia associated with perinatal asphyxia. *Pediatrics* 64:336, 1979.

31. Ballard RA, Vinocur B, Reynolds JW, et al: Transient hyperammonemia of the preterm infant. *N Engl J Med* 299:920, 1978.

32. Ellison PH, Cowger ML: Transient hyperammonemia in prematures. *Neurology* 31:767, 1981.

33. Thomas DW, Sinatra FR, Hack SL, et al: Hyperammonemia in neonates receiving intravenous nutrition *JPEN* (in press).

34. Bessman SP: Blood ammonia. *Adv Clin Chem* 2:135, 1959.

35. Beddis IR, Hughes EA, Rosser E, et al: Plasma ammonia levels in newborn infants admitted to an intensive care baby unit. *Arch Dis Child* 55:516, 1980.

36. Batshaw ML, Brusilow SW: Asymptomatic hyperammonemia in low birth weight infants. *Pediatr Res* 12:221, 1978.

37. Stegink LD, Baker GL: Infusion of protein hydrolysates in the newborn infant: Plasma amino acid concentrations. *J Pediatr* 78:595, 1971.

38. Abitol CL, Feldman DP, Ahmann P, et al: Plasma amino acid patterns during supplemental intravenous nutrition of low-birth-weight infants. *J Pediatr* 86:766, 1975.

39. Anderson GH, Bryan H, Jeejeebhoy KN, et al: Dose-response relationships between amino acid intake and blood levels in newborn infants. *Am J Clin Nutr* 30:1110, 1977.

40. Lindblad BS, Settergren G, Feychting H, et al: Total parenteral nutrition in infants. Blood levels of glucose, lactate, pyruvate, free fatty acids, glycerol, p-β-hydroxybutyrate, triglycerides, free amino acids and insulin. *Acta Paediatr Scand* 66:409, 1977.

41. Winters RW, Heird WC, Dell RB, et al: Plasma amino acids in infants receiving parenteral nutrition, in Greene HL, Holliday MA, Munro HN, (eds): *Symposium on Clinical Nutrition Update—Amino Acids.* Chicago, American Medical Association, 1977, p 147.

42. Filer LJ, Jr, Stegink LD, Chandramouli B: Effect of diet on plasma aminograms of low birth weight infants. *Am J Clin Nutr* 30:1036, 1977.

43. Lindblad BS, Alfven G, Zetterstrom R: Plasma free amino acid concentrations of breastfed infants. *Acta Paediatr Scand* 67:659, 1978.

44. Snyderman SE: The protein and amino acid requirements of the premature infant, in Jonxis JHP, Visser HKA, Troelstra JA (eds): *Metabolic Processes in the Fetus and Newborn Infant.* Leiden, Stenfert Kroese, 1971, p 128.

45. Heird WC: Panel report on nutritional support of pediatric patients. *Am J Clin Nutr* 34:1223, 1981.

46. Olney JW, Ho OL, Rhee V: Brain damaging potential of protein hydrolysates. *N Engl J Med* 289:39, 1973.

47. Bürger U, Fritsch U, Bauer M, et al: Comparison of two amino acid mixtures for total parenteral nutrition of premature infants receiving assisted ventilation. *JPEN* 4:290, 1980.

48. Goldstein AS, Hoogenraad NJ, Johnson JD, et al: Metabolic and genetic studies of a family with ornithine transcarbamylase deficiency. *Pediatr Res* 8:5, 1974.

7
Fat Requirements

John A. Kerner, Jr.

With the development of a stable lipid emulsion, Intralipid, for intravenous use, it became possible to provide a more balanced nutritional regimen not only for infants and children, but for the premature infant as well. In addition, the greater caloric content of fat has decreased the need for concentrated glucose solutions, thus frequently allowing physicians to avoid cannulating large caliber central veins (1–3). Administration of nutrients by peripheral vein virtually eliminates the complications that have occurred with central catheter placement, including thrombosis of major vessels, hemorrhage, and septicemia.

Historical Background

A great deal of experience has been accumulated regarding the use of intravenous fat emulsions (IVF). In fact, an entire symposium devoted to experience gained with a single IVF (Lipomul) was published (*Metabolism* 6:591–831, 1957). A recent review provides a detailed summary of the development of fat emulsions (4).

Lipomul, made from cottonseed oil, was the first IVF introduced in the United States but was withdrawn from the market in 1965 following several reports of a "fat overloading syndrome" characterized by anemia, coagulation abnormalities with hemorrhagic diathesis, thrombocytopenia, peptic ulceration, and liver damage (5–7). For the next 10 years no IVF was commercially available in the United States. Intralipid, distributed by Cutter Laboratories, was approved for use in the United States in 1975 after extensive use in Europe. In 1979 Liposyn, a second IVF, was marketed in the United States by Abbott Laboratories. More recently, a third fat preparation, Travamulsion, was released by Travenol Laboratories. When administered in recommended volumes, these three IVFs have not exhibited the cumulative toxicities reported with Lipomul. The toxic fat accumulation observed with Lipomul has been attributed to one or more of the following factors: a nonextractable substance in cottonseed oil; its large particle size (approximately 1 μm in diameter); and the synthetic emulsifying agent, "pluronic F-68" (8,9).

Intralipid and Travamulsion contain soybean oil as a base, whereas Liposyn is made from safflower oil (Table 1). Each product contains purified egg phospholipids as an emulsifier. Water is added to make a 10% emulsion. Glycerin, a

Table 1. 10% Intravenous Fat Emulsions

	Intralipid	Liposyn	Travamulsion
Base	Soybean oil	Safflower oil	Soybean oil
Egg phospholipids (emulsifier)	1.2%	1.2%	1.2%
Glycerin	2.25%	2.5%	2.25%
Fatty acids			
Linoleic[a]	54%	77%	56%
Oleic	26%	13%	23%
Palmitic	9%	7%	11%
Linolenic[a]	8%	<0.5%	6%
Supplied as	100, 500 ml containers	50, 100, 200, 500 ml containers	500 ml container
Osmolarity	280 mOsm/liter	300 mOsm/liter	270 mOsm/liter
Emulsified fat particle size	0.5 μ	0.4 μ	0.4 μ
Caloric value	1.1 cal/ml	1.1 cal/ml	1.1 cal/ml

[a]Major differences between Liposyn and the other two products

water soluble substance, is added to make fat emulsions isotonic. Each product delivers 1.1 calories per milliliter since fat, phospholipid, and glycerol contribute to the total calories. Whereas the 10% emulsions have been used widely in the United States, experience with the 20% emulsions has emanated from Europe (10). Intralipid and Liposyn are now also available as 20% emulsions. The fatty acid composition of the three U.S. products is shown in Table 1. Liposyn has a substantially greater concentration of linoleic acid than does Intralipid or Travamulsion, but the daily requirements of linoleic acid are easily attained with any of the three preparations.

Intralipid and Travamulsion contain linolenic acid in substantial amounts as compared to Liposyn. Initially, this difference appeared to be of only theoretical interest because the physiological importance of linolenic acid in humans was unknown (11); linolenic-acid-deficient trout exhibit a shocklike syndrome and poor appetite (12), and defects in learning (13) and rod function (14) have been associated with linolenic deficiency in rats. Recently, however, a six-year-old girl on total parenteral nutrition (with Liposyn as the fat source) for 5 months developed episodes of numbness, paresthesia, weakness, inability to walk, pain in the legs, and blurring of vision (15). Diagnostic analysis of her fatty acid pattern revealed a *significant deficiency of linolenic acid*. When her regimen was changed to a fat preparation containing linolenic acid (Intralipid), *her neurologic symptoms disappeared*. Interestingly, analysis of the fatty acid pattern revealed a correction of the linolenic acid deficiency, but a worsening of the linoleic acid deficiency in the patient. Until more data become available, Liposyn as the sole source of fatty acids should be used with caution in patients on long-term total parenteral nutrition (11). Holman and coworkers estimated the human requirements of linolenic acid to be about 0.54% of the total calories delivered (15). Their data suggest that the linolenic concentration of Intralipid may be higher than optimal and may interfere with proper utilization of linoleic acid; however, they cannot recommend an optimum intake of linoleic and linolenic acid. This must be the subject of future research.

Each fat emulsion has a slightly different chemical composition and, therefore, a potential for unique complications. For example, the cottonseed oil emulsions have produced more complications than those containing soybean oil (4). In addition to the three products available in the United States, two additional soybean oil base products are available—Intrafat (Daigo, Osaka, Japan) and Lipofundin S (Braun, Melsungen, Germany); there is also one cottonseed oil preparation currently available in France, Lipiphysan (Egic, Loiret, France). The most extensive investigations have been with Intralipid. From 1965 to 1979 there were 1.6 million units of Intralipid administered in Sweden with only eight reports of suspected adverse reaction, and in only one of the eight cases was a causal relationship probable (4).

Metabolic Clearance

Figure 1 illustrates the natural digestion and absorption of dietary fats, which are predominantly in the form of triglycerides. These are hydrolyzed initially by pharyngeal (lingual) lipase, an enzyme that is especially important in the preterm and term infant, since these infants have relatively little pancreatic lipase.

The ingested triglycerides are emulsified in the stomach by the continuous shearing action of gastric muscular contractions. The emulsion passes into the duodenum, where pancreatic lipase hydrolyzes the triglycerides to β-monoglycerides and fatty acids. These products are then solubilized into micelles with the aid of bile acids. The fatty acids and β-monoglycerides are absorbed across the brush border and then reesterified to once again form triglycerides. The triglyceride is coated with cholesterol, phospholipids, and a protein to form a chylomicron that is excreted into the lymphatics and subsequently in the blood stream. IVF has a metabolic fate similar to that of naturally occurring chylomicrons (16) (Fig. 2). Its clearance from the bloodstream is dependent upon lipoprotein lipase activity, the rate-limiting enzymatic step in the hydrolysis of circulating protein-bound triglyceride (17). This reaction takes place at or near capillary endothelial cells primarily in muscle and adipose tissue. Free fatty acids generated during the hydrolysis of Intralipid enter adipose tissue where they are reesterified to triglycerides and then

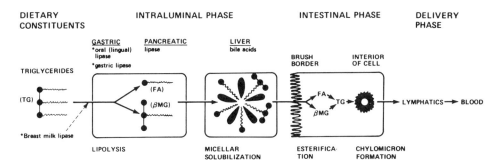

Figure 1 The natural digestion and absorption of dietary fats.

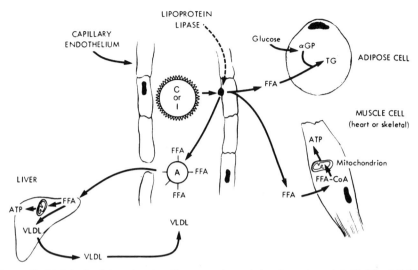

Figure 2 Metabolic fate of naturally occurring chylomicrons or Intralipid particles. (Bryan H, Shennan A, Griffin E, et al: Intralipid—Its rational use in parenteral nutrition of the newborn. *Pediatrics* 58:788, 1976; Copyright © 1976, American Academy of Pediatrics. Reproduced with permission.)

stored. A portion of the released free fatty acids can recirculate, having bound to albumin, and are readily utilizable as metabolic fuel in the liver, heart, or skeletal muscles. In the liver, circulating free fatty acids are also converted to very low density lipoprotein (VLDL or pre-β-lipoprotein) and secreted into the plasma. Both dietary chylomicrons and IVF particles, which are similarly metabolized, as well as VLDL particles all contribute to plasma turbidity or lipemia (Table 2).

Lipid clearance may be accelerated in severely catabolic patients (e.g., burns, surgery, trauma, cachexia, starvation patients) (18). Lipid clearance can also be enhanced with the concurrent use of heparin (explained later in this chapter), dextrose, or insulin.

During the simultaneous infusion of dextrose and IVF, in both premature infants and adults the disappearance rate of free fatty acids from the serum is more rapidly accelerated with 10% than with 5% dextrose solutions (19–21). Adequate dextrose calories are necessary for the body to oxidize free fatty acids from the citric acid cycle (Fig. 3). All nutrient metabolites involved in energy production ultimately

Table 2. Contributors to Plasma Turbidity (Lipemia)

1. Chylomicrons of exogenous (dietary) origin
2. Intravenous fat particles (0.4–0.5 microns—the same size as naturally occurring chylomicrons)
3. Pre-β-lipoproteins (VLDL) which are 65% triglycerides and are converted in the liver from free fatty acids (liberated by metabolism of natural or intravenous fat chylomicrons—see Fig. 2)

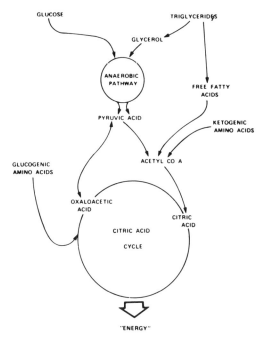

Figure 3 Interrelation of carbohydrate, protein, and fatty acids. (Pelham LD: Rational use of intravenous fat emulsions. *Am J Hosp Pharm* 38:200, 1981. Reproduced with permission.)

enter the citric acid cycle. Oxaloacetic acid is the necessary carbohydrate fuel to maintain this process. With insufficient oxaloacetic acid from carbohydrate to maintain the cycle efficiently, acetyl CoA from fat is not used properly and is diverted to form ketone bodies (18).

Insulin decreases the release of free fatty acids from adipose tissue. This anabolic hormone also enhances serum triglyceride clearance and tissue uptake through lipogenesis (22,23).

Glucose utilization is somewhat depressed when IVF is administered. The blood sugar levels of infants receiving Intralipid supplementation in addition to dextrose exceeded baseline concentrations (although the difference was not statistically significant) for 2 hours after the IVF infusion was stopped (24). Recent findings in very low birth weight infants were consistent with these observations (25). Similar persistent elevations of blood sugar were obtained after single bolus injections of Intralipid (0.5 g/kg) in low birth weight infants (26). Das and co-workers (27) postulate that intermediary products of fatty acid oxidation inhibit key enzymes in the glycolytic pathway. They feel the fatty acidemia and its metabolic consequences can be avoided by intermittent IVF at lower rates (0.15 g/kg/hr for 18 hours each day) during total parenteral nutrition (TPN)—this will assure a larger carbohydrate-to-fat calorie ratio. The 6 hour period of interrupted infusion each day will also assure cyclical regeneration of the enzyme systems involved in lipid metabolism (27).

Nitrogen Sparing Effects

Data from adults and animal studies suggest that a fat calorie is not equivalent to a nitrogen calorie with respect to promoting nitrogen retention (28). A controlled study (29) documented that glucose does have a greater water retaining effect than fat, and water retention can be a problem with patients on TPN. The authors concluded that fat in conjunction with glucose may be more effective as an energy source than equicaloric amounts of glucose alone (29).

In a study on neonates and infants (30), administration of glucose infusion alone resulted in negative nitrogen balance. Addition of amino acids with glucose produced marked nitrogen retention. The positive nitrogen balance remained when lipid was substituted for glucose as a nonprotein energy source (30).

James Long III, in a symposium at the Sixth Clinical Congress of the American Society of Parenteral and Enteral Nutrition in February, 1982, updated his earlier study (28) and explained that in the normal state both carbohydrate and fat spare protein equally. However, with increasing stress, especially at levels of maximum stress, a fat calorie spares protein less well than a carbohydrate calorie.

Indications for Intravenous Fat Use

There are two main indications for the use of IVF—to provide a concentrated caloric source and to prevent essential fatty acid deficiency.

CONCENTRATED CALORIC SOURCE

IVF enables the physician to provide a highly concentrated calorie source (1.1 cal/ml for the 10% solution as compared to 0.17 cal/ml for 5% dextrose, 0.34 cal/ml for 10% dextrose, and 0.68 cal/ml for 20% dextrose). Furthermore, IVF has a low osmolality (280–300 mOsm/liter) compared to that of dextrose 5%/sodium chloride 0.45% (400 mOsm/liter) and dextrose 10%/4.25% amino acids (925 mOsm/liter). The concentrated calories and low osmolality of IVF make it ideal for peripheral parenteral nutrition.

PREVENTION OF ESSENTIAL FATTY ACID DEFICIENCY

All animals, including humans, require a dietary source of certain essential poylunsaturated fatty acids, which have multiple functions in the body. The primary dietary essential fatty acid for humans is linoleic acid. In the body, linoleic acid is converted to longer chain fatty acids with three to five double bonds, which are essential components of membranes. Most experts also consider arachidonic acid an "essential" fatty acid, since it is also a vital component of cell membranes, even though it can be synthesized in the body from linoleic acid. Linolenic acid has essential fatty acid properties in animals, but in most species is not as effective as linoleic acid in alleviating the many abnormalities of essential fatty acid deficiency.

Table 3. Clinical Problems Associated
with Essential Fatty Acid Deficiency[37-39]

Reduced growth rate
Dermatitis (scaly)
Thrombocytopenia
Decreased capillary resistance
Increased fragility of erythrocytes
Increased susceptibility to infections

As mentioned earlier, the role of linolenic acid in human nutrition has not yet been completely elucidated.

Essential fatty acids (EFA) are necessary for a variety of physiological functions such as platelet function (31), prostaglandin synthesis (31,32), wound healing (33,34), immunocompetency (35), and integrity of skin, hair, and nerve linings (34,36). The clinical problems associated with EFA deficiency are shown in Table 3 (37–39). Growing tissues require a greater supply of dietary EFA since the utilization rate is higher. In the postnatal period EFA deficiency may prevent the central nervous system from developing normally (40–42).

Adults have two sources of linoleic acid for their daily nutritional requirements: dietary intake and lipolysis of adipose tissues, which are approximately 10% linoleic acid in composition (43). In comparison, total body weight of a 1 kg premature infant is only about 1% fat, of which only a small percentage is linoleic acid (44). For an extensive review of essential fatty acids and their importance, see Friedman's excellent review (45).

The clinical picture of isolated EFA deficiency is unclear because experimental depletion, by feeding formulas deficient in EFA to otherwise healthy and calorically satisfied infants, has only been attempted in one study, which was terminated after approximately 12 weeks (39). A flaky skin condition appeared over the dorsal surface of the infants 1 week into the trial. Poor hair growth, thrombocytopenia, failure to thrive, and increased susceptibility to infection, and syrupy diarrhea also developed.

A deficiency of EFA in adult humans was unknown until recently. A deficiency has been produced inadvertently in infants and adults who were hospitalized, received nothing by mouth, and received fat-free intravenous nutrition (46–53). In preterm infants and nutritionally depleted infants, EFA deficiency can develop very quickly. Biochemical evidence of EFA deficiency has been noted in serum of neonates as early as 2 days after initiating fat-free parenteral nutrition (53).

EFA deficiency may be detected biochemically before clinical signs appear. There are two current biochemical criteria for the assessment of EFA status: (1) the determination in plasma lipids of linoleic ($18:2\omega6$),* arachidonic ($20:4\omega6$), and 5,8,11-eicosatrienoic ($20:3\omega9$) acid levels; (2) the determination of the ratio of eicosatrienoic to arachidonic acid (triene/tetraene ratio). A ratio of greater than 0.4 is

---

*The abbreviated formula indicates the number of carbon atoms before the colon and the number of double bonds after the colon; the position of the double bond nearest to the methyl terminus is indicated by the Greek letter ω.

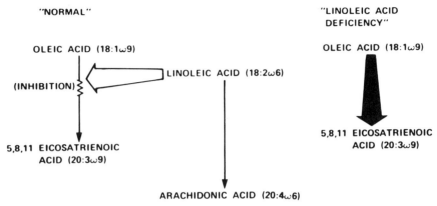

Figure 4 Essential fatty acid deficiency (Pelham LD: Rational use of intravenous fat emulsions. *Am J Hosp Pharm* 38:202, 1981. Reproduced with permission.)

generally assumed to be an early indicator of EFA deficiency (37,54). See Figure 4 for a graphic depiction of the mechanics in EFA deficiency.

The amount of dietary linoleic acid found to prevent both biochemical and clinical evidence of deficiency in humans is 1–2% of the dietary calories (37) (see Appendix I for Recommended Dietary Allowances, 1980). Medium-chain triglyceride (MCT) oils do not provide EFAs, and Hirono et al. (55) described the development of EFA deficiency in infants on a formula whose only fat source was MCT oil. The previous recommendation to prevent or treat EFA deficiency with twice weekly infusions of 10 ml/kg of plasma (56) has not been reliable. In infants and adults neither exchange transfusion nor multiple blood transfusions were able to prevent or correct EFA deficiency (48,53).

Tashiro and co-workers (57) demonstrated in experiments on puppies and two newborn infants that providing 4% of total calories as Intralipid (2% of total calories would be as linoleic acid, since half of the fatty acid composition of Intralipid is linoleate) prevented or improved EFA deficiency. Tashiro et al. (46) showed that although fat emulsion providing 4% of total calories (2% as linoleic acid) cured EFA deficiency, fat emulsion supplying 2% of total calories neither improved nor prevented the deficiency. Bivins observed that providing linoleic acid as 4% of calories every other day in the form of Liposyn also prevented EFA deficiency (58). For the adult patient, three 500 ml units of 10% emulsion are usually infused during the first week to correct an existing deficiency; while one to two units per week thereafter may prevent recurrence (47,48). In pediatrics, the prevention of EFA deficiency requires 0.5–1.0 g/kg/day of IVF (59).

Interestingly, 30 ml of corn oil, sunflower seed oil, or safflower oil provide as much linoleic acid as 150 ml of 10% fat emulsion at less than 5% of the cost. Many parenteral nutrition patients not on complete bowel rest tolerate oral fat-containing solutions in divided doses of 15 ml twice a day. The linoleic acid content is 72% in safflower oil, 61% in sunflower seed oil, and 54% in corn oil (18). Since acalculous cholecystitis has been shown to develop during TPN (60), oral supplementation with small volumes of vegetable oils may not only prevent EFA deficiency but may also stimulate gallbladder contractions to prevent acalculous cholecystitis (18).

Cutaneous application of sunflower seed oil rapidly reversed clinical and biochemical manifestations of EFA deficiency in two newborn infants on long-term fat-free TPN (61). Hunt et al. (62) failed to correct EFA deficiency in nine out of 10 neonates who received topical sunflower seed oil, irrespective of the amount applied. Cutaneous application of safflower oil alleviated the skin manifestations of EFA deficiency but did not correct the triene/tetraene ratio of total plasma fatty acids in a study of 28 surgical patients aged newborn to 66 years (52). Thus, the benefits of cutaneous application of EFA-rich oils have not been conclusively demonstrated.

Use of Intravenous Fat in the EFA Deficiency of Cystic Fibrosis

Patients with cystic fibrosis (CF) have a relative EFA—primarily linoleic acid— deficiency (63–66). However, CF patients without malabsorption appear to be unaffected (67). The deficiency of linoleic acid is secondary to both pancreatic insufficiency and reduced dietary intake of fats containing linoleic acid. Patients with CF who have significant liver disease may develop decreased production of bile acids which would further worsen the fat malabsorption (68).

Chase et al. (69) pointed out the importance of linoleic acid in the control of prostaglandin synthesis. In patients with CF and low linoleic acid levels, there was an increase in prostaglandin $F_{2\alpha}$ production, but the concentrations decreased following supplementation with linoleic acid (66). Since prostaglandin $F_{2\alpha}$ is associated with bronchoconstriction and pulmonary vasoconstriction, its increased production may be casually related to chronic pulmonary disease in CF.

Treatment of linoleic acid deficiency in CF has been attempted by Elliott using IVF (Intralipid) in seven children; IVF infusions of 20 ml/kg of 10% emulsion were administered approximately every 3 weeks for 1 year (70). Weight percentiles and sweat tests improved in all patients, and pancreatic function improved in some patients. In the four patients whose linoleic and arachidonic acid levels were measured initially, there was a significant rise in both EFAs after treatment. Rosenlund et al. (71) gave 20 CF patients oral corn oil for 1 year with resultant improvement in linoleic and arachidonic acid as well as decreased sweat test values and variable pancreatic function improvement. Unfortunately, neither study was double-blind.

Chase and co-workers (72) performed a double blind study in patients with CF comparing twice monthly infusions of IVF to isocaloric infusions of 10% dextrose. Two weeks after each infusion, plasma and red blood cell linoleic acid levels were not increased in the IVF group, although this group did show greater clinical improvement (72).

The experience of Chase et al. (69) and dietary recall records of the CF clinic at the Children's Hospital at Stanford document that CF patients have inadequate caloric intake. EFA supplementation given in the presence of inadequate caloric intake will most likely be used for calories rather than for EFA repletion. Our pilot study demonstrated that over 2 months linoleic acid deficiency was corrected in 16 out of 20 patients with CF by (1) providing adequate oral calories or (2) providing adequate oral calories plus Myveral (Eastman Kodak, Rochester, New York)—a form of linoleic acid not requiring digestion by pancreatic lipase (73).

Further studies are needed to define whether adequate calories alone or in combination with either oral linoleic acid monoglyceride or IVF will be able to maintain normal EFA levels in CF patients. Long-term follow-up studies will then be necessary to determine if maintaining normal EFA levels in CF patients has a significant impact on the course of the disease.

Major Stimulus to Use IVF in Premature Infants

Cashore and co-workers (74) described 23 infants, all weighing less than 1500 g, who received peripheral intravenous supplementation with glucose, casein hydrolysate, and Intralipid. These infants regained their birth weight by 8–12 days of life and achieved growth rates that approximated the intrauterine rates of growth. The infants had an unusually low incidence of hyperbilirubinemia (two of 19 survivors) and a decreased incidence of apneic spells. It appears that such a regimen would be beneficial and would prevent the development of EFA deficiency in infants receiving TPN. Cashore's (74) and other studies (2,75) suggest that IVF is safe for premature infants when used correctly but that there are many theoretical problems regarding the use of IVF in these infants.

Impaired Tolerance

While the clearance rates of Intralipid in newborn infants are similar to those of adults (76,77), decreased tolerance has been noted in preterm infants of 27–32 weeks gestation (78–80). Infants of 25–26 weeks gestation have an even greater intolerance since they have less than one third of the postheparin lipolytic activity of infants above 27 weeks gestation (81). The incidence of hyperlipidemia in infants less than 33 weeks gestation and those weighing less than 1500 g is three to four times that of larger and more mature neonates (79). Recently, it has been shown that infants of less than 32 weeks gestation and appropriate for gestational age (AGA) increases their capacity to tolerate IVF after the first week of extrauterine life (82,83).

The ability of infants who are small for gestational age (SGA) to metabolize Intralipid is often much more impaired than that found in small premature infants. Concentrations of triglycerides and free fatty acids following the infusion of Intralipid in SGA infants are often two to three times higher than those noted in preterm infants who are AGA (77,80,84,85). In addition, Bryan et al. (86) suggested that sepsis and acute illness may decrease tolerance for Intralipid infusion at rates previously tolerated, resulting in hyperlipidemia.

AGA infants can clear IVF at a rate of 0.15 g/kg/hr, a maximum of 3.6 /kg/day (84). SGA babies receiving IVF at this rate will accumulate plasma lipids, and slower rates of infusion are required in these infants (84).

Impaired IVF clearance has been noted in a marasmic child (87) as well as in very premature infants and SGA infants, suggesting that a critical mass of adipose tissue may be necessary for normal metabolism of circulating triglycerides. Additional causes for impaired IVF tolerance may be hepatic immaturity and reduced lipoprotein lipase activity (79,81).

Heparin has been shown to decrease total lipid levels and turbidity when given as a single injection of 50–100 IU/kg to SGA infants (84). The immediate lipolytic effect of heparin administered as a bolus in doses of 50–150 IU/kg has also been described in studies of newborn dogs and infants (88,89). Heparin stimulates the release of the enzyme lipoprotein lipase (90–92). Based on the above data it was initially recommended that heparin be used during the intravenous feeding of fat to infants and children to enhance IVF clearance (3,20). Subsequently, Coran et al. (93) demonstrated that heparin administered chronically at 150 IU/kg/day does *not* significantly influence the clearance of fat from the blood stream of infants receiving IVF. The relatively high concentrations of heparin that would be necessary to establish a long-lasting effect cast doubt on the feasibility of this practice (81), and routine addition of heparin to patients receiving IVF is no longer recommended.

Complications

Immediate or early adverse effects with IVF occur in less than 1% of patients. These side effects include dyspnea, cyanosis, allergic reactions, hyperlipemia, hypercoagulability, nausea, vomiting, headache, flushing, increase in temperature, sweating, sleepiness, dizziness, slight pressure over the eyes, chest and back pain, irritation at the infusion site and, rarely, thrombocytopenia in neonates. Gram-negative sepsis has been reported (94) with the use of IVF given both by central venous catheter and by scalp vein. It is likely these episodes were due to extrinsic contamination of the lipid emulsion (94). Extreme care must be exercised in the preparation and delivery of all parenteral nutrition solutions to avoid such problems.

If the rate of IVF administration exceeds its maximal clearance rate, plasma IVF levels rise and visible lactescence and hyperlipidemia occur. The consequences of hyperlipidemia during the use of IVF are unknown but may be responsible for the following potential complications: (1) alteration of pulmonary function, (2) deposition of pigmented material in macrophages, (3) displacement of albumin-bound bilirbuin by plasma free fatty acids, (4) possible risk of coronary artery disease, and (5) "overloading" syndrome.

Altered Pulmonary Function

Hyperlipidemia following the infusion of Intralipid has been reported to decrease pulmonary diffusing capacity in healthy adults (95) and to alter blood flow through the microcirculation (96). Rabbits infused with Intralipid have been shown to have erythrocytes in their lung coated with lipid particles (95), and two low birth weight premature infants who had received Intralipid had fat globules in alveolar macrophages and capillaries at necropsy (97). In addition, Barson and co-workers (98) reported four cases of "fat embolism" in infants receiving prolonged intravenous infusion of 20% Intralipid. These infants had refractile globules of unstained fat blocking capillaries in the periphery of the lung. Frozen section of the lung stained with oil red O showed fat emboli present within the capillaries. In all four of these infants the maximum rate of IVF exceeded 0.15 g/kg/hr (the recommendation of Gustafson et al. (84) for AGA infants). In one case the infusion rate was as high as 0.7 g/kg/hr. One of the infants was also SGA; theoretically, that child would not even be able to metabolize the 0.15 g/kg/hr infusion. Levine and co-workers (99) described eight preterm infants. All had received Intralipid and all had fat accumulation in the lung when examined at autopsy. The maximum rate of IVF administration in seven of the eight patients had exceeded 0.15 g/kg/hr. Levine's data has been questioned by Andersen et al. (100) because lungs of control infants who had not been treated with IVF were not examined histologically. In Andersen and coworkers' study of 21 infants weighing less than 1500 g who had died, nine had received Intralipid for an average of 5 days with a mean dosage of 1.77 ± 0.74 g/kg/day. The other 12 had received intravenous carbohydrate and mother's milk but no Intralipid. Their patients were similar to Levine's series regarding clinical conditions. Of the nine infants receiving Intralipid, seven had lipid in alveolar cells, lung macrophages, and pulmonary capillaries. Of the 12 receiving no IVF, six had lipid in alveolar cells, seven had lipid-filled lung macrophages, and two had lipid in pulmonary capillaries. Their results appear to demonstrate that pulmonary fat accumulation is not caused by IVF infusion per se but may be accentuated by IVF infusion. They could not explain the pulmonary fat accumulation in the infants who had not received Intralipid (100).

Dahms and Halpin (101) described three newborns with a distinctive pulmonary arterial lipid lesion characterized by a wide, foamy layer of intima partially occluding the lumen of small muscular pulmonary arteries. Lipid stains indicated lipid infiltration of the walls of these arteries involving not only the intimal layer, but the media and adventitia as well. All three infants had received IVF. The infants also had histologic evidence of pulmonary hypertension. A retrospective study of long-term neonatal ICU dwellers revealed eight infants who had received IVF and had no pathologic signs of pulmonary hypertension and no evidence of pulmonary arterial lipid. Two additional infants with pulmonary hypertension had fat deposition in pulmonary artery walls while seven other infants with pulmonary hypertension who had received IVF did not have pulmonary artery lesions. The authors speculated that the distinctive lipid deposits seen in pulmonary arteries were derived from Intralipid but were dependent on antecedent or concurrent vascular damage from pulmonary hypertension. They further speculated that increased pulmonary arterial pressure damaged vessel walls and facilitated passage of high blood levels of Intralipid through the endothelium. They cautioned that infants likely to have significant pulmonary hypertension, such as those with chronic pulmonary disease or congenital heart disease, should receive IVF with caution, and serum lipid values, especially triglycerides, should be monitored daily to be sure values are not excessive.

Sun and co-workers (102) have demonstrated that 1 g/kg of 10% Intralipid given over 15 minutes to eight preterm infants caused greater than a 10 mm Hg reduction in oxygen tension of umbilical arterial blood in six of the eight infants. These reductions correlated with elevated triglyceride concentrations. Pereira et al. (83) also demonstrated significant decrease in PO_2 levels in AGA premature infants less than 1 week of age. There were no changes in other pulmonary function parameters. A direct correlation between PO_2 changes and increased plasma triglycerides could not be demonstrated. In addition, the younger infants had lower PO_2 levels that persisted for 4 hours after the IVF infusion, a time when plasma triglyceride levels had already returned to normal (83).

The reduction in arterial PO_2, which may occur with IVF infusions, is apparently not secondary to hyperlipidemia. McKeen and co-workers (103) found that administering the same IVF doses used in humans to sheep caused: (1) an increase in pulmonary artery pressure, (2) a decrease in arterial oxygen tension (PaO_2), and (3) an increase in transvascular fluid filtration, reflected by an increase in lung lymphatic flow. Heparin treatment of the sheep did not change these findings, although it did clear the serum of triglycerides. The pulmonary hypertension and hypoxemia caused by the IVF infusion were, therefore, *not* caused by hyperlipidemia. Treatment of the sheep with indomethacin, a potent prostaglandin inhibitor, blocked the rise in pulmonary artery pressure, the increase in lymphatic flow, and the fall in arterial PO_2. Since the effects were blocked with indomethacin, they may be prostaglandin mediated (103).

Deposition of Pigmented Material in the Reticuloendothelial System

A pigmented material has been noted at autopsy in the macrophages of the reticuloendothelial system (RES) in some infants and children who had received IVF (104–106). A number of investigators were concerned that this fat deposition might impair immune function.

Fat emulsions were noted to markedly impair neutrophil function, according to a number of in vitro chemotaxis and bactericidal assays (107–111). More recent studies failed to confirm these observations.

Palmblad et al. (112) reported that neutrophils from blood of adult volunteers given Intralipid at rates used clinically (500 ml/6 hours) were *not* inhibited in their bactericidal and chemotactic functions. English and co-workers, (113) demonstrated *no* inhibition of four neutrophil function tests even by very high concentrations of normalized fat emulsions. The authors concluded that "host defense considerations would not be an adequate justification for withholding intravenous lipid therapy" (113).

Displacement of Albumin-Bound Bilirubin by Plasma Free Fatty Acids

Potential problems may arise not from IVF per se but from the free fatty acids released during the hydrolysis of the IVF. In jaundiced newborns the use of IVF may be hazardous, since these fatty acids can displace bilirubin from albumin producing unbound (free) bilirubin, which may increase the risk of kernicterus (Fig. 2) (114–118).

Previous studies have shown that fatty acids do not begin to displace bilirubin from albumin (in the process generating free bilirubin) until the fatty acid to serum albumin molar ratio (FA/SA) is greater than four in vitro (114,115) or greater than six in vivo (118). In the latter study, Andrew et al. (118) administered 1 g/kg of IVF over 4 hours to low birth weight infants in the first two days of life. Their study is the only one that provides a specific guideline for a "safe" FA/SA in newborn infants—recommending that the FA/SA not exceed six. They went on to show that SGA infants receiving 1 g/kg of IVF over four hours in the first two days of life had mean FA/SA in excess of 10, putting such infants at risk for kernicterus.

In our laboratories at Stanford, we developed a convenient method to measure the FA/SA (119). We then monitored our use of IVF in neonates with the FA/SA to determine if we were placing premature infants at risk for kernicterus. We concluded that continuous IVF, given over 24 hours whenever possible and started during the second week of life when the bilirubin level was less than half of the potential exchange level for the individual infant, did not place neonates at risk for kernicterus. Our mean FA/SA in 29 premature infants on IVF, with doses ranging from 0.5–3.3 g/kg/day (with a mean dose of 1.5 g/kg/day), was only 1.1 (infants on oral feedings alone had a mean of 0.7), which is well within the safe range (120). Intensive care nurseries administering IVF by bolus or in the first week of life should closely monitor the FA/SA since bolus IVF infusion at day two of life resulted in a FA/SA of greater than 10 in SGA infants, as previously mentioned.

Possible Risk of Coronary Artery Disease

Earlier in this chapter it was shown that infants receiving IVF can have a rise in plasma triglycerides and free fatty acids, which is especially marked in SGA infants. Franklin and co-workers (121) have shown elevations in cholesterol in all 14 low birth weight infants studied within 1–3 weeks of beginning Intralipid. Since hyperlipidemia is recognized as a risk factor in the development of premature coronary artery disease, it is important to avoid hyperlipidemia during long-term use of IVF preparations.

"Overloading Syndrome"

Classic delayed "overloading" syndrome is caused, presumably, by presenting the patient with a fat load that exceeds metabolic capacity. The syndrome is characterized by hyperlipemia, fever, lethargy, liver damage, and coagulation disorders; it has been reported in adults, but has been recognized very rarely in children (122,123).

Miscellaneous Problems

Additional problems include (1) the potential risk of substitution of phytosterols (plant sterols), present in small amounts (0.1%) in soybean oil, for cholesterol in the developing central nervous system, which could lead to changes in myelin configuration and function (86); (2) altered prostaglandin synthesis rate and turnover (124); (3) increased concentrations of IVF in plasma that can interfere with biochemical tests—leading to spurious hyperbilirubinemia when determined by certain direct spectrophotometric methods (125) and spurious hyponatremia caused by the space-occupying effect of fat (these inaccurate readings can be corrected by prior ultracentrifugation) (125); (4) accidental injection of IVF into extradural, subdural, and subarachnoid spaces (126); (5) transient sinus bradycardia (127); (6) acute hypersensitivity reaction (128); (7) arachidonic acid deficiency, which may occur in spite of the high linoleic acid content of IVF (129); (8) abnormal platelet function, reduced platelet count (130); (9) interference with the determination of hemoglobin levels (131); (10) hemolysis, reported in three patients receiving IVF (132); and (11) pulmonary vasculitis induced by *Malassezia furfur*, a fungus of low pathogenicity (133).

Monitoring

If the IVF infusion exceeds its maximal clearance rate, plasma IVF levels rise and visible lactescence and hyperlipidemia occur. This excessive accumulation of IVF can be recognized by (1) "turbidity checks"—increase in plasma turbidity noted on visual inspection of plasma; (2) nephelometry—a measurement of plasma light scattering activity—which provides an IVF level; (3) chemical determination of plasma triglycerides, cholesterol, and fatty acids.

Recent data reveal that visual inspection of centrifuged hematocrit tubes is not reliable for monitoring patients receiving IVF (134). Bryan and co-workers suggest using the micronephelometer as a routine method for monitoring IVF levels; when the level exceeds 100–150 mg/dl, the rate of lipid infusion must be reduced (135). This recommendation is based on Forget and co-workers' observation that Intralipid concentrations greater than 100 mg/dl, as determined by nephelometry, are associated with hyper-pre-β-lipoproteinemia, hypercholesterolemia, hypertriglyceridemia, and hyperphospholipidemia (136). In one study using a common laboratory fluorometer set up as a nephelometer, "nephelometry" (light scattering index) levels did not correlate well with triglycerides, cholesterol, or free fatty acids (134).

Twenty-three infants in our intensive care nursery receiving 0.25–2.5 g/kg/day IVF by continuous infusion were tested simultaneously for IVF levels by micronephelometry as recommended by Bryan (86) (n = 58, range 18–150 mg/dl), serum free fatty acid–albumin molar ratios (n = 58, range 0–5.18), serum triglycerides (n = 54, range 33–305 mg/dl), serum cholesterol (n = 36, range 85–304 mg/dl), and serum turbidity (137). We found a positive correlation between IVF level and triglycerides (r = 0.406, p < .01), but the IVF level did not reliably predict elevated triglycerides. Of seven triglyceride determinations above 200 mg/dl, only two had elevated IVF levels. No correlation was found between IVF level and cholesterol or free fatty acid–albumin molar ratio. Serum turbidity was also a poor predictor of hyperlipidemia (137). We, like Schreiner (134), concluded that monitoring IVF use with either IVF levels or turbidity checks does not accurately provide information regarding hyperlipidemia; therefore, one must regularly monitor serum triglycerides, cholesterol, and fatty acids when using IVF.

The Importance of Carnitine in Fat Metabolism

For optimum oxidation of fatty acids carnitine is necessary. Carnitine, in the form of acyl-carnitine, transfers free fatty acids into mitochondria where they are recombined with CoA to form acyl-CoA. Carnitine is known to be present in equal concentrations in human milk and Similac (1 mg/dl), and recently has been shown to be absent in soybean-based formulas (138,139). Schiff and co-workers showed that PN solutions commonly used for intravenous feeding in newborn infants contain no carnitine (140).

Plasma levels of carnitine rapidly decrease in premature newborns during the first 3 days of life if no exogenous carnitine is given, whereas no significant changes of total carnitine were detected in adult patients on TPN for 1 week. This difference indicates fewer carnitine depots or limited capacity for carnitine biosynthesis in neonates (141). Thus, premature infants are not able to synthesize enough carnitine to maintain blood levels, and carnitine deficiency can occur following TPN (142).

As yet, there has been no clinical problem described secondary to a lack of carnitine while on TPN or soy formulas. Nevertheless, since premature infants and SGA infants have a relative inability to utilize lipids, their problem may, in part, be related to lack of exogenous carnitine. Thus, a number of investigators raise the question of the possible benefits of supplementing carnitine in the intravenously alimented child (140,141). In older children and adults it has been hypothesized that exogenous carnitine may enhance the use of endogenous fat under hypocaloric conditions and increase hepatic fatty acid oxidation, thereby minimizing fat deposition and facilitating the use of IVF emulsion as part of a TPN regimen (143). As yet there are no specific recommendations for the use of exogenous carnitine supplementation.

Future Research

Dr. Harry Greene recently summarized an expert panel's recommendation for needed research.

> Further research is needed on the safety and efficacy of intravenously administered lipid emulsions. In particular, we need to know more about: 1) pathways by which intravenously administered lipids are metabolized, as well as the factors regulating metabolism; 2) alterations in lipid metabolism secondary to immaturity or pathological conditions; 3) deleterious effects of impairment in lipid clearance, incident to immaturity or disease; and 4) the influence of intravenous fat on cell membrane structure, prostaglandin synthesis and platelet function. Such studies are of utmost importance in the stressed LBW infant. (144).
>
> A recent pilot study* shows that intravenous carnitine supplementation for premature infants receiving TPN maintains blood carnitine levels and may have a beneficial effect on the utilization of exogenously administered fat in infants <34 weeks gestation. Additional studies in this area should be pursued.

Practical Guidelines

PEDIATRIC DOSE

IVF may be administered either by peripheral or central vein.

1. Initial rate in a pediatric patient should be 0.1 ml/min for the first 10–15 minutes for patients over 5 kg, and 1 ml/kg over 1 hour for patients under 5

---

*Penn D, Schmidt-Sommerfeld E, Wolf H: L-carnitine supplementation in parenterally alimented premature infants. *Clinical Nutrition* 1 (Special Supplement): 60, 1982.

kg. If the patient tolerates the test dose (with no allergic reaction, respiratory distress, fever, etc.) the first daily dose may then be administered. In infants, the volume given in the test dose should be calculated as part of the first day's infusion.

2. Initial daily dose and guidelines for progression of the dosage, plus maximum dosages are shown for various ages in Table 4. (Example in a premature infant: day 1, 0.5 g/kg/day; day 2, 0.75 g/kg/day; day 3, 1 g/kg/day . . . to a maximum of 3 g/kg/day on day 11.)

3. IVF should make up no more than 60% of total caloric input.

ADMINISTRATION

1. Since IVF contains emulsified fat particles of 0.4–0.5 μ, filters should not be used.

2. IVF must be infused separately from any other intravenously administered solution, since these solutions may "crack" (disturb) the fat emulsion.

3. IVF may be infused in the same vein as dextrose–amino acid solutions using a Y connector near the infusion site and beyond the filter. When administered in this way, the fat emulsion will remain stable.

4. The flow rates of each solution should be controlled separately using infusion pumps.

5. IVF should be infused over 24 hours whenever possible. It should not exceed a rate of 0.15 g/kg/hr (3.6 g/kg/day) in AGA premature infants. Slower infusion rates, if any at all, are required for SGA infants. Eighteen hour infusions at a rate of 0.15 g/kg/hr with "6 hours off," as recommended by Das et al. (27), is an alternative regimen.

6. IVF should not be given if the total bilirubin level exceeds half of the exchange level (e.g., in a 1200 g infant whose exchange level is a total bilirubin of 12, IVF should not be given if the total bilirubin is greater than six).

CAUTIONS

1. IVF is contraindicated in patients with abnormal fat metabolism (e.g., pathologic hyperlipidemia, pancreatitis with hyperlipidemia).

2. IVF should be used cautiously in patients with pulmonary disease, hyperbilirubinemia, or infection.

Table 4. Use of Intravenous Fat (10% Solutions)

	Premature or SGA Infants	Full-term AGA Infants	Older Children
Initial dose	0.5 g/kg/day (5 ml/kg/day)	1 g/kg/day (10 ml/kg/day)	1 g/kg/day (10 ml/kg/day)
Increase daily dose by	0.25 g/kg/day (2.5 ml/kg/day)	0.5 g/kg/day (5 ml/kg/day)	0.5 g/kg/day (5 ml/kg/day)
Maximum dose	3 g/kg/day (30 ml/kg/day)	4 g/kg/day (40 ml/kg/day)	2 g/kg/day (20 ml/kg/day)

3. Do not use a bottle that appears to have oiling out of the emulsion.

MONITORING

1. Lab specimens for total bilirubin, sodium, and calcium should be *ultracentrifuged* to avoid spurious lab values.
2. During 24-hour infusions of IVF, serum turbidity must be checked at least once daily. At no time should there be any turbidity. If the serum is turbid, the IVF dose should be decreased or temporarily discontinued, and a serum triglyceride obtained.
3. All patients receiving IVF should have triglyceride, cholesterol, and free fatty acid (or FA/SA) levels drawn at least weekly. If any of these values is elevated, the IVF dose must be adjusted appropriately.
4. A serum triglyceride should be obtained 24 hours after an incremental increase in IVF dose to be sure the patient can tolerate this new dose.

EFA DEFICIENCY

To prevent EFA deficiency, the IVF dose is only 0.5–1.0 g/kg/day.

THE USE OF 20% IVF

20% IVF is indicated when there is a drastic need to restrict fluid volume (e.g., renal or cardiac compromise, chronic lung disease). Because of limited experience with this concentration of IVF in this country, it should be administered with great care.

1. A dose of 20% IVF should not exceed 0.15 g/kg/hr in AGA infants; slower rates, if any at all, should be attempted in SGA infants.
2. A serum triglyceride should be obtained 24 hours after each change in IVF dose to determine the patient's tolerance.

References

1. Coran AG: The long-term total intravenous feeding of infants using peripheral veins. *J Pediatr Surg* 8:801, 1973.
2. Deitl M, Kaminsky V: Total nutrition by peripheral vein—The lipid system. *Can Med Assoc J* 111:1, 1974.
3. Coran AG: Total intravenous feeding of infants and children without the use of a central venous catheter. *Ann Surg* 179:445, 1974.
4. Wretlind A: Development of fat emulsions. *JPEN* 5:230, 1981.
5. Levenson SM, Upjohn HL, Sheehy TW: Two severe reactions following the long term infusion of large amounts of intravenous fat emulsion. *Metabolism* 6:807, 1957.
6. Watkin DM: Clinical, chemical, hematologic and anatomic changes accompanying repeated intravenous administration of fat emulsion to man. *Metabolism* 6:785, 1957.

7. Alexander CS, Zieve L: Fat infusions. *Arch Intern Med* 197:514, 1961.

8. Meng HC: Use of fat emulsions in parenteral nutrition. *Drug Intelligence and Clinical Pharmacy* 6:321, 1972.

9. Waddell WR, Geyer RP, Olsen FR, et al: Clinical observations on the use of non-phosphatide (pluronic) fat emulsions. *Metabolism* 6:815, 1957.

10. Wretlind A: Parenteral nutrition. *Surg Clin North Am* 58:1055, 1978.

11. Byrne WJ: Intralipid[R] or Liposyn[R]—Comparable products? *Journal of Pediatric Gastroenterology and Nutrition* 1 (1):7, 1982.

12. Yu TC, Sinnhuber RO, Hendricks JD: Reproduction and survival of rainbow trout (*Salmo gairdneri*) fed linolenic acid as the only source of essential fatty acids. *Lipids* 14:572, 1979.

13. Lamptey MS, Walker BL: A possible essential role for dietary linolenic acid in the development of the young rat. *J Nutr* 106:86, 1976.

14. Wheeler TG, Anderson R: Visual membranes: Specificity of fatty acid precursors for the electrical response to illumination. *Science* 188:1312, 1975.

15. Holman RT, Johnson SB, Hatch TF: A case of human linolenic acid deficiency involving neurologic abnormalities. *Am J Clin Nutr* 35:617, 1982.

16. Hallberg D: Studies on the elimination of exogenous lipids from the bloodstream. *Acta Physiol Scand* 65 (Suppl 254):1, 1965.

17. Boberg J, Carlson LA: Determination of heparin-induced lipoprotein lipase activity in human plasma. *Clin Chem Acta* 10:420, 1964.

18. Pelham LD: Rational use of intravenous fat emulsions. *Am J Hosp Pharm* 38:198, 1981.

19. McFayden B, Dudrick S, Tagudar A, et al: Triglyceride and free fatty acid clearance in patients receiving complete parenteral nutrition using 10% soybean emulsion. *Surg Gynecol Obstet* 137:813, 1973.

20. Coran AG: The intravenous use of fat for the total parenteral nutrition of the infant. *Lipids* 7:455, 1976.

21. Rubecz I, Mestyan J, Horvath M, et al: The elimination of free fatty acids, free glycerol, and triglycerides from plasma of low birth weight infants receiving intravenous fat emulsions. *Acta Paediatr Acad Sci Hung* 17:65, 1976.

22. Brunzell J, Chait A, Bierman E: Pathophysiology of lipoprotein transport. *Metabolism* 27:1109, 1978.

23. Flatt JP, Blackburn GL: Metabolic fuel regulatory system: Implication for protein sparing therapies during caloric deprivation and disease. *Am J Clin Nutr* 27:175, 1974.

24. Mestyan J, Rubecz I, Soltesz G: Changes in blood glucose, free fatty acids and amino acids in low birth weight infants. *Biol Neonate* 30:74, 1976.

25. Vileisis RA, Cowett RM, Oh W: Glycemic response to lipid infusion in the premature neonate. *J Pediatr* 100:108, 1982.

26. Gustafson A, Kjellmer I, Olegard R, et al: Nutrition in low birth weight infants. I. Intravenous injection of fat emulsion. *Acta Paediatr Scand* 61:149, 1972.

27. Das JB, Joshi ID, Philippart AI: Depression of glucose utilization by Intralipid[R] in the post-traumatic period: An experimental study. *J Pediatr Surg* 15:739, 1980.

28. Long JM III, Wilmore DW, Mason AD Jr, et al: Effect of carbohydrate and fat intake on nitrogen excretion during total intravenous feeding. *Ann Surg* 185:417, 1977.

29. Macfie J, Smith RC, Hill GL: Glucose or fat as a nonprotein energy source? A controlled clinical trial in gastroenterological patients requiring intravenous nutrition. *Gastroenterology* 80:103, 1981.

30. Rubecz I, Mestyan J, Varga P, et al: Energy metabolism, substrate utilization, and nitrogen balance in parenterally fed postoperative neonates and infants: The effect of

glucose, glucose and amino acids, lipid and amino acids infused in isocaloric amounts. *J Pediatr* 98:42, 1981.

31. Marcus AJ: The role of lipids in platelet function: With particular reference to the arachidonic acid pathway. *J Lipid Res* 19:793, 1978.

32. Robertson RP: Prostaglandins as modulators of pancreatic islet function. *Diabetes* 28:943, 1979.

33. Jelenko C, Wheeler ML, Anderson AP, et al: Studies in burns: Healing in burn wounds treated with ethyl linoleate alone or in combination with selected topical antibacterial agents. *Ann Surg* 182:562, 1975.

34. Essential fatty acids and water permeability of the skin. *Nutr Rev* 35:303, 1977.

35. Heird WC, Winters RW: Total parenteral nutrition: The state of the art. *J Pediatr* 86:2, 1975.

36. Goodgame J, Lowry S, Brennan M: Essential fatty acid deficiency in total parenteral nutrition: Time course of development and suggestions for therapy. *Surgery* 84:271, 1978.

37. Holman RT: Essential fatty acid deficiency, in Holman RT (ed): *Progress in the Chemistry of Fats and Other Lipids.* Elmsford, NY, Pergamon Press Inc, 1968, Vol 9, pp 275–348.

38. Holman RT: Essential fatty acid deficiency in humans, in Recheigl M (ed): *Handbook of Nutrition and Foods.* Cleveland, CRC Press, 1977.

39. Hansen AE, Wiese HF, Boelsche AN, et al: Role of linoleic acid in infant nutrition: Clinical and chemical study of 428 infants fed on milk mixtures varying in kind and amount of fat. *Pediatrics* 31:171, 1963.

40. Sinclair AJ, Crawford MA: The effect of a low-fat maternal diet on neonatal rats. *Br J Nutr* 29:127, 1973.

41. Paoletti R, Galli C: Effects of essential fatty acid deficiency on the central nervous system in the growing rat, in Elliott K, Knight J (eds): *Lipids, Malnutrition and the Developing Brain.* CIBA Foundation Symposium, Amsterdam, Assoicated Scientific Publishers, 1972, pp 121–132.

42. Sun GY, Sun AY: Synaptosomal plasma membranes: Acyl group composition of phosphoglycerides and (Na^+ plus K^+) ATPase activity during fatty acid deficiency. *J Neurochem* 22:15, 1974.

43. Gellhorn A, Marks PA: The composition and biosynthesis of lipids in human adipose tissues. *J Clin Invest* 40:925, 1961.

44. Sinclair JC, Driscoll JM, Heird WC, et al: Supportive management of the sick neonate. *Pediatr Clin North Am* 17:863, 1970.

45. Friedman Z: Essential fatty acids revisited. *Am J Dis Child* 134:397, 1980.

46. Tashiro T, Ogata H, Yokoyama H, et al: The effects of fat emulsion (Intralipid[R]) on essential fatty acid deficiency in infants receiving intravenous alimentation. *J Pediatr Surg* 11:505, 1976.

47. Riella MC, Broviac JW, Wells M, et al: Essential fatty acid deficiency in human adults during total parenteral nutrition. *Ann Intern Med* 83:786, 1975.

48. Faulkner WJ, Flint LM: Essential fatty acid deficiency associated with total parenteral nutrition. *Surg Gynecol Obstet* 144:665, 1977.

49. Sailer D, Berg G: Essential fatty acid deficiency syndrome in the adult. *Nutr Metab* 21:101, 1977.

50. McCarthy DM, May RJ, Maher M, et al: Trace metal and essential fatty acid deficiency during total parenteral nutriton. *Dig Dis Sci* 23:1009, 1978.

51. Richardson TJ, Sgoutas D: Essential fatty acid deficiency in four adult patients during total parenteral nutrition. *Am J Clin Nutr* 28:258, 1975.

52. O'Neill JA, Caldwell MD, Meng HC: Essential fatty acid deficiency in surgical patients. *Ann Surg* 185:536, 1977.

53. Friedman Z, Danon A, Stahlman MT, et al: Rapid onset of essential fatty acid deficiency in the newborn. *Pediatrics* 58:640, 1976.

54. Holman RT: The ratio of trienoic:tetraenoic acids in tissue lipids as a measure of essential fatty acid requirement. *J Nutr* 70:405, 1960.

55. Hirono H, Suzuki H, Igarashi Y, et al: Essential fatty acid deficiency induced by total parenteral nutrition and by medium-chain triglyceride feedings. *Am J Clin Nutr* 30:1670, 1977.

56. Filler RM, Eraklis AJ, Rubin VG, et al: Long-term parenteral nutrition in infants. *N Engl J Med* 281:589, 1969.

57. Tashiro T, Ogata H, Yokoyama H, et al: The effect of fat emulsion on essential fatty acid deficiency during intravenous hyperalimentation in pediatric patients. *J Pediatr Surg* 10:203, 1975.

58. Bivins BA: Effectiveness of a parenteral safflower oil emulsion (Liposyn[R] 10%) in preventing essential fatty acid deficiency in surgical patients, in: *Liposyn Research Conference Proceedings*. North Chicago, Abbott Laboratories, 1979.

59. Levy JS, Winters RW, Heird WC: Total parenteral nutrition in pediatric patients. *Pediatrics in Review* 2:99, 1980.

60. Peterson SR, Sheldon GF: Acute acalculous cholecystitis: A complication of hyperalimentation. *Am J Surg* 138:814, 1979.

61. Friedman Z, Shochat SJ, Maisels MJ, et al: Correction of essential fatty acid deficiency in newborn infants by cutaneous application of sunflower seed oil. *Pediatrics* 58:650, 1976.

62. Hunt CE, Engel RR, Modler S, et al: Essential fatty acid deficiency in neonates: Inability to reverse deficiency by topical application of EFA rich oil. *J Pediatr* 92:603, 1978.

63. Rosenlund ML, Kim H, Kritchewsky D: Essential fatty acids in cystic fibrosis. *Nature* 251:719, 1974.

64. Kuo PT, Huang NN, Bassett DR: The fatty acid composition of the serum chylomicrons and adipose tissue of children with cystic fibrosis of the pancreas. *J Pediatr* 60:395, 1962.

65. Bennet MJ, Medwadowski BF: Vitamin A, vitamin E, and lipids in children with cystic fibrosis or congenital heart defects compared to normal children. *Am J Clin Nutr* 20:415, 1967.

66. Chase HP, Dupont J: Abnormal levels of prostaglandin and fatty acids in blood of children with cystic fibrosis. *Lancet* ii:236, 1978.

67. Hubbard VS, Dunn GD, di Sant'Agnese PA: Abnormal fatty acid composition of plasma lipids in cystic fibrosis: A primary or a secondary defect? *Lancet* ii:1302, 1977.

68. Goodchild MC, Murphy GM, Howell AM, et al: Aspects of bile acid metabolism in cystic fibrosis. *Arch Dis Child* 50:769, 1975.

69. Chase HP, Long MA, Lavin MH: Cystic fibrosis and malnutrition. *J Pediatr* 95:337, 1979.

70. Elliott RB: A therapeutic trial of fatty acid supplementation in cystic fibrosis. *Pediatrics* 57:474, 1976.

71. Rosenlund ML, Selekman JA, Kim HK, et al: Dietary essential fatty acids in cystic fibrosis. *Pediatrics* 59:428, 1977.

72. Chase HP, Cotton EK, Elliott RB: Intravenous linoleic acid supplementation in children with cystic fibrosis. *Pediatrics* 64:207, 1979.

73. Landon C, Kerner JA, Castillo R, et al: Oral correction of essential fatty acid deficiency in cystic fibrosis. *JPEN* 5:501, 1981.

74. Cashore WJ, Sedaghatian MR, Usher RH: Nutritional supplements with intravenously administered lipid, protein hydrolysate, and glucose in small premature infants. *Pediatrics* 56:8, 1975.

75. Cohen IT, Dahms B, Hays DM: Peripheral total parenteral nutrition employing a lipid emulsion (Intralipid^R): Complications encountered in pediatric patients. *J Pediatr Surg* 12:837, 1977.

76. Boberg J, Carlson LA, Halberg D: Application of a new intravenous fat tolerance test in the study of hypertriglyceridemia in man. *Journal of Atherosclerosis Research* 9:159, 1967.

77. Gustafson A, Kjellmer I, Olegard R, et al: Nutrition in low birth weight infants. I. Intravenous injection of fat emulsion. *Acta Paediatr Scand* 61:149, 1972.

78. Shennan AT, Bryan MH, Angel A: The effect of gestational age on Intralipid^R tolerance in newborn infants. *J Pediatr* 91:134, 1977.

79. Filler RM, Takada Y, Carreras T, et al: Serum Intralipid^R levels in neonates during parenteral nutrition: The relation of gestational age. *J Pediatr Surg* 15:405, 1980.

80. Andrew G, Chan G, Schiff D: Lipid metabolism in the neonate. I. The effects of Intralipid^R infusion on plasma triglyceride and free fatty acid concentrations in the neonate. *J Pediatr* 88:273, 1976.

81. Dhanireddy R, Hamash M, Sivasubraimanian KN, et al: Postheparin lipolytic activity and Intralipid^R clearance in very low birth weight infants. *J Pediatr* 98:617, 1981.

82. Pereira GR, Stanley CA, Fox WW, et al: The effect of postnatal age on the metabolism of intravenous fat emulsion. *Pediatr Res* 12:440, 1978.

83. Pereira GR, Fox WW, Stanley CA, et al: Decreased oxygenation and hyperlipemia during intravenous fat infusions in premature infants. *Pediatrics* 66:26, 1980.

84. Gustafson A, Kjellmer I, Olegard R, et al: Nutrition in low-birth-weight infants. II. Repeated intravenous injections of fat emulsion. *Acta Paediatr Scand* 63:177, 1974.

85. Olegard R, Gustafson A, Kjellmer I, et al: Nutrition in low-birth-weight infants. III. Lipolysis and free fatty acid elimination after intravenous administration of fat emulsion. *Acta Paediatr Scand* 64:745, 1975.

86. Bryan H, Shennan A, Griffin E, et al: Intralipid^R—Its rational use in parenteral nutrition of the newborn. *Pediatrics* 58:787, 1976.

87. Gurson CT, Saner G: Lipoprotein lipase activity in a marasmic type of protein–calorie malnutrition. *Arch Dis Child* 44:765, 1969.

88. Borresen HC, Coran AG, Knutrud O: Metabolic results of parenteral feeding program based on a synthetic 1-amino acid solution and a commercial fat emulsion. *Ann Surg* 172:291, 1970.

89. Coran AG, Nesbakken R: The metabolism of intravenously administered fat in adult and newborn dogs. *Surgery* 66:922, 1969.

90. Havel RJ: Metabolism of lipids in chylomicrons and very low density lipoproteins, in Renold AE, Cahill CF, Jr (eds): *Handbook of Physiology*. Washington, DC, American Physiological Society, 1965, Sec 5, p 499.

91. Cherkes A, Gordon RS: The liberation of lipoprotein lipase by heparin from adipose tissue incubated in vitro. *J Lipid Res* 1:97, 1959.

92. Michajlik A, Bragdon JG: Effects of intravenous heparin on oxidation of fat. *J Lipid Res* 1:164, 1960.

93. Coran AG, Edwards B, Zaleska R: The value of heparin in the hyperalimentation of infants and children with a fat emulsion. *J Pediatr Surg* 9:725, 1974.

94. McKee KT, Melly MA, Greene HL, et al: Gram-negative bacillary sepsis associated with the use of lipid emulsion in parenteral nutrition. *Am J Dis Child* 133:649, 1979.

95. Greene HL, Hazlett D, Demares R: Relationship between Intralipid[R] induced hyper-lipemia and pulmonary function. *Am J Clin Nutr* 29:127, 1976.

96. Branemark PI, Lindstrom J: Microcirculatory effects of emulsified fat infusions. *Circ Res* 15:124, 1964.

97. Friedman Z, Marks KH, Maisels J, et al: Effect of parenteral fat emulsion on the pulmonary and reticuloendothelial systems in the newborn infant. *Pediatrics* 61:694, 1978.

98. Barson AJ, Chiswick ML, Doig CM: Fat embolism in infancy after intravenous fat infusions. *Arch Dis Child* 53:218, 1978.

99. Levine MJ, Wigglesworth JS, Desai R: Pulmonary fat accumulation after Intralipid[R] infusion in the preterm infant. *Lancet* ii:815, 1980.

100. Andersen GE, Hertel J, Tygstrup I: Pulmonary fat accumulation in preterm infants. *Lancet* i:441, 1981.

101. Dahms B, Halpin TC: Pulmonary arterial lipid deposit in newborn infants receiving intravenous lipid infusion. *J Pediatr* 97:800, 1980.

102. Sun SC, Ventura C, Verasestakul S: Effect of Intralipid-induced lipemia on the arterial oxygen tension in preterm infants. *Resuscitation* 6:265, 1978.

103. McKeen CR, Brigham KL, Bowers RE, et al: Pulmonary vascular effects of fat emulsion infusions in unanesthetized sheep. *JCI* 61:1291, 1978.

104. Koga Y, Swanson VL, Hays DM: Hepatic "intravenous fat pigment" in infants and children receiving lipid emulsion. *J Pediatr Surg* 10:641, 1975.

105. Passwell JH, David R, Katznelson D, et al: Pigment deposition in the reticuloendothelial system after fat emulsion infusion. *Arch Dis Child* 51:366, 1976.

106. van Haelst UJ, Sengers RC: Effects of parenteral nutrition with lipids on the human liver. An electron-microscopic study. *Virchows Arch* (Cell Path) 22:323, 1976.

107. Tovar JA, Mahour GH, Miller SW, et al: Endotoxin clearance after Intralipid infusion. *J Pediatr Surg* 11:23, 1976.

108. Fischer GW, Hunter KW, Wilson SR, et al: Inhibitory effect of Intralipid on reticuloen-dothelial function and neutrophil bactericidal activity. *Pediatr Res* 13:494, 1979.

109. Fischer GW, Wilson SR, Hunter KW, et al: Diminished bacterial defenses with In-tralipid. *Lancet* ii:819, 1980.

110. Nordenstrom J, Jarstrand C, Wiernik A: Decreased chemotactic and random migration of leukocytes during Intralipid infusion. *Am J Clin Nutr* 32:2416, 1979.

111. Cleary TG, Getz SL, Pickering LK: Effect of Intralipid on oxidative metabolism and functional activities of polymorphonuclear leukocytes. *Pediatr Res* 15:529, 1981.

112. Palmblad J, Bronstrom O, Uden AM, et al: *Lancet* ii:1138, 1980 (letter).

113. English D, Roloff JS, Lukens JN, et al: Intravenous lipid emulsions and human neut-rophil function. *J Pediatr* 99:913, 1981.

114. Starinsky R, Shafrir E: Displacement of albumin-bound bilirubin by free fatty acids: Implications for neonatal hyperbilirubinemia. *Clin Chim Acta* 29:311, 1970.

115. Thiessen H, Jacobsen J, Brodersen R: Displacement of albumin-bound bilirubin in fatty acids. *Acta Paediatr Scand* 61:285, 1972.

116. Berde C, Rasmussen F, Benitz W, et al: Binding of bilirubin and fatty acids in the sera of neonates. *Clinical Research* 27:134A, 1979.

117. Chan G, Schiff D, Stern L: Competitive binding of free fatty acids and bilirubin to albumin: Differences in HBABA dye method and Sephadex G-25 interpretation of results. *Clin Biochem* 4:208, 1971.

118. Andrew G, Chan G, Schiff D: Lipid metabolism in the neonate. II. The effect of Intralipid on bilirubin binding in vitro and in vivo. *J Pediatr* 88:279, 1976.

119. Berde CB, Kerner JA, Johnson JD: Use of the conjugated polyene fatty acid, parinaric acid, in assaying fatty acids in serum or plasma. *Clin Chem* 26:1173, 1980.

120. Kerner JA, Cassani C, Hurwitz R, et al: Monitoring intravenous fat emulsions in neonates with the fatty acid/serum albumin molar ratio. *JPEN* 5:517, 1981.

121. Franklin F, Watkins JB, Heafitz L, et al: Serum lipids during total parenteral nutrition with Intralipid. *Pediatr Res* 10:354, 1976.

122. Belin RP, Bivins BA, Jona JZ, et al: Fat overload with a 10% soybean emulsion. *Arch Surg* 111:1391, 1976.

123. Monnens L, Smuldero Y, Dekker W: Lipid overloading due to Intralipid infusion in an infant with intractable diarrhea. *Z Kinderchir* 19:1, 1976.

124. Friedman Z, Lamberth EL, Frolich JC, et al: The effect of parenteral fat emulsions (PFE) on tissue fatty acid composition, the major urinary metabolites of E prostaglandins (PGE-M) and lung histology. *Pediatr Res* 11:443, 1977.

125. Shennan AT, Cherian AG, Angel A, et al: The effect of Intralipid on the estimation of serum bilirubin in the newborn infant. *J Pediatr* 88:285, 1976.

126. Black VD, Little GA, Marin-Padilla M: Failure of inflammatory response to accidental intracranial lipid infusion. *Pediatrics* 62:839, 1978.

127. Sternberg A, Gruenevald T, Deutsch AA, et al: Intralipid-induced transient bradycardia. *N Engl J Med* 304:422, 1981.

128. Kamath KR, Berry A, Cummins G: Acute hypersensitivity reaction to Intralipid. *N Engl J Med* 304:360, 1981.

129. Friedman Z, Frolich JC: Essential fatty acids and major urinary metabolites of the E prostaglandins in thriving neonates and infants receiving parenteral fat emulsions. *Pediatr Res* 13:932, 1979.

130. Lipson AH, Pritchard J, and Thomas G: Thrombocytopenia after Intralipid infusion in a neonate. *Lancet* i:1462, 1974.

131. Harris P, Thomson S, Inwood MJ: The effect of intravenous emulsified lipid (Intralipid^R) on hematologic results in infants. *Canadian Journal of Medical Technology* 39:123, 1977.

132. Marks LM, Patel N, Kurtides ES: Hematological abnormalities associated with intravenous lipid therapy. *Am J Gastroenterol* 73:490, 1980.

133. Redline RW, Dahms BB: Malassezia pulmonary vasculitis in an infant on long-term Intralipid therapy. *N Engl J Med* 305:1395, 1981.

134. Schreiner RL, Glick MR, Nordschow CD: An evaluation of methods to monitor infants receiving intravenous lipids. *J Pediatr* 94:197, 1979.

135. Bryan H, Shennan A, Griffin E, et al: Intralipid—Its rational use in parenteral nutrition of the newborn. *Pediatrics* 58:787, 1976.

136. Forget PP, Fernandes J, Begemann PH: Utilization of fat emulsion during total parenteral nutrition in children. *Acta Paediatr Scand* 64:377, 1975.

137. D'Harlingue A, Stevenson DK, Shahin SM, et al: Monitoring the use of intravenous fat (IVF) in neonates. *Pediatr Res* 16(4):160A, 1982.

138. Novak M, Wieser PB, Buch M, et al: Acetylcarnitine and free carnitine in body fluids before and after birth. *Pediatr Res* 13:10, 1979.

139. Schmidt-Sommerfeld E, Novak M, Penn D, et al: Carnitine in the development of newborn adipose tissue. *Pediatr Res* 12:660, 1978.

140. Schiff D, Chan G, Seccombe D, et al: Plasma carnitine levels during intravenous feeding of the neonate. *J Pediatr* 95:1043, 1979.

141. Novak M, Monkus EF, Chung D, et al: Carnitine in perinatal metabolism in lipids. I.

Relationship between maternal and fetal plasma levels of carnitine and acylcarnitines. *Pediatrics* 67:95, 1981.

142. Penn D, Schmidt-Sommerfeld E, Wolf H: Carnitine deficiency in premature infants receiving total parenteral nutrition. *Early Hum Dev* 4:23, 1980.

143. Tao RC, Yoshimura NN: Carnitine metabolism and its application in parenteral nutrition. *JPEN* 4:469, 1980.

144. Heird WC, Greene HL: Panel report on nutritional support of pediatric patients. *Am J Clin Nutr* 34:1223, 1981.

8

Electrolyte and Mineral Requirements

Robert L. Poole

There are numerous recommendations in the literature for the daily addition of appropriate amounts of electrolytes and minerals to parenteral nutrient infusates. The following electrolytes and minerals are addressed in this chapter: sodium, potassium, chloride, acetate, magnesium, phosphorus, and calcium. The usual requirements of these elements during the course of parenteral nutrition (PN) have been outlined for low birth weight infants (1,2), neonates (3–5), and children (6–12). Actual requirements of the elements vary with each patient's clinical condition, and factors such as renal function, state of hydration, cardiovascular status, concurrent use of diuretics, and nutritional status must be evaluated regularly. The recommended daily intake of electrolytes and minerals is shown in Table 1 (trace mineral recommendations appear in Chapter 10).

When these electrolytes and minerals are delivered in either insufficient or excessive amounts, physiological complications ensue. A summary of the potential electrolyte and mineral abnormalities associated with parenteral nutrition is listed in Table 2.

Electrolytes

SODIUM

The major function of sodium is osmotic regulation. Hypernatremia and hyponatremia result from an inappropriate sodium intake in relation to concurrent water intake. Management of common electrolyte problems in pediatrics is discussed at length in an excellent article by Perkin and Levin (11).

Heird and Anderson (2) reported that the minimal daily sodium requirement for the low birth weight infant is approximately 1.6 mEq/kg. Depending on the maturity of the kidneys and their ability to retain sodium, daily requirements may be increased. The following factors can increase the amount of sodium necessary to maintain a normal serum sodium concentration (135–140 mEq/liter): glycosuria,

Table 1. Recommended Daily Intake of Electrolytes and Minerals for PN Solutions

Element	Daily Amount
Sodium	2–4 mEq/kg
Potassium	2–3 mEq/kg
Chloride	2–3 mEq/kg
Magnesium	0.25–0.5 mEq/kg
Calcium gluconate[a]	100–500 mg/kg
Phosphorus	1–2 mmol/kg

[a]Gluconate is the recommended calcium salt for use in PN solutions (see section on calcium in this chapter).

use of diuretics, diarrhea or other excessive losses through the gastrointestinal tract, and increased fluid losses that may occur postoperatively. Excluding the above factors, 2–4 mEq/kg/day of sodium is usually adequate. *Very* low birth weight infants may require large quantities of sodium to compensate for excessive urinary loss of this element. However, sodium intakes of up to 9 mEq/kg/day have been tolerated by infants without causing significant changes in compensatory mechanisms (13).

POTASSIUM

Potassium is the primary intracellular cation, and its major function involves enzyme activity. The usual causes of potassium imbalance are mentioned briefly in Table 2. The pathophysiology and management of potassium disorders are discussed in detail by Perkin and Levin (11).

"Hyperkalemia" is a common problem in the nursery where serum electrolytes are drawn frequently by heelstick. The squeezing of the heel may cause hemolysis of red blood cells, resulting in a falsely high potassium measurement.

The minimal potassium requirement for the low birth weight infant is approximately 1.4 mEq/kg/day (2). Even though adequate nutrition may be supplied to promote anabolism, hypokalemia may develop as the extracellular supply is used to build new cells. Sodium, glycosuria, the use of diuretics, diarrhea or other excessive gastrointestinal tract losses, and postoperative fluid loss all contribute to an increase in the daily potassium requirements. However, 2–3 mEq/kg/day is the usual potassium requirement to maintain a normal serum concentration (3.5–5.0 mEq/liter) (4). Although unusual, the very low birth weight infant may require as much as 8–10 mEq/kg/day of potassium (4).

CHLORIDE

The primary function of chloride is osmotic regulation. Hyperchloremic metabolic acidosis was a common finding when crystalline amino acid solutions were first introduced (14). The incidence of this acidosis can be prevented or treated by altering the amounts of chloride salts in the parenteral nutrition solutions (15). By supplying some of the sodium and potassium requirements as acetate or phosphate

Table 2. Electrolyte and Mineral Abnormalities Associated with Parenteral Nutrition

Abnormality	Manifestations	Usual Causes
Hyponatremia	Weakness, hypotension, oliguria, tachycardia	Inadequate sodium intake relative to water intake
Hypernatremia	Edema, hypertension, thirst, intracranial hemorrhage	Inappropriate sodium intake in relation to water intake especially with abnormal losses, e.g., diarrhea, diuretic use
Hypokalemia	Weakness, alkalosis, cardiac abnormalities	Insufficient potassium intake associated with protein anabolism
Hyperkalemia	Weakness, paresthesias, cardiac arrythmias	Acidosis, renal failure, excessive potassium intake
Hyperchloremia	Metabolic acidosis	Excessive chloride intake with sodium and potassium administration. Amino acid solutions with high chloride content
Hypocalcemia	Tetany, seizures, demineralization of bone, rickets	Inadequate calcium, phosphorus and/or vitamin D intake
Hypercalcemia	Renal failure, aberrant ossification	Inadequate phosphorus intake, Excess vitamin D intake
Hypophosphatemia	Weakness, bone pain, demineralization of bone	Insufficient phosphorus intake in relation to calcium intake
Hypomagnesemia	Seizures, neuritis	Inadequate intake

salts, the amount of chloride can be reduced in PN solutions. Also, the reformulation of synthetic amino acid solutions (e.g., Freamine III, Aminosyn, Travasol) by commercial manufacturers has helped to avoid this serious complication.

The usual chloride requirement during PN therapy is 2–3 mEq/kg/day (4), while the minimal requirement for the low birth weight infant is approximately 1.1 mEq/kg/day (2).

ACETATE

There are no specific requirements for the use of acetate in parenteral nutrition solutions. However, in vivo acetate is rapidly metabolized to bicarbonate; therefore, sodium acetate and potassium acetate can be employed in the treatment or prevention of hyperchloremic metabolic acidosis. Acetate salts are compatible with all other common PN components and are therefore ideal to use when acidosis is present. Sodium bicarbonate cannot be used in PN solutions containing calcium, since a calcium carbonate precipitate forms readily. The use of acetate salts not only increases the serum bicarbonate but also decreases the amount of chloride delivered to the patient.

Minerals

Daily requirements for sodium, potassium, and chloride in PN solutions are well established for all age groups (2,4–8). The daily needs of magnesium, calcium, and phosphorus for various age groups are not as well defined. The following are recommendations from exisiting data.

MAGNESIUM

Magnesium is an essential component of numerous intracellular enzyme systems. More specifically, magnesium is required as a catalyst for many enzymatic reactions relating to carbohydrate metabolism and adenosine triphosphate (ATP). Wacker and Parisi (16) provide an extensive review of magnesium metabolism. Hypomagnesemia has been demonstrated in studies of protein–calorie malnutrition (17,18). Magnesium deficiency can also occur during PN therapy (19,20).

Usual recommendations for magnesium requirements during a course of PN are 0.25–0.5 mEq/kg/day (2–4,8). These requirements are altered by impaired renal function, diuretic use. inflammatory bowel diseases, anabolism, and so on. A recommended amount of magnesium to be used in the treatment of symptomatic hypomagnesemia is 0.2 mEq/kg given intramuscularly or intravenously every 6 hours until symptoms resolve and the serum magnesium returns to normal (11). Hypotension can occur with rapid intravenous administration of magnesium; therefore, the magnesium should be diluted and administered over several hours.

PHOSPHORUS

Phosphate is an essential element of any parenteral nutrition regimen. It is an important intracellular anion and is required for the formation of energy-transfer enzymes such as ATP and ADP. Phosphorus is also necessary for bone metabolism and normal skeletal mineralization.

Severe hypophosphatemia has been reported in patients requiring prolonged intravenous alimentation (21–23). The consequences of acute hypophosphatemia include the following: rhabdomyolysis; a reduction in 2,3-diphosphoglycerate (2-3-DPG) and ATP (which may depress P50* values or shift the oxygen–hemoglobin saturation curve to the left such that oxygen release to peripheral tissues is dimin-

---

*P50 is the value for oxygen tension of mixed venous blood at 37°C, pH 7.4, at which hemoglobin is 50% saturated.

ished); myocardial dysfunction; depressed chemotactic, phagocytic and bactericidal activity of granulocytes; central nervous system symptoms compatible with metabolic encephalopathy; metabolic acidosis; and osteomalacia (24).

Phosphorus can be provided as either potassium or sodium phosphate salts. Most commercial preparations of potassium phosphate contain 4.4 mEq potassium/ml and 3 mmol phosphorus/ml. Sodium phosphate contains 4 mEq sodium/ml and 3 mmol phosphorus/ml. Phosphorus is also present in the phospholipid portion of intravenous fat emulsion. However, Tovey et al. (22) cast doubt upon the bioavailability of the phosphorus contained in fat emulsions when they reported that patients developed hypophosphatemia while receiving intravenous nutrition that included fat emulsion.

Recommendations for maintenance requirements of phosphorus range between 0.5 and 2.0 mmol/kg/day, (1,3,4,8,11,21). For the treatment of severe hypophosphatemia, an initial dose of 0.15–0.3 mmol/kg administered intravenously over 6 hours is recommended (11). Phosphorus must be ordered in millimoles rather than milliequivalents since the milliequivalent content changes with pH, and changes in pH may occur with each PN solution additive.

Administration of phosphate has been associated with hyperphosphatemia, hypocalcemia, deposition of calcium–phosphate crystals, hypotension, cation toxicity from phosphate salts, and dehydration (11). Serum phosphorus should be determined frequently during acute phosphorus repletion. Calcium supplements may be required during phosphate administration, but the administration of concentrated calcium solutions added to phosphate-containing solutions may result in precipitation. Phosphorus and calcium can be provided in the same solution if certain criteria are met—if the concentrations of each do not exceed critical amounts and if the pH, temperature, and dextrose and amino acid concentrations of the solutions are appropriate (see Chapter 11).

CALCIUM

The major functions of calcium involve bone metabolism and neural transmission. Calcium is also an important cofactor in blood coagulation, enzyme function, and other cellular activities (25). While calcium imbalance is frequent during the neonatal period, it is much less common in older children and adolescents. Hypocalcemia, bone demineralization, and rickets have all been reported in patients receiving total parenteral nutrition (TPN) (26–29). Although hypercalcemic disorders are rare in children, hypercalciuria with nephrolithiasis has been reported as a potential complication of TPN (30).

Precise calcium requirements for normal growth and development for the various pediatric age groups are not well understood at present. The Committee on Nutrition of the American Academy of Pediatrics has made a statement on the oral dietary calcium requirements in infancy and childhood (31) (Table 3). However, this statement does not address parenteral calcium requirements. Other authors have presented recommendations for the amount of calcium to be added to PN solutions (1,3,4,6–8,32). Unfortunately, these recommendations are primarily intended for preterm infants, neonates, and older infants. During the final weeks of gestation, the fetus normally receives approximately 150 mg/kg/day of elemental

Table 3. Recommended Calcium Intakes[a]

	Calcium (mg/day)		
Subject	FAO/WHO	NAS	Fomon[b]
Infants	500–600[c]	360–540[c]	300–450
Children	400–500	800	
Adolescent boy	600–700	1,200	
Adolescent girl	600–700	1,200	
Lactating women	1,000–1,200	1,200	

SOURCE: Committee on Nutrition, American Academy of Pediatrics: *Pediatrics* 62:832, 1978. Copyright © 1978, American Academy of Pediatrics. Reprinted with permission.
[a]The Committee on Nutrition suggests 335 mg of calcium per liter as the minimum for infant formulas. The European Society of Paediatric Gastroenterology and Nutrition suggests 400 mg of calcium per liter.
[b]"Advisable intakes"; estimated requirements are 84% of these values.
[c]Not breast-fed.

calcium* transplacentally (32). Calcium requirements for older children and adolescents on PN therapy are less clear. Filler (33) has recommended parenteral calcium intakes for all pediatric age groups using standard solutions with fixed amounts of calcium: premature infants, 13 mEq/liter; infants and young children ages 0–7 years, 18 mEq/liter; children and adolescents ages 7–18 years, 10 mEq/liter.

Based upon available data, maintenance calcium* requirements during pediatric PN range between 100 and 500 mg/kg/day of calcium gluconate. Gluconate is the recommended calcium salt for use in PN solutions since this salt dissociates less than the chloride salt (34). This fact allows more calcium and phosphorus to remain soluble in PN solutions, thus making it possible to give more of these two minerals to premature infants with high requirements of both. Maintenance calcium should be given daily even though the serum calcium may be in the normal range. The serum calcium can be normal or even high when hypophosphatemia is present. Also, the serum calcium can be normal at the expense of bone demineralization (27–29). Administering a dose of 200 mg/kg of 10% calcium gluconate given intravenously over at least 1 hour, while monitoring the cardiac rate for bradycardia, has been recommended for the treatment of symptomatic hypocalcemia (11).

The maximum amounts of calcium and phosphorus that can be given in the same solution are limited by their solubilities. Usually 20 mEq of calcium (approximately 4000 mg calcium gluconate) and 20 mmol of phosphate per liter of solution are the maximum quantities that can be mixed without causing precipitation (see Chapter 11). This limiting factor may render it impossible to prevent or treat osteoporosis or rickets in very low birth weight infants that are fluid restricted (29,32).

References

1. Shaw JCL: Parenteral nutrition in the management of sick low birthweight infants. *Pediatr. Clin North Am* 20:333, 1973.

---

*Twenty milligrams of elemental calcium is equivalent to approximately 1 mEq of calcium, and 1 mEq of calcium is approximately equal to 200 mg of calcium gluconate.

2. Heird WC, Anderson TL: Nutritional requirements and methods of feeding low birth weight infants, in Gluck L (ed): *Current Problems in Pediatrics*. Chicago, Year Book Medical Publishers, 1977, vol 7, p 26.

3. Jacobs WC, Lazzara A, Martin DJ: *Parenteral Nutrition in the Neonate*. Chicago, Abbott Laboratories, 1980.

4. Kerner JA, Sunshine P: Parenteral alimentation. *Semin Perinatol* 3:417, 1979.

5. Lorch V, Lay SA: Parenteral alimentation in the neonate. *Pediatr. Clin North Am* 24:547, 1977.

6. Reimer SL, Michener WM, Steiger E: Nutritional support of the ciritically ill child. *Pediatr Clin North Am* 27:647, 1980.

7. Heird WC, MacMillan RW, Winters RW: Total parenteral nutrition in the pediatric patient, in Fischer JE (ed): *Total Parenteral Nutrition*. Boston, Little, Brown and Co, 1976, p 253.

8. Heird WC, Winters RW: Total parenteral nutrition—The state of the art. *J Pediatr* 86:2, 1975.

9. Jewett TC, Lebenthal E: Intravenous hyperalimentation—Surgical impact and outcome, in Gluck L (ed): *Current Problems in Pediatrics*. Chicago, Year Book Medical Publishers, 1978, vol 9, p 15.

10. Forlaw L: Parenteral nutrition in the critically ill child. *Critical Care Quarterly* 3:1, 1981.

11. Perkin RM, Levin DL: Common fluid and electrolyte problems in the pediatric intensive care unit. *Pediatr Clin North Am* 27:567, 1980.

12. Feliciano DU, Telander RL: Total parenteral nutrition in infants and children. *Mayo Clin Proc* 51:647, 1976.

13. Committee on Nutrition, American Academy of Pediatrics: Sodium intake of infants in the United States. *Pediatrics* 68:444, 1981.

14. Heird WC, Dell RB, Driscall JM, et al: Metabolic acidosis resulting from intravenous alimentation mixtures containing synthetic amino acids. *N Engl J Med* 287:293, 1972.

15. Quinby GE, Nowak MM, Andrews BF: Parenteral nutrition in the neonate. *Clin Perinatol* 2:59, 1975.

16. Wacker WEC, Parisi AF: Magnesium metabolism. *N Engl J Med* 278:658–663, 712–717, 772–776, 1968.

17. Caddell JL, Goddard DR: Studies in protein–calorie malnutrition. I. Chemical evidence for magnesium deficiency. *N Engl J Med* 276:533, 1967.

18. Caddell JL: Studies in protein–calorie malnutrition. II. A double-blind clinical trial to assess magnesium therapy. *N Engl J Med* 276:535, 1967.

19. Grand RJ, Colodny AH: Increased requirement for magnesium during parenteral therapy for granulomatous colitis. *J Pediatr* 81:788, 1972.

20. Main ANH, Morgan RJ, Russell RI, et al: Mg deficiency in chronic inflammatory bowel disease and requirements during intravenous nutrition. *JPEN* 5:15, 1981.

21. Ricour C, Millot M, Balsan S: Phosphorus depletion in children on long-term total parenteral nutrition. *Acta Paediatr Scand* 64:385, 1975.

22. Tovey SJ, Benton KGF, Lee HA: Hypophosphatemia and phosphorus requirements during intravenous nutrition. *Postgrad Med J 53:299, 1977*.

23. Aladjem M, Lotan D, Biochis H, et al: Changes in the electrolyte content of serum and urine during total parenteral nutrition. *J Pediatr* 97:437, 1980.

24. Knochel JP: Hypophosphatemia (Nutrition in Medicine). *West J Med* 134:15, 1981.

25. Root AW, Harrison HE: Recent advances in calcium metabolism. II. Disorders of calcium homeostasis. *J Pediatr* 88:177, 1976.

26. Heird WC: Disorders of calcium and phosphorus metabolism, in Winters RW, Hassel-

meyer EG (eds): *Intravenous Nutrition in the High Risk Infant.* New York, John Wiley & Sons, 1975, p 249.

27. Tsang RC, Steichen JJ, Brown DR: Perinatal calcium homeostasis: Neonatal hypocalcemia and bone demineralization. *Clin Perinatol* 4:385, 1977.

28. Geggel RL, Pereira GR, Spackman TJ: Fractured ribs: Unusual presentation of rickets in premature infants. *J Pediatr* 93:680, 1978.

29. Leape LL, Valaes T: Rickets in low birth weight infants receiving total parenteral nutrition. *J Pediatr Surg* 11:665, 1976.

30. Adelman RD, Abern SB, Merten D, et al: Hypercalciuria with nephrolithiasis: A complication of total parenteral nutrition. *Pediatrics* 59:473, 1977.

31. Committee on Nutrition: Calcium requirements in infancy and childhood. *Pediatrics* 62:826, 1978.

32. Knight PJ, Buchanan SB, Clatworthy HW: Calcium and phosphate requirements of preterm infants who require hyperalimentation. *JAMA* 243:1244, 1980.

33. Filler RM: Parenteral support of the surgically ill child, in Suskind RM (ed): *Textbook of Pediatric Nutrition.* New York, Raven Press, 1981, p 381.

34. Henry RS, Jurgens RW, Sturgeon R, et al: Compatibility of calcium chloride and calcium gluconate with sodium phosphate in a mixed TPN solution. *Am J Hosp Pharm* 37:673, 1980.

9
Vitamin Requirements

John A. Kerner, Jr.

Vitamins are essential cofactors in a wide range of metabolic reactions. These functions are summarized in Table 1. The physical findings and biochemical abnormalities associated with the most common vitamin deficiencies are discussed in the Nutritional Assessment chapter. The oral recommended dietary allowances (RDA) of these nutrients are shown in Appendix I. Numerous reviews describe vitamin metabolism more thoroughly (1–9).

Plasma or serum levels of vitamins may not necessarily reflect their content in various tissues or their biologic activity (10), and studies describing only serum levels of various vitamins (11,12) may not be sensitive in assessment of vitamin status. Assays of vitamin dependent enzymes, such as erythrocyte transketolase to assess vitamin B_1 status or erythrocyte glutamic oxaloacetic transaminase to assess vitamin B_6, have proved to be a more convenient, specific, and sensitive index of vitamin status (see Chapter 2 for a list of the enzymes that can be measured to properly assess the status of an individual vitamin). Studies such as that of Kishi and co-workers (13) helped define requirements for thiamine and pyridoxine during total parenteral nutrition (TPN) by using enzymatic methods.

Insufficient intake of a vitamin results in a steplike progression to obvious clinical signs. There is depletion of measurable vitamin content followed by a series of metabolic changes that occur at the cellular level as a consequence of the depleted vitamin coenzymes. After these changes have occurred clinical symptoms begin to appear (14).

The requirements for vitamins in TPN are not well known. The oral RDA can serve as a general guide, but these recommendations clearly have to be modified for TPN use (10). There are several reasons why parenteral vitamin requirements might differ from oral requirements.

Most parenteral vitamins are supplied in multivitamin solutions and are then added to a mixture of substrates and minerals; thus, nutrient–nutrient interactions are likely and may alter the relative effectiveness of a specific vitamin (15).

Parenteral nutrients are generally infused from plastic or glass containers with some admixture of room air; thus, vitamins may adhere to tubing and containers or may be subject to oxidative destruction (15). Adherence of vitamin A to plastic and glass has previously been described (16,17). Howard et al. (18) were the first to report that clinical vitamin A deficiency may result from prolonged use of pre-

Table 1. Vitamins

Name	Characteristics	Biochemical Action	Effects of Deficiency	Effects of Excess	Daily Requirement	Food Sources
Vitamin A (retinol) 1 IU = 0.3 µg retinol	Fat soluble, heat stable; bile necessary for absorption, specific binding protein in plasma; stored in liver	Component of visual purple; integrity of epithelial tissues, bone cell function	Night blindness xerophthalmia, keratomalacia, poor growth, impaired resistance to infection	Hyperostosis, hepatomegaly, alopecia, increased cerebrospinal fluid pressure	Infants—300 µg; adolescents —750 µg; lactation—1,200 µg	Milk fat, egg, liver
Provitamin A: β-carotene; 1/6 activity of retinol	Converted to retinol in liver, intestinal mucosa			Carotenemia		Dark green vegetables, yellow fruits and vegetables, tomato
Biotin	Water soluble; synthesized by intestinal bacteria; deficiency only with large intake of egg white	Coenzyme	Dermatitis, anorexia, muscle pain, pallor	Unknown	Unknown	Liver, egg yolk, peanuts
Cobalamin (vitamin B₁₂)	Slightly soluble in water, heat stable only at neutral pH, light sensitive; absorption (ileum) dependent on gastric intrinsic factor; Co a part of the molecule	Coenzyme component; red blood cell maturation, central nervous system metabolism	Pernicious anemia; neurologic deterioration	Unknown	1-2 µg	Animal foods, only: meat, milk, egg

Vitamin	Properties	Function	Deficiency	Toxicity	Requirement	Sources
Folacin: group of compounds containing pteridine ring, p-aminobenzoic and glutamic acids	Slightly soluble in water, light sensitive, heat stable; some production by intestinal bacteria; ascorbic acid involved in interconversions; interference from oral contraceptives, anticonvulsants	Tetrahydrofolic acid the active form; synthesis of purines, pyrimidines, methylation reactions	Megaloblastic anemia	Only in patients with pernicious anemia not receiving cobalamin	Infants—50 μg; adolescents—400 μg; pregnancy—800 μg	Liver, green vegetables, cereals, orange
Niacin (nicotinic acid, nicotinamide)	Water soluble, heat and light stable; availability from corn enhanced by alkali; synthesized in the body from tryptophan (60:1), some by intestinal bacteria	Components of coenzymes I and II (NAD, NADP), many enzymatic reactions	Pellagra: dermatitis, diarrhea, dementia	Nicotinic acid (not the amide): flushing, pruritus	6.6 mg/1,000 calories	Meat, fish, whole grains, green vegetables
Pantothenic acid	Water soluble, heat stable	Component of coenzyme A; many enzymatic reactions	Observed only with use of antagonists; depression, hypotension, muscle weakness, abdominal pain	Unknown	Unknown; estimated at 5–10 mg	Most foods

Table 1. (Continued)

Name	Characteristics	Biochemical Action	Effects of Deficiency	Effects of Excess	Daily Requirement	Food Sources
Pyridoxine (vitamin B$_6$) also pyridoxal, pyridoxamine	Water soluble, heat and light labile, interference from isoniazid; pyridoxal is the active form	Cofactor for many enzymes	Dermatitis, glossitis, cheilosis, peripheral neuritis. Infants—irritability, convulsions, anemia	Unknown	Infants—0.2–0.3 mg; adults—2 mg	Liver, meat, whole grains, corn, soybeans
Riboflavin	Water soluble, light labile, heat stable; ? synthesis by intestinal bacteria	Cofactor for many enzymes	Photophobia, cheilosis, glossitis, corneal vascularization, poor growth	Unknown	0.6 mg/1,000 cal	Meat, milk, egg, green vegetables, whole grains
Thiamine (vitamin B$_1$)	Heat labile; absorption impaired by alcohol, requirements a function of carbohydrate intake; synthesis by intestinal bacteria	Coenzyme for decarboxylation, other reactions	Beriberi: neuritis, edema, cardiac failure, hoarseness, anorexia, restlessness, aphonia	Unknown	0.5 mg/1,000 cal	Liver, meat, milk, whole grains, legumes
Ascorbic acid (vitamin C)	Easily oxidized, especially in presence of copper, iron, high pH; absorption by simple diffusion	Exact mechanism unknown: functions in folacin metabolism, collagen biosynthesis, iron absorption and transport, tyrosine metabolism	Scurvy	Massive doses may lead to temporary increase in requirement	Infants—35 mg; adolescents —45 mg	Citrus fruits, tomatoes, cabbage, potatoes, human milk

Vitamin	Physiology/Metabolism	Deficiency	Recommended Allowance	Sources
Vitamin D (D_2-activated calciferol; D_3-activated dehydrocholesterol 1 IU = 0.025 µg)	D_2 from diet, D_3 from action of ultraviolet on skin; hydroxylated sequentially in liver and kidney to form 1,25-dihydroxycholecalciferol, the active compound; regulated by dietary calcium, PTH; now called a hormone; anticonvulsant drugs interfere with metabolism	Rickets, osteomalacia	All ages 10 µg (400 IU)	Fortified milk, fish liver, salmon, sardines, mackerel, egg yolk, sunlight
Vitamin E (1 IU = 1 mg α-tocopherol acetate)	Stored in adipose tissue, transported with β-lipoproteins; absorption dependent on pancreatic juice and bile (iron may interfere); requirement increased by large amounts of polyunsaturated fats	Formation of calcium transport protein in duodenal mucosa; facilitates bone resorption, phosphorus absorption	Hypercalcemia, azotemia, poor growth, vomiting, nephrocalcinosis	Cereal seed oils, peanuts soybeans, milk fat, turnip greens
Vitamin K (napthoquinones)	Fat soluble, bile necessary for absorption, synthesis by intestinal bacteria	Blood coagulation: factors II, VII, IX, X	Newborn—single dose of 1 mg; thereafter, 5 µg/day; older infants, children—unknown	Cow's milk, green leafy vegetables, pork, liver

Antioxidant, ? role in red blood cell fragility — Hemolytic anemia in premature infants; otherwise, no clearcut deficiency syndrome in man — Unknown — Infants—4 mg; adolescents —15 mg

Hemorrhagic manifestations — Water-soluble analogs only: hyperbilirubinemia

SOURCE: Barness LA: Vitamins, in Committee on Nutrition, *Pediatric Nutrition Handbook*. Evanston, Illinois: American Academy of Pediatrics, 1979. Reprinted with permission.

mixed nutrient solutions. In Howard's study, for which vitamin A was premixed in a standard TPN solution, the vitamin A content was only 23% of the initial concentration after the solution was stored in the dark at 4°C for 2 weeks. The loss was secondary to oxidation and adherence of the vitamin A onto the plastic bags containing the TPN solutions (18). According to the results of in vitro studies, fresh vitamin A should be added to TPN solutions each day.

Parenteral vitamins are delivered systemically, rather than enterally, and this may impair their activation and storage, and allow for their rather rapid excretion in the urine (15).

Underlying disease states may also change vitamin requirements. For example, a burn patient faced with extensive healing may have vitamin requirements comparable to those during phases of rapid growth (15).

Vitamin B_{12} and the fat-soluble vitamins (A, D, E, K) may be stored in body tissues and, therefore, are not needed in full daily amounts for short periods of time.

Water Soluble Vitamins

Intravenous (IV) requirements for water-soluble vitamins are greater than oral requirements because a larger portion is excreted by the kidneys when the vitamins are given IV (19). Vitamin C and the B vitamins are generally added to PN solutions in amounts that will provide two to three times the oral RDA.

Vitamin C is a necessary cofactor in premature infants. Because of decreased activity of hepatic tyrosine transaminase, the ability of the preterm infant to metabolize tyrosine and phenylalanine is limited (20). Supplemental vitamin C allows the infant to metabolize these amino acids normally (21). Premature infants fed high protein diets containing large amounts of threonine excrete parahydroxyphenyllactic acid and parahydroxyphenylpyruvic acid unless given additional vitamin C (22,23).

When water-soluble vitamins are given as described above, no vitamin deficiencies have been observed, with the exception of biotin deficiency (described below). Until recently parenteral vitamin preparations in the United States did not contain biotin.

BIOTIN DEFICIENCY

In 1927 Boas-Fixsen observed that the feeding of raw egg white to rats produced an eczemalike dermatitis accompanied by loss of hair (24). In 1936 it was found that administering biotin could cure this disorder. Next, the protein factor that induced biotin deficiency in animals was isolated and named *avidin*. Avidin bound biotin very strongly, and initially the reaction was felt to be irreversible. Subsequently, it was learned that this binding capacity was lost upon boiling or steaming (24,25). The few human cases of biotin deficiency reported were all caused by excessive intake of raw egg white (24). Biotin deficiency is rare in human beings partly because the vitamin is ubiquitous among foods and partly because it is produced in adequate amounts by bacteria in the intestine (24).

Mock et al. (26) recently reported a child with short bowel syndrome who developed biotin deficiency during TPN. During the third to sixth months of TPN the child developed an exfoliative dermatitis that exuded clear fluid. During the fifth and sixth month of TPN the patient lost all body hair and developed a waxy pallor, irritability, lethargy, and mild hypotonia. Diagnostic studies ruled out zinc deficiency or essential fatty acid deficiency as the cause of the dermatitis. However, biotin concentrations were very low in plasma and whole blood, and urinary biotin was also well below normal. Biotin supplementation resolved the symptoms and corrected the biochemical abnormalities. The child had been receiving antibiotics almost continuously, which suppressed intestinal flora and therefore may have altered biotin synthesis. Whatever biotin was synthesized by bacteria may have been poorly absorbed by the patient's severely shortened gut. Biotin deficiency should be included in the differential diagnosis of rash and alopecia occuring during TPN, particularly if the intestinal flora are suppressed and intestinal absorption is compromised (26).

Fat-Soluble Vitamins

The fat-soluble vitamins (A, D, E, and K) differ from the water-soluble vitamins primarily in four ways: (1) infants and children are particularly prone to deficiency because of a greater tendency to develop steatorrhea with secondary malabsorption of fat-soluble vitamins; (2) Specific deficiency syndromes are often peculiar to infants; (3) requirements are more dependent on age and maturation; (4) since the fat soluble vitamins can be stored in body tissues, excess intake may result in toxicity (14). The reported occurrence of hypervitaminosis A or D is rare. Reported cases have frequently involved the consumption of inappropriately large amounts of vitamins without medical supervision.

VITAMIN A

Lippe et al. (27) recently described a 4-year-old boy and a 2½-year-old boy with chronic vitamin A intoxication. The two children demonstrated symptoms of increased intracranial pressure, edema of the extremities and face, rash, bone pain and tenderness, and hypercalcemia. Both had received extraordinarily high doses of oral vitamin A for some time. Serum vitamin A concentrations were markedly elevated, and serum vitamin D levels were normal. The history of excessive vitamin intake was elicited only after the detection of hypercalcemia (27).

Classic clinical and radiographic findings of hypervitaminosis A including dermatitis, irritability, pain upon ambulation, chelosis, and gingivitis. X-ray films of the extremities show thick periosteal new bone formation, and dense metaphyses in the fibulae, tibiae, and distal femurs have been described in a 4-year-old child on TPN who inadvertently received large doses of vitamin A. Because of gastrointestinal losses of approximately 5 liters per day, the patient received 6 liters per day of fluid parenterally; each liter contained 10,000 IU of vitamin A (28).

Vitamin A is very sensitive to photodecomposition in TPN solutions so that it is essential to protect the solution bottle from sunlight in order to provide the prescribed quantity of vitamin A (29). Concomitant administration of vitamin E is essential to keep the proper level of vitamin A in plasma (29).

VITAMIN D

The known action of vitamin D is to facilitate calcium absorption from the intestine, to deposit and retain calcium in the bones, and to mobilize calcium from bone. A deficiency of this vitamin can contribute to the development of osteomalacia in the adult and can produce rickets in the infant or growing child. (The problem of rickets in low birth weight infants is discussed in detail in Chapter 11.) It might be argued that vitamin D need not be included in TPN since it is not desirable to mobilize bone calcium, and gut absorption of calcium during TPN should be negligible.

METABOLIC BONE DISEASE

Shike and co-workers (30) did a prospective study of calcium and bone metabolism in patients on home TPN. Their studies indicate that patients developed metabolic bone disease as a complication of the treatment. The disease was characterized by hypercalciuria, intermittent hypercalcemia, reduced skeletal calcium, low circulating parathyroid hormone levels, a bone biopsy appearance of osteomalacia, and normal serum levels of 25-OH vitamin D. The metabolic and clinical features greatly improved within 30–60 days after vitamin D was withdrawn (30).

Thus, osteomalacia, hypercalcemia, hypercalciuria, and negative calcium balance developed despite an average daily intake of 250 IU of vitamin D_2, 400 mg calcium, and 500–700 mg phosphate with normal plasma levels of 25-OH vitamin D. Withdrawal of the solution containing vitamin D (MVI-1000) resulted in healing of the osteomalacia, normalization of the serum calcium, decrease in urinary calcium excretion, and reversal to a positive calcium balance (30).

Increased calcium loss in the urine has also been demonstrated in patients who were receiving TPN for short periods when solutions containing vitamin D were added to their TPN regimen (10). Vitamin D is not required for intestinal calcium and phosphate absorption in the parenterally fed patient. Whether it fulfills other roles in bone and calcium metabolism is a subject of current controversy (10). While $1,25(OH)_2$ vitamin D is thought to cause bone resorption, $24,25(OH)_2$ vitamin D has been suggested as an essential factor in bone mineralization. At present, it is not clear whether vitamin D is required in adult TPN regimens; if required, the dose would probably be quite small (10).

Disorders of bone metabolism have also been reported in infants (31,32). This syndrome in the neonate is due, in part, to the problem of providing adequate calcium and phosphate in the small fluid volumes usually allowable (31). Additionally, there is still uncertainty about vitamin D requirements and about the maturity of the vitamin D hydroxylating enzyme systems, especially in preterm infants (33).

Vitamin D requirements will depend on a patient's exposure to sunlight. Shike and co-workers' patients were ambulatory (34). Patients confined to the indoors (i.e., hospitalized patients) may be more likely to require vitamin D. In these patients, the amount of vitamin D necessary will probably vary with the clinical condition (34).

In conclusion, the amount of supplemental vitamin D in pediatric TPN is still a cause for controversy. Jeejeebhoy recommends *no* vitamin D for adult patients on TPN (10). However, premature infants need vitamin D in addition to adequate amounts of calcium and phosphorus to prevent rickets. The skeletal findings in premature infants who had had radiographic findings of rickets while on TPN improved after the quantity of administered vitamin D_2 was increased (35). Careful review of the latest literature will help your hospital design appropriate guidelines for vitamin D use.

VITAMIN E

Infants are born in a relative state of vitamin E deficiency; total body content is about 20 mg in a 3 kg infant. Low birth weight infants generally have substantially less vitamin E—about 3 mg in an infant weighing 1 kg. In 1969 Oski and Barness (36) first described the hemolytic anemia of prematurity associated with insufficient intake of vitamin E.

The erythrocyte life span for the full-term infant is approximately two thirds of that for the normal adult (37). Infants born prematurely have a more rapid and greater fall in hemoglobin (Hgb) values postnatally (38,39). This is probably secondary to an even shorter erythrocyte life span (40), which may be influenced by dietary factors, such as iron supplementation, vitamin E intake, and the proportion of polyunsaturated fatty acids (PUFA) in the diet (36,41–43). The nadir of Hgb values normally occurs at about 2–3 months of age. Although some iron supplementation of the diet would appear to be indicated in premature infants in view of their low iron stores at birth, iron may act as a catalyst in the oxidative breakdown of the red blood cell membrane lipids, thereby accelerating hemolysis (41,43,44). Vitamin E, on the other hand, may limit the peroxidation of membrane lipids, specifically of their PUFA component, thereby mitigating, to some extent, the oxidant effect of iron. The elucidation of the antioxidant effects of vitamin E on the PUFA component of cell membranes, and its potential role in the anemia of prematurity, prompted changes in the composition of infant formulas, including increased fortification with vitamin E and attention to the vitamin E:PUFA ratio. Melhorn and Gross (42) demonstrated that in very low birth weight infants, the daily administration of 7–10 mg/kg of iron accelerated the postnatal decline in Hgb levels, especially in the presence of vitamin E deficiency. Daily supplementation with iron at lower doses 2–2.5 mg/kg from 2 weeks of age), however, has not been found to adversely affect Hgb levels by 2 months of age in low birth weight infants (45,46).

Bell and Filer have recently reassessed the role of vitamin E in the nutrition of premature infants (47). Their critical analysis reveals that published controlled studies of vitamin E supplementation do not agree on the degree or even the existence of vitamin E's protective effect against anemia. Their analysis of commonly used feeding practices suggests that the dietary ratio of vitamin E (α-tocopherol) to PUFA is generally sufficient to prevent manifestations of vitamin E deficiency without supplementation. The protective effects of large parenteral doses of vitamin E for bronchopulmonary dysplasia (BPD) and retrolental fibroplasia (RLF) were shown in early studies (48–53) but not substantiated in subsequent reports (54–58).

Hittner et al. (59) recently reported the results of a double-blind study in 101 premature infants weighing less than 1500 g at birth who had respiratory distress to evaluate the efficacy of oral vitamin E in preventing the development of RLF. The treatment group received 100 mg/kg/day of vitamin E whereas the "control" group received 5 mg/kg/day. The overall incidence of RLF was not reduced (65% of the controls, 64% of the treatment group), but the treatment group had a significantly decreased incidence of *severe* RLF. Thus, most intensive care nurseries now recommend that all their premature infants with respiratory distress receive 100 mg/kg/day of vitamin E by mouth. An important warning appeared in an editorial discussing the article of Hittner et al. Weiter stated that "vitamin E in large doses should not be assumed to be as innocuous as oxygen was considered to be in the early 1940's" (60). Future research can be expected to further clarify the approach to prevention and treatment of RLF.

Bell and Filer concluded that infants who are being fed parenterally with regimens that include 10% lipid emulsion (Intralipid or Liposyn) in doses up to 2 g/kg/day plus 1 ml/day of MVI concentrate will receive adequate amounts of vitamin E. Above 2 g/kg/day Intralipid or above 2.5 g/kg/day Liposyn, the vitamin E to PUFA ratio diminishes with increasing lipid dose, unless additional vitamin E is given orally or parenterally (an adequate vitamin E to PUFA ratio for premature infants is greater than 0.6 mg/g) (47).

The other manifestations that have been linked to vitamin E deficiency both in animals and humans include the following:

1. Creatinuria, reversed by vitamin E administration (61)
2. Ceroid pigment deposition in smooth muscle (ceroid represents peroxidized polyunsaturated fatty acids; vitamin E may act to prevent the formation of ceroid by its antioxidant properties) (62,63)
3. Multifocal degeneration of striated muscle (64)
4. Central nervous system findings of axonal "dystrophic" lesions in gracile and cuneate nuclei of patients with biliary atresia and cystic fibrosis (65,66)

Clinical correlates of these biochemical and histologic abnormalities have not been established. The above disturbances have been observed in patients with prolonged steatorrhea and low serum vitamin E levels (e.g., patients with biliary atresia or cystic fibrosis) (67). Therefore, it is recommended that vitamin E supplementation be administered to such patients.

VITAMIN K

Vitamin K is essential in blood coagulation; it maintains normal plasma levels of prothrombin (factor II) and factors VII, IX, and X. The chief dietary source of vitamin K is green leafy vegetables; vitamin K is also synthesized by intestinal bacteria. Because the amount of vitamin K derived from intestinal flora is not known, and because pure dietary deficiency of vitamin K is rare, the exact human requirement for vitamin K has not been established (67). (See Appendix I for Recommended Dietary Allowances.)

Vitamin K supplementation is required (67)

1. Prophylactically in the newborn period—a newborn initially has *no intestinal flora* to produce vitamin K

2. For malabsorption of vitamin K associated with diarrhea (e.g., biliary atresia, cystic fibrosis, other causes of obstructive jaundice)

3. In the presence of impaired liver function (inability to produce clotting factors)

4. For impaired synthesis of vitamin K—*secondary to use of antibiotics* or to diarrhea itself

The Committee on Nutrition recommends 1 mg vitamin K, parenterally, once a month for infants and children with fat malabsorption (68).

Use of Antibiotics.   Frick et al. (69) were unable to produce vitamin K deficiency in adults by total starvation over 5 weeks. In contrast, only 3 to 4 weeks of antibiotic therapy was required to produce deficiency. Pineo and co-workers (70) described 27 vitamin K-deficient adults; 22 of 27 were taking antibiotics while all 27 had little or no food intake for several days prior to diagnosis. Ansell et al. (71) described a similar experience.

Based on our experience, all babies in our intensive care nursery receiving antibiotics receive supplemental vitamin K. Infants less than 1000 g receive 0.25 mg intramuscularly twice weekly; infants over 1000 g receive 0.5 mg intramuscularly twice weekly. Older infants and children generally receive 0.5 mg intramuscularly twice weekly.

Use of Total Parenteral Nutrition.   When there is no enteral intake, supplemental vitamin K is required. Specific recommendations appear in the Practical Guidelines section.

Practical Guidelines

NEED FOR SUPPLEMENTATION

An infant or child who is also receiving some oral feedings with a *complete* oral vitamin supplementation does not need additional parenteral vitamins.

SUPPLEMENTATION FOR INFANTS

1. MVI concentrate. *The standard recommendation is to provide 1 ml MVI concentrate/day* (72–76). See Table 2 for the contents of MVI concentrate. The vitamin D content *may* be too low for growing premature infants and needs special consideration—up to 600 additional IU/day may be needed (74). Please see the section on rickets in Chapter 13 for further discussion of vitamin D needs. The amount of vitamin A recommended is slightly on the high side while the vitamin D dose is slightly low. Ideally, there should be a separate preparation of each of the fat-soluble vitamins and a separate preparation of water-soluble vitamins.

2. Folate vitamin B_{12}, vitamin K

   a. Vitamin K is required for the synthesis of coagulation factors. Normally, it is derived from the diet (mainly vegetables) and from the gut bacteria. In the patient receiving TPN the gut bacteria may be a sufficient source

Table 2. MVI Concentrate: Vitamin in 1 ml

Vitamin A	2000 IU
Thiamine (B_1)	10 mg
Riboflavin (B_2)	2 mg
Pyridoxine (B_6)	3 mg
Niacinamide	20 mg
Ascorbic acid (C)	100 mg
Ergocalciferol (D)	200 IU
Vitamin E	1 IU
Panthothenic acid	5 mg

of vitamin K. However, since changes may occur in the flora of the nonactive gut (especially if a child is receiving antibiotics), supplementation with vitamin K seems reasonable (10). Vitamin B_{12} and folate are necessary to prevent megaloblastic anemia (76,77).

b. A number of authors recommend adding folate, vitamin B_{12}, and vitamin K daily to the TPN solution in the following dosages:

Folate	50 µg/day (73–75)
Vitamin B_{12}	5 µg/day (75)
Vitamin K	0.5 mg/day (74,75)

Although a 10–15% deterioration may be expected over 24 hours when exposed to fluorescent light, vitamin K (Aquamephyton), appears to be stable in amino acid solutions and may be included with other additives in PN solutions (WC Jacobs: Personal communication with Merck, Sharp, and Dohme Laboratories, 1978) (73).

c. Other authors recommend adding folate, vitamin B_{12}, and vitamin K separately (78–80). They base this recommendation on reports that these three vitamins may be oxidized in glucose–amino acid solutions (81). Vitamin B_{12} may deteriorate on standing when included in an aqueous solution with vitamin C (82). Vitamin B_{12} and vitamin K are incompatible in the same solution (see Chapter 11).

d. Alternative recommended dosages:

Folic acid:	1–2 mg IM every 2 wk (80)
	50 µg IV daily in a solution other than the TPN solution (72)
Vitamin B_{12}:	50 µg IM monthly (80)
	50 µg IM twice monthly (72)
Vitamin K:	1 mg IM every 2 weeks (80)
	0.25–0.5 mg IM twice weekly (72)

e. Tiny premature infants have little or no muscle mass and for these patients we definitely recommend giving the vitamins *intravenously* in the doses described above. We have seen no evidence of vitamin deficiency when these nutrients are provided intravenously; we have actually demonstrated rises in levels of serum B_{12} and serum folic acid while on TPN. Ideally, controlled studies need to be performed to determine the most effective route to deliver these three vitamins.

SUPPLEMENTATION FOR OLDER CHILDREN (THROUGH AGE 10)

1. MVI concentrate: 2 ml/day IV
2. Folic acid: 1 mg/day IV
3. Vitamin K—give IM on a *weekly* basis:
   < 2 yr—2 mg IM
   2–5 yr—5 mg IM
   > 5 yr—10 mg IM
4. Vitamin B_{12}—give 100 µg IM at the beginning of parenteral nutrition and then *monthly*.

SUPPLEMENTATION FOR CHILDREN 11 YEARS AND OLDER

1. *One daily dose of MVI-12* (USV Laboratories)—5 ml of Vial 1 + 5 ml of Vial 2; *or one daily dose of MVC 9 + 3* (Lypho-Med Inc)—5 ml of Vial 1 + 5 ml of Vial 2.
2. Vitamin K: 10 mg IM *weekly*

FORMULATIONS

Tables 3 and 4 present data from a statement by The American Medical Association Nutrition Advisory Group (AMA/NAG). No preparation to date meets the recommendations for infants and children (although a preparation is expected soon). Two preparations meet the AMA/NAG recommendations for children aged 11 and older and for adults (see Table 5).

The major difference between MVI and MVI-12 (or MVC 9 + 3) is that the latter two products contain smaller amounts of vitamin A and D, and they contain biotin, B_{12}, and folic acid which are not present in MVI.

Vitamins A and D are included at a lower dosage because they are fat-soluble and may accumulate in adipose tissue. A metabolic bone disease (30), described earlier, occurs in some TPN patients and may be related to excessive vitamin D intake. Whether this bone disease will occur with daily use of MVI-12 or MVC 9 + 3 is not yet known. Patients receiving long term TPN should be closely monitored for early signs of this bone disease with serum and urinary calcium determinations if daily MVI-12 or MVC 9 + 3 is used.

Biotin deficiency has occurred during TPN (26), but no data exist for biotin requirements.

Folic acid and B_{12} have been added to the formulation, eliminating the need to add them separately to the patient's regimen. Additional ascorbic acid may need to be given to stressed patients and can be added to the same or separate PN bottles.

MVI is still stocked in our hospital for children under age 11 years, using the doses described above. When the new "pediatric MVI-12" is released, our nutritional support team will review its revised contents to determine if it better fits

Table 3. Formulations for Infants and Children Under 11 years[a]

Vitamins	RDA			AAP[b] minimum/ 100 kcal orally	Suggested Formulations	
	Range—Infants (/kg body wt 0.0-0.5 and 0.5-1.0 yr)	Mean—Infant	Range—Children Under 11 yr		Multivitamin[c] for Intravenous Use for Under 11 yr	Water-Soluble Vitamins for Intramuscular Use
A (retinol), IU	233–222	227.0	2,000–3,300	250.0	2,300.0[d]	
D, IU	66-44	55.0	400	40.0	400.0[e]	
E (α tocopherol), IU	0.66–0.55	0.6	7–10	0.3	7.0	
K$_1$ (phylloquinone), mg					0.2	
Ascorbic acid, mg	6–4	5.0	40	8.0	80.0	80.0
Folacin, μg	8–6	7.0	100–300	4.0	140.0	140.0
Niacin, mg	0.9–0.8	0.85	9–16	0.25	17.0	17.0
Riboflavin, mg	0.07	0.07	0.8–1.2	0.06	1.4	1.4
Thiamin, mg		0.053	0.7–1.2	0.025	1.2	1.2
B$_6$ (pyridoxine), mg	0.055–0.05	0.045	0.6–1.2	0.035	1.0	1.0
B$_{12}$ (cyanocobalamin), μg	0.05–0.04	0.035	1–2	0.15	1.0	1.0
Pantothenic acid, mg	0.04–0.03			0.3	5.0[f]	5.0
Biotin, μg					20.0[f]	20.0

SOURCE: Nutrition Advisory Group of Department of Food and Nutrition, AMA: Multivitamin preparations for parenteral use—A statement by the Nutrition Advisory Group. *JPEN*, 3:260, 1979. Copyright© 1975, *American Medical Association*. Reprinted with permission.

[a]Adapted from Tables 1, 2, and 4, Guidelines for Multivitamin Preparations for Parenteral Use, AMA, 1975.

[b]American Academy of Pediatrics.

[c]May be provided in appropriate salt or ester form in equivalent potency.

[d]700 μg of retinol.

[e]As ergocalciferol or cholecalciferol.

[f]RDA not established; amount = 20 × 100 kcal human milk.

Table 4. Suggested Formulations for Children Age 11 yr and Above, and Adults[a] (Results do not include requirements for pregnancy or lactation.)

Vitamins	RDA Adult Range	Multivitamin Formulation for IV Use	Water-Soluble Vitamin Formulation for IM Use
A, IU	4,000–5,000[b]	3,300	
D, IU	400	200	
E, IU	12–15	10.0	
Ascorbic acid, mg	45	100.0	100.0
Folacin, μg	400	400.0	400.0
Niacin, mg	12–20	40.0	40.0
Riboflavin, mg	1.1–1.8	3.6	3.6
Thiamin, mg	1.0–1.5	3.0	3.0
B$_6$ (pyridoxine), mg	1.6–2.0	4.0	4.0
B$_{12}$ (cyanocobalamin), μg	3	5.0	5.0
Pantothenic acid, mg	5–10[c]	15.0	15.0
Biotin, μg	150–300[c]	60.0	60.0

SOURCE: Nutrition Advisory Group of Department of Food and Nutrition, AMA: Multivitamin preparations for parenteral use—A statement by the Nutrition Advisory Group. *JPEN* 3:260, 1979; Copyright© 1975, American Medical Association. Reprinted with permission.

[a]Adapted from Tables 1, 2, and 4, Guidelines for Multivitamin Preparations for Parenteral Use, AMA, 1975.

[b]Assumes 50% intake as carotene, which is less available than vitamin A.

[c]RDA not established, amount considered adequate in usualy dietary intake.

Table 5 Vitamin Content Per Package of Selected TPN Preparations

Products	Units A	Units D	Units E	mg B$_1$	mg B^2	mg Ni[a]	mg PA[b]	mg B$_6$	mg C	μg FA[c]	μg B$_{12}$	μg Bi[d]
AMA/NAG[e]	3300	200	10	3	3.6	40	15	4	100	400	5	60
M.V.I.-12	3300	200	10	3	3.6	40	15	4	100	400	5	60
MVC 9 + 3[f]	3300	200	10	3	3.6	40	15	4	100	400	5	60
M.V.I.	10,000	1,000	5	50	10	100	25	15	500	—	—	—
Berocca-C	—	—	—	10	10	80	20	20	100	—	—	200
Betalin Complex F.C.	—	—	—	25	6	100	5	10	150	—	—	—
Folbesyn	—	—	—	10	10	75	10	15	300	1,000	15	—
Solu-B with Ascorbic Acid	—	—	—	10	10	250	50	5	500	—	—	—
Vi-Cert	—	—	—	25	10	100	20	20	500	—	—	—
Bejectal-C	—	—	—	200	30	750	50	50	1,000	—	20	—
Solu-B- forte	—	—	—	250	50	1,250	500	50	1,000	—	—	—

SOURCE: Product information. Courtesy of USV Laboratories, Tuckahoe, New York, 1982.

[a]Ni—Niacinamide

[b]PA—Pantothenic acid

[c]FA—Folic acid

[d]Bi—Biotin

[e]Recommendations for children age 11 yr and above, and adults (AMA/NAG = the American Medical Association Nutrition Advisory Group)

[f]Does not require refrigeration

the needs of these patients, based on the most current data present in the literature.

VITAMIN B$_{12}$ ASSAY

Standard assays for vitamin B$_{12}$ (cobalamin) deficiency may be unreliable. Two recent reports make suggestions to help your hospital's laboratory improve its ability to identify true vitamin B$_{12}$ deficiency (83,84).

References

1. Goldbloom RB: Fat-soluble vitamins, in Oliver K, Cox BG, Johnson TR, et al (eds): *Developmental Nutrition.* Columbus, Ohio, Ross Laboratories, 1979, p 45.

2. LeLeiko NS, Suskind RM: Water soluble vitamins, in Oliver K, Cox BG, Johnson TR, et al (eds): *Developmental Nutrition.* Columbus, Ohio, Ross Laboratories, 1979, p 55.

3. Herman RH: Disorders of fat soluble vitamins A, D, E, and K, in Suskind RM (ed): *Textbook of Pediatric Nutrition.* New York, Raven Press, 1981, p 65.

4. Greene HL: Disorders of the water soluble vitamin B-complex and vitamin C, in Suskind RM (ed): *Textbook of Pediatric Nutrition.* New York, Raven Press, 1981, p 113.

5. Caldwell MD, Kennedy-Caldwell C: Normal nutritional requirements. *Surg Clin North Am* 61:489, 1981.

6. Moran JR, Greene HL: The B vitamins and vitamin C in human nutrition. I. General consideration and "obligatory" B vitamins. *Am J Dis Child* 133:192, 1979.

7. Moran JR, Green HL: The B vitamins and vitamin C in human nutrition. II. "Conditional" B vitamins and vitamin C. *Am J Dis Child* 133:308, 1979.

8. Schwarz KB, Olson RE: Requirements and absorption of fat-soluble vitamins during infancy, in Lebenthal, E (ed): *Textbook of Gastroenterology and Nutrition in Infancy.* New York, Raven Press, 1981. p 563.

9. Greene HL: Water-soluble vitamins, in Lebenthal, E (ed): *Textbook of Gastroenterology and Nutrition in Infancy.* New York, Raven Press, 1981, p 585.

10. Shike M, Jeejeebhoy KN: Trace elements and vitamins in total parenteral nutrition. Postgraduate course of ASPEN 5th Clinical Congress, February, 1981.

11. Lowry SF, Goodgame JT, Maher MM, et al: Parenteral vitamin requirements during intravenous feeding. *Am J Clin Nutr* 31:2149, 1978.

12. Ricour C, Navarro J, Duhamel JF: Trace elements and vitamins in infants on total parenteral nutrition (T.P.N.) *Acta Chir Scand* (Suppl) 498:67, 1980.

13. Kishi H, Nishii S, Ono T, et al: Thiamin and pyridoxine requirements during intravenous hyperalimentation. *Am J Clin Nutr* 32:332, 1979.

14. Greene HL: Vitamins and trace minerals. Nutritional care of high risk obstetrical patients and high risk infants. Postgraduate course, Department of Pediatrics, Stanford University, Stanford, Calif, June 18, 1980.

15. Howard LJ: Vitamins in TPN. Postgraduate course of ASPEN 5th Clinical Congress, February, 1981.

16. Moorhatch P, Chiou WL: Interactions between drugs and plastic intravenous fluid bags. *Am J Hosp Pharm* 31:149, 1974.

17. Hartline JV, Zachman RD: Vitamin A delivery in total parenteral nutrition solutions. *Pediatrics* 58:448, 1976.

18. Howard L, Chu R, Feman S, et al: Vitamin A deficiency from long-term parenteral nutrition. *Ann Int Med* 93:576, 1980.

19. Greene HL: Vitamins in total parenteral nutrition. *Drug Intel Clin Pharm* 6:355, 1972.

20. Gordon H, Levin SZ: The metabolic basis for the individualized feeding of infants, premature and full-term. *J Pediatr* 25:464, 1944.

21. Sunshine P: Nutrition of the low birthweight infant, in Quilligan EJ, Kretchmer N (eds): *Fetal and Maternal Medicine.* New York, John Wiley & Sons, 1980, p 637.

22. Scriver CR, Rosenberg LE: *Amino Acid Metabolism and Its Disorders.* Philadelphia, WB Saunders Co, 1973, p 345.

23. LeLeiko NS, Suskind RM: Water soluble vitamins, in Oliver K, Cox BG, Johnson TR, et al (eds): *Developmental Nutrition.* Columbus, Ohio, Ross Laboratories, 1979, p 55.

24. Robinson FA: *The Vitamin Co-factors of Enzyme Systems.* New York, Pergammon Press, 1966, p 497.

25. Tanaka K: New light on biotin deficiency. *N Engl J Med* 304:839, 1981.

26. Mock DM, DeLorimier AA, Liebman WM, et al: Biotin deficiency: An unusual complication of parenteral alimentation. *N Engl J Med* 304:820, 1981.

27. Lippe B, Hensen L, Mendoza G, et al: Chronic vitamin A intoxication. *Am J Dis Child* 135:634, 1981.

28. Seibert JJ, Byrne WJ, Golladay ES: Development of hypervitaminosis A in a patient on long-term parenteral hyperalimentation. *Pediatr Radiol* 10:173, 1981.

29. Kishi H, Yamaji A, Kataoka K, et al: Vitamin A and E requirements during total parenteral nutrition. *JPEN* 5:420, 1981.

30. Shike M, Harrison JE, Sturtridge WC, et al: Metabolic bone disease in patients receiving long-term parenteral nutrition. *Ann Int Med* 92:343, 1980.

31. Knight PJ, Buchanan S, Clatworthy HW Jr: Calcium and phosphate requirements of preterm infants who require prolonged hyperalimentation. *JAMA* 243:1244, 1980.

32. Klein GL, Cannon RA, Ament ME, et al: Rickets and osteopenia with normal 25-OH vitamin D in infants on parenteral nutrition, abstracted. *Clin Res* 28:596A, 1980.

33. Hillman LS, Haddad JG: Vitamin D metabolism and bone mineralization in premature and small-for-gestational-age infants, in DeLuca HF, Anast CS (eds): *Pediatric Diseases Related to Calcium.* Amsterdam, Elsevier/North Holland, 1980, p 355.

34. Allam BF, Dryburgh FJ, Shenkin A: Metabolic bone disease during parenteral nutrition. *Lancet I*: 385, 1981.

35. Klein GL, Cannon RA, Ament M, et al: Vitamin D-resistant rickets associated with long-term parenteral nutrition, in Howard AN (ed): *Recent Advances in Clinical Nutrition.* London, John Libbey & Co, vol 1 (in press).

36. Oski FA, Barness LA: Vitamin E deficiency: A previously unrecognized cause of hemolytic anemia in the premature infant. *J Pediatr* 70:211, 1967.

37. Pearson HA: Life span of the fetal red blood cell. *J Pediatr* 70:166, 1967.

38. Sisson TRC, Whalen LE, Telek A: The blood volume of infants. II. The premature infant during the first year of life. *J Pediatr* 55:430, 1959.

39. Matoh Y, Zaizov R, Varsano I: Postnatal changes in some red cell parameters. *Acta Pediatr Scand* 60:317, 1971.

40. O'Brien RT, Pearson HA: Physiologic anemia of the newborn infant. *J Pediatr* 79:132, 1971.

41. Melhorn DK, Gross S: Vitamin E-dependent anemia in the premature infant. I. Effects of large doses of medicinal iron. *J Pediatr* 79:569, 1971.

42. Melhorn DK, Gross S: Vitamin E-dependent anemia in the premature infant. II. Relationships between gestational age and absorption of vitamin E. *J Pediatr* 79:581, 1971.

43. Williams ML, Shott RJ, O'Neal PL, Oski FA: Role of dietary iron and fat on vitamin E deficiency anemia of infancy. *N Engl J Med* 292:887, 1975.

44. Smith KA, Mengel CE: Associatin of iron-dextran-induced hemolysis and lipid peroxidation in mice. *J. Lab Clin Med* 72:505, 1968.

45. Rudolph N, Preis O, Bitzos EI, Reale MM, Wong SL: Hematologic and selenium status of low-birth-weight infants fed formulas with and without iron. *J Pediatr* 99:57, 1981.

46. Lundstrom V, Siimes MA, Dallman PR: At what age does iron supplementation become necessary in low-birth-weight infants? *J Pediatr* 91:878, 1977.

47. Bell EF, Filer LJ: The role of vitamin E in the nutrition of premature infants. *Am J Clin Nutr* 34:414, 1981.

48. Ehrenkranz RA, Bonta BW, Ablow RC, et al: Amelioration of bronchopulmonary dysplasia after vitamin E administration: A preliminary report. *N Engl J Med* 299:564, 1978.

49. Johnson L, Schaffer D, Boggs TR Jr: The premature infant, vitamin E deficiency and retrolental fibroplasia. *Am J Clin Nutr* 27:1158, 1974.

50. Johnson LH, Schaffer DB, Rubinstein D. et al: The role of vitamin E in retrolental fibroplasia. *Pediatr Res* 10:425, 1976.

51. Johnson L, Schaffer D, Boggs T, et al: Vit E Rx of retrolental fibroplasia grade III or worse. *Pediatr Res* 14:601, 1980.

52. Phelps DL, Rosenbaum AL: Vitamin E in kitten oxygen-induced retinopathy: Kitten model. *Pediatrics* 59:998, 1977.

53. Phelps DL, Rosenbaum AL: Vitamin E in kitten oxygen-induced retinopathy. II. Blockage of vitreal neovascularization. *Arch Ophthalmol* 97:1522, 1979.

54. Curran JS, Cantolino SJ: Vitamin E (injectable) administration in the prevention of retinopathy of prematurity: Evaluation with fluorescein angiography and fundus photography. *Pediatr Res* 12:404, 1978.

55. McClung HJ, Backes C, Lavin A, Kerzner B: Prospective evaluation of vitamin E therapy in premature infants with hyaline membrane disease. *Pediatr Res* 14:604, 1980.

56. Ehrenkranz RA, Ablow RC, Warshaw JB: Prevention of bronchopulmonary dysplasia with vitamin E administration during the acute stages of respiratory distress syndrome. *J Pediatr* 95:873, 1979.

57. Abbasi S, Johnson L, Boggs T: Effect of vit E by infusion in sick small premature infants at risk for BPD. *Pediatr Res* 14:638, 1980.

58. Saldanha RL, Cepeda EE, Poland RL: Effect of prophylactic vitamin E on the development of bronchopulmonary dysplasia in high-risk neonates. *Pediatr Res* 14:650, 1980.

59. Hittner HM, Godio LB, Rudolph AJ, et al: Retrolental fibroplasia: Efficiency of vitamin E in a double-blind clinical study of preterm infants. *N Engl J Med* 305:1365, 1981.

60. Weiter JJ: Retrolental fibroplasia: An unsolved problem. *N Engl J Med* 305:1404, 1981.

61. Nitowsky HM, Tildon JT, Levin S, et al: Studies of tocopherol deficiency in infants and children. VII. The effect of tocopherol on urinary, plasma, and muscle creatine. *Am J Clin Nutr* 10:368, 1962.

62. Blanc WA, Reid JD, Anderson DH: Avitaminosis E in cystic fibrosis of the pancreas. *Pediatrics* 22:494, 1958.

63. Kerner I, Goldbloom RB: Investigations of tocopherol deficiency in infancy and childhood: Studies of ceroid pigment disposition. *Am J Dis Child* 99:597, 1960.

64. Oppenheimer EH: Focal necrosis of striated muscle in an infant with cystic fibrosis of the pancreas and evidence of lack of absorption of fat-soluble vitamins. *Bulletin of Johns Hopkin Hospital* 98:353, 1956.

65. Sung JH, Park SH, Mastri AR, et al: Axonal dystrophy in the gracile nucleus in con-

genital biliary atresia and cystic fibrosis (mucoviscidosis): Beneficial effect of vitamin E therapy. *J Neuropathol Exp Neurol* 39:584, 1980.

66. Towfighi J: Effects of chronic vitamin E deficiency on the nervous system of the rat. *Acta Neuropath* (Berl) 54:261, 1981.

67. Goldbloom RB: Fat soluble vitamins, in Oliver K, Cox BG, Johnson TR, et al (eds): *Developmental Nutrition.* Columbus, Ohio, Ross Laboratories, 1979, p 45.

68. American Academy of Pediatrics, Committee on Nutrition: Vitamin K supplementation for infants receiving milk substitute infant formulas and for those with fat malabsorption. *Pediatrics* 48:483, 1971.

69. Frick PG, Riedler G, Brogli H: Dose response and minimal daily requirement for vitamin K in man. *J Appl Physiol* 23:387, 1967.

70. Pineo GF, Gallus AS, Hirsh J: Unexpected vitamin K deficiency in hospitalized patients. *Can Med Assoc J* 109:880, 1973.

71. Ansell JE, Kumor R, Deykin D: The spectrum of vitamin K deficiency. *JAMA* 238:40, 1977.

72. Kerner JA, Sunshine P: Parenteral alimentation. *Semin Perinatol* 3:417, 1979.

73. Jacobs WC, Lazzara A, Martin DJ: *Parenteral Nutrition in the Neonate.* Chicago, Abbott Laboratories, 1980, p 19.

74. Wesley JR, Saran PA, Khalidi N, et al: *Parenteral and Enteral Nutrition Manual.* Chicago, Abbott Laboratories, 1980, p 45.

75. Heird WC: Total parenteral nutrition, in *Pediatric Nutrition Handbook,* Evanston, Ill, American Academy of Pediatrics, 1979, p 395.

76. Denburg J, Bensen W, Ali MAM, et al: Megaloblastic anemia in patients receiving total parenteral nutrition without folic acid or vitamin B_{12} supplementation. *Can Med Assoc J* 117:144, 1977.

77. Green PJ: Folate deficiency and intravenous nutrition. *Lancet* I:814, 1977.

78. Seashore JH: Metabolic complications of parenteral nutrition in infants and children. *Surg Clin North Am* 60:1239, 1980.

79. Filler RM: Parenteral support of the surgically ill child, in Suskind RM (ed): *Textbook of Pediatric Nutrition.* New York, Raven Press, 1981, p 345.

80. Levy JS, Winters RW, Heird WC: Total parenteral nutrition in pediatric patients. *Pediatrics in Review* 2:99, 1980.

81. Fischer JE: Parenteral and enteral nutrition. *Disease-a-Month* 24:2, 1978.

82. *M.V.I.* Tuckahoe, New York, USV Laboratories, 1973, p 9.

83. England JM: Problems with the serum vitamin B_{12} assay. *Lancet* II:1072, 1980.

84. Cohen KL, Donaldson RM: Unreliability of radiodilution assays as screening tests for cobalamin (vitamin B_{12}) deficiency. *JAMA* 244:1942, 1980.

10

Trace Element Requirements

John A. Kerner, Jr.

The eleven *major elements* (carbon, hydrogen, oxygen, nitrogen, sodium, potassium, calcium, magnesium, phosphorus, sulfur, and chlorine) make up more than 99.7% of the total body weight. The remaining weight comprises many other elements, each contributing less than 0.01% to the total body weight (1). Since these elements are present in tissues only in minute quantities, each occurring in the adult human body in amounts of less than 5 grams, they are arbitrarily designated *trace elements*. A growing number of these trace elements have been recognized to be of nutritional importance to mammals (2)—vanadium, chromium, manganese, iron, cobalt, nickel, copper, zinc, silicon, selenium, molybdenum, tin, iodine, arsenic, and possibly flourine, cadmium, and lead. Chromium, manganese, iron, cobalt, copper, zinc, selenium, molybdenum, and iodine are already recognized to be of physiological importance to humans and nutritional requirements probably exist for most of the other trace elements (3).

Biological Functions of Trace Elements

The trace elements have been shown to influence a number of biochemical and physiological processes. Some have a specific physiological role; for example, there is an atom of cobalt at the center of the vitamin B_{12} molecule and molybdenum is required as a component of xanthine oxidase. The two major recognized functions of trace elements are to act as cofactors for metal-ion-activated enzymes or to form such a tight complex with the protein that the two are isolated together as a unit called a *metalloenzyme*. Molybdenum, iron, copper, zinc, selenium, and manganese all are specific constituents of metalloenzymes (3). Trace elements play a part in the synthesis and structural stabilization of both proteins and nucleic acids (4). They are also constituents of proteins and hormones, for example, iodine in thyroxin and chromium as a cofactor for insulin (3). In addition, they are involved in the function of subcellular systems such as mitochondria, as well as in membrane transport, nerve conduction, and muscle contraction (4).

The nutritional importance of iron and iodine has been known for years, but until very recently little attention was given to the other trace elements. It is now apparent that *specific nutritional deficiencies* of these elements do occur, and that these deficiencies can be detrimental to health, growth, and development. The problem of trace element deficiencies is of special concern in pediatric patients since deficiency states are often most severe during prenatal and postnatal development, and because the infant and growing child are most susceptible to such deficiencies (1). This is not surprising since it is known that nutritional requirements for trace elements are relatively high in young animals (2).

Advances in technology, especially the development of atomic absorption spectroscopy, have enhanced the appreciation of the importance of trace elements in childhood nutrition (5). The marked progress in defining elements "essential" to mammalian life has resulted from the use of technically demanding metal-deprivation studies during which animals were housed under metal-free conditions (6).

General facts about the metabolism of four of the major trace elements are shown in Table 1. Detailed reviews regarding the biochemistry, physiology, and metabolism of the trace elements are available, but beyond the scope of this chapter (1–3,5,7–12).

COPPER

Copper is an essential component of a number of metalloenzymes (Table 2). Ceruloplasmin, a glycoprotein that contains eight copper atoms per molecule, accounts for more than 95% of the copper present in the blood plasma. This cuproprotein plays a major role in copper transport and has ferroxidase activity (2). Ceruloplasmin is necessary for the optimal rate of oxidation of Fe^{2+} from body stores in the liver and bone marrow to Fe^{3+}; this is a necessary step before iron can attach to transferrin for transport to and uptake by the erythrocyte precursors in the bone marrow (3). In copper deficiency, lack of ferroxidases contributes to the hypochromic anemia which is unresponsive to oral iron therapy (13).

Approximately 40% of ingested copper is absorbed by the stomach and small intestine (see Table 1). Absorbed copper is attached to albumin and transported to the liver. The liver has a central role in copper metabolism and homeostasis. Approximately 80% of the absorbed copper is excreted by the biliary system (1) (see Table 1).

ZINC

Zinc is an essential component of more than 40 metalloenzymes, including carbonic anhydrase (involved in carbon dioxide metabolism), alkaline phosphatase, lactic acid dehydrogenase (important for the interconversions between pyruvate and lactate) and some peptidases (important in protein digestion) (14). These metalloenzymes are involved in the metabolism of lipids, carbohydrates, proteins, and nucleic acids. Hence, zinc is crucial to growth and development. Other zinc-containing proteins include nerve growth factor and gustin, a salivary protein that is thought to play an important role in taste perception.

Table 1. Metabolism of Selected Trace Elements in Adults

	Zinc	Copper	Selenium	Chromium
Total-body content	2–3 g	100–150 µg	6–10 mg (estimated)	Less than 6 mg
Plasma concentrations	70–200 µg/dl	80–155 µg/dl	5–15 µg/dl	0.5–1.0 µg/dl
Transport/Binding	40% on an α_2 globulin 60% on albumin	94% bound to ceruloplasmin 6% on albumin and AAs	Plasma proteins (?)	Transferrin
Dietary intake	10–15 mg/day	1–2 mg/day	100–200 µg/day	50–100 µg/day
Site of absorption	Duodenum, jejunum	Stomach, duodenum	Small intestine	Small intestine
Maximum absorption	40–50%	90%	60% for inorganic Se 90 + % for selenomethionine	0.5% for inorganic Cr^{3+} 25–40% for organic "GTF" Cr
Major route of excretion	intestinal/pancreatic secretion	biliary secretion	urine	urine
Daily urinary excretion	500 µg	30 µg	50–100 µg	10–20 µg

SOURCE: Modified from Solomons NW: Trace minerals in digestive diseases. Postgraduate course, American Gastroenterological Association, May 18, 1980.

159

Table 2. Metalloenzymes Containing Copper as an Essential Component

Enzyme	Key Biochemical Function	Signs of Deficiency of the Enzyme
Cytochrome oxidase (present in electron transport chain)	Production of most energy for metabolism (oxidative metabolism)	Impaired synthetic processes dependent on ATP, including myelinogenesis
Amine oxidases such as lysine oxidase	Necessary for the cross-link bonding of elastin[5]	Fragmentation of the internal elastic lamina in blood vessels (may lead to rupture of a major artery)
	Stability of collagen in connective tissue and bone	Skeletal lesions
Tyrosinase	Synthesis of melanin	Decreased pigmentation of skin and hair

Zinc is absorbed by the small intestine by a specific active transport process. Usually 20–30% of the dietary intake of zinc is absorbed. Certain dietary components like phytate and fiber decrease zinc absorption (15,16). The major excretory route for zinc is via the feces (see Table 1).

CHROMIUM

Chromium is essential for normal glucose metabolism. Trivalent chromium is an essential ingredient of the "glucose tolerance factor," an organic chromium complex that occurs naturally in brewer's yeast and mammalian tissues and is a dietary constituent required for optimal glucose metabolism. The role of chromium is to potentiate the effects of insulin (it acts as a cofactor for insulin); therefore, chromium deficiency results in reduced insulin sensitivity in peripheral tissues (5,17).

MANGANESE

Manganese has a role in several enzyme systems (2). Pyruvate carboxylase is a manganese metalloenzyme. Two enzymes required for the synthesis of mucopolysaccharides are now known to be manganese dependent (18). Lack of these enzymes is responsible for the extensive skeletal abnormalities in manganese deficient animals and birds. It also explains the ataxia that occurs in the offspring of manganese deficient animals, which is due to faulty development of the inner ear—mucopolysaccharides compose the inner ear membrane. Abnormalities of glucose tolerance, lipid metabolism, growth, brain function, and oxidative phosphorylation have been reported in manganese deficient animals. Manganese is poorly absorbed from the intestine and is excreted primarily in the bile.

SELENIUM

Glutathione peroxidase in erythrocytes is a selenium containing enzyme (19). This enzyme catalyzes the reduction of hydrogen peroxide to water, thereby protecting the cell membrane and hemoglobin from oxidative damage and hemolysis. The actions of selenium are linked closely to those of vitamin E and have a sparing effect on vitamin E requirements.

MOLYBDENUM

In mammaliam systems, molybdenum is a component of enzymes participating in oxidation–reduction reactions involving organic sulfur (sulfite oxidase) and metabolites of degraded nucleic acid (xanthine oxidase). Molybdenum is readily absorbed from the intestinal tract and excreted chiefly in urine.

IODINE

Iodine is necessary for synthesis of the thyroid hormones thyroxine (T_4) and triiodothyronine (T_3). It is readily absorbed from the intestine and excreted mainly in urine.

IRON

Iron is a constituent of hemoglobin, myoglobin, the cytochromes, and a number of other proteins that function in the transport, storage, and utilization of oxygen. It is absorbed in ferrous form according to body need; its absorption is hindered by fiber, phytic acid, and steatorrhea.

Causes of Trace Element Deficiency

A disturbance of the complex interrelationships between trace elements may lead to a nutritional deficiency. For example, increased exposure to cadmium (secondary to environmental pollution) may lead to enhanced requirement for zinc (5).

Individuals may be at particular risk for a deficiency of one or more trace elements from either absorption abnormalities or excessive excretion. Zinc deficiency may occur with fat malabsorption syndromes. Excessive urinary loss of zinc is observed after trauma, surgery, and burns (5).

Prematurity causes low copper and chromium levels as well as reduced iron stores in the newborn. The term neonate accumulates copper extensively during the last 8–12 weeks of gestation; chromium also appears to be accumulated quite extensively in late fetal life. Although the fetus stores copper and iron, it does not particularly store zinc during late pregnancy. Nevertheless, there is a marked increase in total body zinc content during this time (3). Positive zinc balance is difficult to achieve in the premature infant in early postnatal life (20). Meinel et al. (21) recently found that fetal liver contains significantly less copper, zinc, selenium, magnesium, and molybdenum than healthy adult livers, which suggests that preterm infants may be at greater risk for deficiency.

COPPER

Human copper deficiency has been reported

1. In association with generalized malnutrition and prolonged diarrhea in older infants and children (22)
2. In association with intestinal malabsorption syndromes (23)
3. In Menke's kinky hair syndrome—as a result of a genetic defect in copper absorption (24)
4. In premature infants since the majority of fetal copper stores are accumulated during the last 3 months of gestation, and therefore, the premature infant is born with decreased copper stores as compared to term infants (25,26)
5. In patients maintained on prolonged parenteral nutrition (PN) without copper supplements (see below)

ZINC

Human zinc deficiency occurs with

1. Inadequate dietary intake
2. Malabsorption syndromes associated with steatorrhea (27)
3. Acrodermatitis enteropathica, a genetic defect in zinc absorption (28)
4. Dietary factors such as excess phytate and fiber, which may impair zinc absorption (16)
5. Prematurity since about two thirds of the zinc in the fetal body at term is accumulated during the last 10–12 weeks of gestation (1)
6. Patients maintained on prolonged PN without adequate zinc supplementation (see below)

Trace Element Deficiencies in Patients on Total Parenteral Nutrition

Base solutions used for total parenteral nutrition (TPN) are not routinely supplemented with trace minerals. Variable amounts of zinc have been found in different solutions (29); generally, however, they are not sufficient to provide the estimated parenteral requirements for this mineral. Concentrations of copper, selenium, and chromium are universally deficient in TPN solutions (29,30). Prospective studies have shown progressive decreases in circulating levels of both copper and zinc in patients on TPN (31). Premature infants appear to be particularly susceptible to precipitous decreases in plasma zinc during parenteral alimentation (32). Interestingly, in a study analyzing fresh frozen plasma, the authors documented the presence of high levels of zinc and physiological amounts of copper and selenium (30).

Table 3. Copper Deficiency[1,3,36]

Clinical Manifestations
Anorexia
Failure to grow
Diarrhea
Pallor
Depigmentation of hair and skin
Dilated superficial veins
Defective elastin formation (aneurysm)
Central nervous system abnormalities
Hypothermia
Laboratory Manifestations
Anemia (hypochromic) ⎫
Neutropenia   ⎬ Mild, early findings
Osteoporosis   ⎭
Periosteal reactions[a]
Cupping and flaring of long bones[a]
Flaring of anterior ribs[a]
Submetaphyseal fractures[a]

[a]These findings often resemble those of scurvy.

Since the amount of trace elements varies tremendously in TPN solutions, these solutions cannot be relied on for the delivery of required amounts of trace elements. The presence of trace elements in TPN solutions as contaminants and their presence in blood products, along with a modest oral intake, may provide enough of these metals to at least delay onset of clinical deficiency states. Clinical signs of deficiency are usually not thought to occur until after 4 weeks of TPN therapy. In order to prevent trace element deficiencies, prescribed amounts of trace elements must be delivered to patients receiving PN.

COPPER

Copper deficiency has been noted in infants receiving prolonged TPN that was not supplemented with copper (33–35). Clinical and laboratory manifestations of copper deficiency in childhood are shown in Table 3. The anemia of copper deficiency is initially hypochromic but does not respond satisfactorily to oral iron therapy. Later, when the copper deficiency is so severe that iron metabolism within the developing red cell is disturbed and there is defective red cell production, the anemia will not respond to parenteral iron therapy. Bone marrow exam reveals vacuolization of the red cell series as well as a noticeable maturation arrest of the white cell series (1,35,36).

ZINC

Zinc deficiency has been well documented in patients on TPN without adequate zinc supplementation. Kay and Tasman-Jones reported an acquired syndrome of dermatitis, diarrhea, and alopecia that occurred during TPN using solutions low in

Table 4. Zinc Deficiency[1,3,11,36,43]

Clinical Manifestations
  Growth failure
  Diarrhea
  Perineal and perioral skin lesions (vesicobullous or eczematoid)
  Impaired wound healing
  Alopecia
  Increased susceptibility to infections
  Delayed sexual maturation
  Severe anorexia
  Impaired taste perception
  Lethargy, irritability
  Mental depression, behavioral disturbances
  Adynamic intestinal motility
  Night blindness

zinc (37). Arakawa and associates (38) described zinc deficiency in two male infants receiving TPN for chronic diarrhea; clinical symptoms, beginning on day 22 and day 25 of treatment, included fever, lesions of the skin and mucous membranes, and development of pustules containing *Staphylococcus aureus*. Treatment with zinc sulfate dramatically improved clinical signs within a few days. Numerous other reports on zinc deficiency now exist (39–43). The clinical findings of zinc deficiency appear in Table 4.

Table 5. Deficiency States for Other Trace Elements

Chromium deficiency[44,45]
  Glucose intolerance
  Peripheral neuropathy
  Metabolic encephalopathy
  Increased susceptibility to cardiovascular disease
Manganese deficiency[46]
  Depressed vitamin K-dependent clotting factors
  Mild dermatitis
Selenium deficiency
  Muscle pain and muscle tenderness (secondary to
    prolonged TPN)[51]
  Cardiomyopathy (secondary to prolonged TPN)[53]
  Possible increased incidence of cancer
  Possible increased red blood cell fragility
Molybdenum deficiency[54]
  Tachycardia, tachypnea
  Headache
  Night blindness
  Central scotomas
  Lethargy, disorientation, and coma
  Elevated levels of plasma methionine
  Low serum uric acid levels

Table 6. Deficiencies of Iodine and Iron

Iodine
Hypothyroidism
Iron
Fatigue, listlessness, exertional dyspnea
Headache
Pallor
Irritability, anorexia, poor weight gain
Atrophy of the papillae of the tongue
Hypochromic microcytic anemia

OTHER TRACE ELEMENTS

Chromium deficiency has been reported in two patients receiving long-term TPN (44,45); the signs of the deficiency are shown in Table 5. There is only one tentative report of human manganese deficiency in an adult fed an experimental diet accidentally deficient in this nutrient (46).

Human selenium deficiency has not been clearly demonstrated. Low levels of selenium have been observed in the blood and urine of adults in New Zealand— apparently secondary to low levels of selenium in the soil (47). Low levels of selenium in the soil have been associated with a high incidence of some forms of cancer in humans (48). In addition, the incidence of Keshan disease (a fatal cardiomyopathy in children who live in a region of China where selenium levels are low in staple foods) can be reduced by supplementing the diet with sodium selenite (49,50). A patient on long-term TPN developed incapacitating muscular pain that disappeared after selenium was added to the intravenous solutions (51). Several studies have shown a common tendency for circulating selenium levels to decline during TPN (51,52). It was reported that a 43 year-old man on two years of TPN without selenium supplementation developed a cardiomyopathy that had histiologic features of Keshan disease (53). Selenium deficiency was confirmed with biochemical assessment of glutathione peroxidase and direct selenium measurements (53).

A case of possible molybdenum deficiency was seen in a patient on long-term TPN who developed a complex of clinical symptoms (54) (see Table 5) which resolved with the administration of molybdenum salts. Clinical symptoms associated with iodine and iron deficiency are depicted in Table 6.

Requirements of Trace Elements in Total Parenteral Nutrition

The requirements of trace elements are not well established. The oral recommended daily allowances of these nutrients can provide general guidelines, but they must be modified to apply to TPN. A major problem in determining requirements is that serum levels of these nutrients may not reflect their content in body tissues, their biologic activity, or the state of balance of the nutrients. Therefore, detailed balance studies are needed to determine the requirements of the trace elements. An expert panel of the American Medical Association has made recommendations for intravenous administration of trace elements (Table 7) (55).

The recommendations are based on limited data; larger doses of some elements may be required in some cases (43,56). With prolonged intravenous feeding, the quantity of copper may need to be cautiously increased above the AMA panel guidelines for a rapidly growing premature infant; the quantity of zinc may also need to be increased if there are excessive losses from the kidneys or gastrointestinal tract. Balance studies, such as those by James and co-workers (57), may result in revision of the expert panel's recommendations and may determine guidelines for use of the remaining trace elements. It is known that the requirements for iodine are 5 µg/kg/day in children and 100–140 µg/day in adults (58).

IRON

More is known about iron than about any other trace element. Growing infants and children require approximately 1–1.5 mg/kg/day of elemental iron. Iron is not usually added to TPN solutions because of concerns regarding physical incompatibility and the risk of anaphylaxis using available iron–dextran preparations (59). Hence, the occurrence of iron deficiency anemia is not uncommon in patients requiring TPN.

Three reports have demonstrated that iron–dextran (Imferon) *is* compatible with standard TPN solutions and have suggested guidelines for its addition in the therapy for selected patients (60–62). In addition, a preliminary evaluation of its clinical use in adults at an average dose of 0.5 mg/day showed no adverse effects (62). Some pediatric centers now routinely add iron to standard TPN solutions (63); however, many centers replenish iron stores with an occasional blood tranfusion.

Halpin and co-workers (64–66) have treated hospitalized iron deficient infants and children receiving TPN with a single dose of iron–dextran (Imferon) intravenously. Intravenous Imferon was indicated for (1) children with inadequate muscle mass for deep intramuscular injection, (2) chronically ill children with digestive tract disorders who could not tolerate oral iron, (3) children unable to eat for an extended period of time. Use of intravenous Imferon also avoided the potentital risk of sarcomas arising in areas of previous intramuscular injections (67).

It was critical that intravenous iron–dextran be given after serum proteins returned to normal and the patient was no longer catabolic (64,66). The single dose given by Halpin and co-workers was that required to restore hemoglobin and replenish iron stores:

$$0.3 \times \text{body weight in lbs} \times \left(100 - \frac{\text{Hgb observed}}{\text{Hgb desired}} \times 100\right) = \text{mg of iron}$$

For children weighing less than 13.6 kg, the manufacturers of Imferon recommend using the table provided in the package insert or the *Physician's Desk Reference*. Halpin administered a test dose of 25 mg of elemental iron over 15 minutes (66); if the test dose was tolerated the remainder of the total dose was diluted either in 5% dextrose or in normal saline (total volume approximately 200 ml) and administered over 2 hours through a central or peripheral venous catheter (66). In 3 years of such use, Halpin has experienced no immediate or late reactions. Hemoglobin values became normal in 3 weeks (64). It was concluded that the use of intravenous

Table 7. Suggested Daily Intravenous Intake of Essential Trace Elements

	Pediatric Patients, µg/kg[a]	Stable Adult	Adult in Acute Catabolic State[b]	Stable Adult with Intestinal Losses[b]
Zinc	300[c]	2.5–4.0 mg	Additional 2.0 mg	Add 12.2 mg/l of small-bowel fluid lost; 17.1 mg/kg of stool or ileostomy output[e]
	100[d]			
Copper	20	0.5–1.5 mg		
Chromium	0.14–0.2	10–15 µg		20 µg[f]
Manganese	2–10	0.15–0.8 mg		

SOURCE: Nutrition Advisory Group of the American Medical Association: Guidelines for essential trace element preparations for parenteral nutrition use. *JAMA* 241:2053, 1979. Copyright © 1979, American Medical Association. Reproduced with permission.

[a]Limited data are available for infants weighing less than 1500 g. Their requirements may be more than the recommendations because of their low body reserves and increased requirements for growth.

[b]Frequent monitoring of blood levels in these patients is essential to provide proper dosage.

[c]Premature infants (weight less than 1500 g) up to 3 kg of body weight. Thereafter, the recommendations for full-term infants apply.

[d]Full-term infants and children up to 5 years old. Thereafter, the recommendations for adults apply, up to a maximum dosage of 4 mg/day.

[e]Values derived by mathematical fitting of balance data from a 71-patient-week study in 24 patients.

[f]Mean from balance study.

iron-dextran in hospitalized, sick patients requiring TPN is both safe and efficacious (64–66).

Monitoring Trace Elements

Serum levels of trace elements, especially of zinc and copper, are the mainstay of monitoring trace element status. A number of recent studies have helped to define "normal values" for serum zinc and copper, especially in preterm infants (57,68–71). Ability to monitor urinary and gastrointestinal losses further helps to facilitate calculations of optimal intake.

ZINC

Although zinc is most frequently assessed from plasma or serum—which *must* be collected in zinc-free syringes—this determination has a number of pitfalls. A false increase in levels occurs with external contamination, hemolysis, and prolonged fasting; a false decrease occurs with corticosteroid use, infection and inflammation, and postprandial sampling (36). Nevertheless, with *serial* monitoring of a given patient on TPN, a *progressive* fall in zinc concentration usually reflects inadequate intake of the nutrient (36). Some investigators have reported that a decline in serum alkaline phosphatase activity often signals the onset of zinc deficiency (38,57).

COPPER

As with zinc, the determination of serum and plasma copper levels is subject to pitfalls. Therefore, serial determinations during the course of parenteral nutrition are useful. Approximately 94% of circulating copper can be accounted for by copper in ceruloplasmin. Measuring serum ceruloplasmin can help define the patient's copper status.

OTHER TRACE ELEMENTS

Selenium levels can be monitored in serum (51). Plasma or serum chromium assessment is technically difficult to perform, but neutron activation analysis offers the most precise method (36).

Danks has recently proposed a method of diagnosing trace element deficiency (72). He recommended measurement of an appropriate metalloprotein before and after administration of a physiologic replenishment dose to distinguish low levels due to metal deficiency from those due to other mechanisms. His recommendation was to use ceruloplasmin for copper assessment and serum alkaline phosphatase and red cell carbonic anhydrase for zinc assessment (72).

The following sequence of changes occurs in iron deficiency anemia: (1) ferritin levels decrease to less than 10 ng/ml; (2) serum iron decreases while total iron binding capacity increases, with saturation under 15%; (3) there is a progressive increase in free erythrocyte protoporphyrin; (4) a progressively hypochromic and microcytic anemia develops (36,73).

Practical Guidelines

1. Based on the AMA expert panel guidelines, our pharmacy has formulated a trace element solution (TES) for use in pediatrics. Our pediatric TES preparation contains

zinc	100 μg/ml
copper	20 μg/ml
chromium	0.17 μg/ml
manganese	6 μg/ml

The dose we recommend is 1 ml/kg/day to a maximum of 20 ml/day.

2. Premature infants weighing less than 3 kg require an *additional* 200 μg/kg/day of zinc (for a total of 300 μg/kg/day) to provide amounts suggested by the AMA expert panel.

3. Children weighing 20 kg or more can receive 5 ml/day of the adult TES preparation which contains

zinc	4 mg	
copper	1 mg	per 5 ml
chromium	10 μg	
manganese	0.8 mg	

4. The solutions recommended above can be easily prepared by the pharmacy since Abbott Laboratories, American Quinine, USV, and Travenol Laboratories manufacture individual vials of zinc, copper, manganese, and chromium.

5. Since copper and manganese are excreted primarily in the bile, *in patients with obstructive jaundice* the *dose* of these metals *must be decreased or temporarily discontinued* to avoid liver toxicity.

6. For patients on long-term TPN, monitoring should include monthly determinations of serum copper and zinc.

7. *Patients with large volumes of intestinal fluid loss are at increased risk for zinc deficiency*, since a large proportion of zinc excretion from the body is normally through the gastrointestinal tract.

   a. In three term infants on parenteral nutrition following gastrointestinal surgery, zinc deficiency developed in spite of recommended supplementation of intravenous zinc. These infants were *found to require doses of zinc two to four times* the recommended dose to raise serum zinc levels to normal (74).

   b. In adult balance studies (75) it has been shown that the following *additional zinc replacement* is required:

   (1) 17.1 mg of zinc per kg of stool or ileostomy output

   (2) 12.2 mg of zinc per kg of small bowel fluid lost through fistula or stoma.

References

1. Hambidge KM: Trace elements in pediatric nutrition. *Adv Pediatr* 24:191, 1977.

2. Underwood EJ: *Trace Elements in Human and Animal Nutrition*. New York, Academic Press, 1971.

3. Hambidge KM: Trace element deficiencies in childhood, in Suskind RM (ed): *Textbook of Pediatric Nutrition*. New York, Raven Press, 1981, p 163.

4. Ulmer DD: Trace elements. *N Engl J Med* 297:318, 1977.

5. Hambidge KM, O'Brien D: Trace Elements, in Oliver K, Cox BG, Johnson TR, et al (eds): *Developmental Nutrition*. Columbus, Ohio, Ross Laboratories, 1979, p 101.

6. Schwarz K: Recent dietary trace element research, exemplified by tin, fluorine, and silicon. *Fed Proc* 33:1748, 1974.

7. Shaw JCL: Trace elements in the fetus and young infant. I. Zinc. *Am J Dis Child* 133:1260, 1979.

8. Shaw JCL: Trace elements in the fetus and young infant. II. Copper, manganese, selenium, chromium. *Am J Dis Child* 134:74, 1980.

9. Aggett PJ, Harries JT: Current status of zinc in health and disease states. *Arch Dis Child* 54:909, 1979.

10. Solomons NW: Current knowledge of zinc absorption. *Current Concepts in Gastroenterology* 4:18, 1979.

11. Gordon EF, Gordon RC, Passal DB: Zinc metabolism: Basic, clinical, and behavioral aspects. *J Pediatr* 99:341, 1981.

12. Evans GW: Copper homeostasis in the mammalian system. *Physiol Rev* 53:535, 1973.

13. Hambidge KM: Trace elements, in Committee on Nutrition, *Pediatric Nutrition Handbook*. Evanston, Ill, American Academy of Pediatrics, 1979, p 41.

14. Riordan JF, Vallee BL: Structure and function of zinc metalloenzymes, in Prasad AS (ed): *Trace Elements in Human Health and Disease*. New York, Academic Press, 1976, vol 1, p 227.

15. O'Dell BL: Dietary factors that affect biological availability of trace elements. *Ann NY Acad Sci* 199:70, 1972.

16. Reinhold JG, Faradji B, Abadi P: Binding of zinc to fiber and other solids of wholemeal bread, in Prasad AS (ed): *Trace Elements in Human Health and Disease*. New York, Academic Press, 1976, vol 1, p 163.

17. Mertz W, Toepfer EW, Roginski EE, et al: Present knowledge on the role of chromium. *Fed Proc* 33:2275, 1974.

18. Leach RM, Nuenster AM, Wien EM: Studies on the role of manganese in bone formation: Effect upon chondroitin sulfate synthesis in chick epiphyseal cartilage. *Arch Biochem Biophys*, 133:22, 1969.

19. Rotruck JT, Pope AL, Ganther HE, et al: Selenium: Biochemical role as a component of glutathione peroxidase. *Science* 179:588, 1973.

20. Dauncey MJ, Shaw JCL, Urman J: The absorption and retention of magnesium, zinc, and copper by low birth weight infants fed pasteurized human breast milk. *Pediatr Res* 11:991, 1977.

21. Meinel B, Bode JC, Koenig W, et al: Contents of trace elements in the human liver before birth. *Biol Neonate* 36:225, 1979.

22. Graham GG, Cordano A: Copper depletion and deficiency in the malnourished infant. *John Hopkins Med J* 124:139, 1969.

23. Cordano A, Graham GG: Copper deficiency complicating severe chronic intestinal malabsorption. *Pediatrics* 38:596, 1966.

24. Danks DM, Campbell PE, Stevens BJ: Menkes' kinky hair syndrome. *Pediatrics* 50:188, 1972.

25. Al-Rashid RA, Spangler J: Neonatal copper deficiency. *N Engl J Med* 285:841, 1971.

26. Ashkenazi A, Levin S, Djaldetti M: The syndrome of neonatal copper deficiency. *Pediatrics* 52:525, 1973.

27. Sandstead HH, Vo-Khactu KP, Solomons N: Conditioned zinc deficiencies, in Prasad AS (ed): *Trace Elements in Human Health and Disease*. New York, Academic Press, 1976, vol 1, p 33.

28. Neldner KH, Hambidge KM: Zinc therapy of acrodermatitis enteropathica. *N Engl J Med* 292:879, 1975.

29. Hauer EC, Kaminski MV: Trace metal profile of parenteral nutrition solutions. *Am J Clin Nutr* 31:264, 1978.

30. van Caillie M, Luijendik I, Degenhart H, et al: Zinc content of intravenous solutions. *Lancet* 2:200, 1978.

31. Solomons NW, Layden TJ, Rosenberg IH, et al: Plasma trace metals during total parenteral nutrition. *Gastroenterology* 70:1022, 1976.

32. Michie DD, Wirth H: Plasma zinc levels in premature infants receiving parenteral nutrition. *J Pediatr* 92:798, 1978.

33. Karpel JT, Peden VH: Copper deficiency in long-term parenteral nutrition. *J Pediatr* 80:32, 1972.

34. Heller RM, Kirchner SG, O'Neill JA Jr: Skeletal changes of copper deficiency in infants receiving prolonged total parenteral nutrition. *J Pediatr* 92:947, 1978.

35. Joffe G, Etzioni A, Levy J, et al: A patient with copper deficiency anemia while on prolonged intravenous feeding. *Clin Pediatr* 20:226, 1981.

36. Solomons NW: On the assessment of trace element nutriture in patients on total parenteral nutrition. *Nutritional Support Services* 1:13, 1981.

37. Kay RG, Tasman-Jones C: Acute zinc deficiency in man during intravenous alimentation. *Aust NZ J Surg* 45:325, 1975.

38. Arakawa T, Tamura T, Igarachi Y, et al: Zinc deficiency in two infants during total parenteral nutrition for diarrhea. *Am J Clin Nutr* 29:197, 1976.

39. Bernstein B, Leyden JJ: Zinc deficiency and acrodermatitis after intravenous hyperalimentation. *Arch Dermatol* 114:1070, 1978.

40. Suita S, Ikeda K, Nagasaki A, et al: Zinc deficiency during total parenteral nutrition in childhood. *J Pediatr Surg* 13:5, 1978.

41. Latimer JS, McClain CJ, Shapr HL: Clinical zinc deficiency during zinc-supplemented parenteral nutrition. *J Pediatr* 97:434, 1980.

42. Principi N, Giunta A, Gervasoni A: The role of zinc in total parenteral nutrition. *Acta Paediatr Scand* 68:129, 1979.

43. Weber TR, Sears N, Davies B, et al: Clinical spectrum of zinc deficiency in pediatric patients receiving total parenteral nutrition (TPN). *J Pediatr Surg* 16:236, 1981.

44. Jeejeebhoy KN, Chu RC, Marliss EB, et al: Chromium deficiency, glucose intolerance, and neuropathy reversed by chromium supplementation, in a patient receiving long-term total parenteral nutrition. *Am J Clin Nutr* 30:531, 1977.

45. Freund H, Atamian S, Fisher JE: Chromium deficiency during total parenteral nutrition. *JAMA* 241:496, 1979.

46. Doisy RJ: Human manganese deficiency, in Hemphill DD (ed): *Trace Substances in Environmental Health*. Columbia, University of Missouri Press, 1972, vol 6, p 193.

47. Griffiths NM, Thomson CD: Selenium in whole blood of New Zealand residents. *N Z Med J* 80:199, 1974.

48. Shamberger RJ, Rukovena E, Longfield AK, et al: Antioxidants and cancer. I. Selenium in the blood of normals and cancer patients. *J Nat Cancer Inst* 50:863, 1973.

49. Keshan Disease Research Group of the Chinese Academy of Medical Sciences, Beijing. Epidemiologic studies on the etiologic relationship of selenium and Keshan disease. *Chin Med J* (Engl) 92:477, 1979.

50. Keshan Disease Research Group of the Chinese Academy of Medical Sciences, Beijing. Observations of effect of sodium selenite in prevention of Keshan disease. *Chin Med J* (Engl) 92:471, 1979.

51. Van Rij AM, Thomson CD, McKenzie JM, et al: Selenium deficiency in total parenteral nutrition. *Am J Clin Nutr* 32:2076, 1979.

52. Hankins DA, Riella MC, Scribner BH, et al: Whole blood trace element concentrations during total parenteral nutrition. *Surgery* 79:674, 1976.

53. Johnson RA, Baker SS, Fallon JT, et al: An occidental case of cardiomyopathy and selenium deficiency. *N Engl J Med* 304:1210, 1981.

54. Abumrad NN, Schneider AJ, Steel D, et al: Amino acid intolerance during prolonged total parenteral nutrition reversed by molybdate therapy. *Am J Clin Nutr* 34:2551, 1981.

55. Shils ME, Burke AW, Greene HL, et al: Guidelines for essential trace element preparations for parenteral use—A statement by the nutrition advisory group. *JAMA* 241:2051, 1979.

56. Thorp JW, Boecky RL, Robbins S, et al: A prospective study of infant zinc nutrition during intensive care. *Am J Clin Nutr* 34:1056, 1981.

57. James BE, Hendry PG, MacMahon RA: Total parenteral nutrition of premature infants. 2. Requirement for micronutrient elements. *Aust Paediatr J* 15:67, 1979.

58. Shike M, Jeejeebhoy KN: Trace elements and vitamins in total parenteral nutrition. Postgraduate course, ASPEN 5th Clinical Congress, 1981.

59. Seashore JH: Metabolic complications of parenteral nutrition in infants and children. *Surg Clin North Am* 60:1239, 1980.

60. Figueredo JV, Kaminski MV: Iron-dextran in intravenous hyperalimentation solutions in the treatment of iron-deficiency anemia. *JPEN* 3:509, 1979.

61. Gilbert L, Dean RE, Karaganis A: Iron-dextran administration via TPN solution in malnourished patients with low serum transferrin levels. *JPEN* 3:509, 1979.

62. Wan KK, Tsallas G: Dilute iron dextran formulation for addition to parenteral nutrients solutions. *Am J Hosp Pharm* 37:206, 1980.

63. Filler RM: Parenteral support of the surgically ill child, in Suskind RM (ed): *Textbook of Pediatric Nutrition.* New York, Raven Press, 1981, p 341.

64. Halpin T, Reed M, Bertino J: Intravenous iron-dextran (ivID) in children receiving TPN for nutritional support of inflammatory bowel disease. *JPEN* 4:600, 1980.

65. Reed MD, Bertino JS Jr, Halpin TC Jr: Use of intravenous iron-dextran injection in children receiving total parenteral nutrition. *Am J Dis Child* 135:829, 1981.

66. Halpin TC Jr: Use of intravenous iron dextran in sick patients receiving TPN. *Nutritional Support Services* 2(1):19, 1982.

67. Weinbren K, Salm R, Greenberg G: Intramuscular injections of iron compounds and oncogenesis in man. *Br Med J* 1:683, 1978.

68. Sann L, Rigal D, Galy G, et al: Serum copper and zinc concentrations in premature and small-for-date infants. *Pediatr Res* 14:1040, 1980.

69. Manser JI, Crawford CS, Tyrola EE, et al: Serum copper concentrations in sick and well preterm infants. *J Pediatr* 97:795, 1980.

70. Hillman LS: Serial serum copper concentrations in premature and SGA infants during the first 3 months of life. *J Pediatr* 98:305, 1981.

71. Hillman LS, Martin L, Fiore B: Effect of oral copper supplementation on serum copper and ceruloplasmin concentrations in premature infants. *J Pediatr* 98:311, 1981.

72. Danks DM: Diagnosis of trace element deficiency—with emphasis on copper and zinc. *Am J Clin Nutr* 34:278, 1981.

73. Pearson HA: Iron, in Oliver K, Cox BG, Johnson TR, et al (eds): *Developmental Nutrition.* Columbus, Ohio, Ross Laboratories, 1979, p 81.

74. Palma PA, Denson SE, Adcock EW III: TPN for the neonate. Part II: Major minerals and micronutrients. *Nutritional Support Services* 2(1)8, 1982.

75. Wolman SL, Anderson H, Marliss EB, et al: Zinc in total parenteral nutrition: Requirements and metabolic effects. *Gastroenterology* 76:458, 1979.

Part III
Complications

11
Problems with Preparation of Parenteral Nutrition Solutions

Robert L. Poole

The preparation of parenteral nutrition (PN) solutions presents a number of problems to the hospital pharmacist. It is essential for the pharmacist to possess a working knowledge of *in vitro* physical and chemical reactions in order to recognize those factors that may affect the stability and compatibility of the solution components. Additional factors that may lead to problems in PN solution preparation include component mixing sequence, microbial contamination, incomplete or inappropriate solution orders, and product selection. Available data to assist the pharmacist in solving many of these problems is continually expanding and requires constant review.

The development of PN solutions designed specifically for pediatric conditions requiring nutritional support is a challenge. In order to tailor the solutions to the patient's particular needs, the pharmacist must be familiar with the metabolic requirements of the patient and with the biochemical pathways involved in nutrient utilization.

This chapter reviews the literature on the preparation of PN solutions and specifically addresses the following: (1) quality assurance, (2) microbial contamination, and (3) PN solution stability and component compatibilities.

Quality Assurance

The necessity for quality assurance (QA) programs for hospital pharmacy intravenous admixture services is well established (1–5). The objectives of QA are to insure that compounded intravenous products are: therapeutically and pharmaceutically appropriate for the patient; free from pyrogens and microbial contaminants; void of undesirable amounts of particulate or toxic contaminants; and labeled, stored, and distributed according to principles of quality control (6). Detailed guidelines describing the various aspects of QA programs for intravenous admixture services have been published by the National Coordinating Committee on Large Volume Parenterals (NCCLVP) (7–12).

The Joint Commission on Accreditation of Hospitals (JCAH) requires pharmacy departments to adhere to a QA program when compounding parenteral products. The QA program as outlined by JCAH should include: the monitoring of personnel qualifications, training, and performance; the testing of equipment and facilities; and the examination of the final product on a regular basis.

Quality control and the monitoring safeguards exercised in PN solution preparation should incorporate the following standard procedures:

1. All solutions should be prepared in the pharmacy under a laminar flow hood.
2. The work area should be isolated from heavy traffic and separated from contaminated supplies.
3. Laminar flow hoods should run continuously, or at least be allowed to warm up for 30 minutes prior to use.
4. All solutions should be visually inspected for particulate matter.
5. Periodic pH testing, electrolyte concentration determination, pyrogen testing, and microbiological testing should be performed on compounded solutions (13–20).

"Adherence to procedure is the key to assuring the quality of admixture products. In developing a QA program, the highest priority should be given to the education and training of admixture personnel, particularly with respect to aseptic technique and pharmaceutical calculations" (6).

Microbial Contamination of PN Solutions

The potential for developing infection from contaminated intravenous fluids is well recognized (21–23). The true incidence of septicemia caused by contaminated infusates is unknown at the present time. However, in a review based on over 20 published studies, Maki estimates that one case of septicemia results from contaminated intravenous fluid for every 1000 infusions, that is, 0.1% of all infusions (24). *In vitro* studies (25–27) of the growth of microorganisms in PN solutions have shown that *Candida albicans* is the only microorganism to undergo significant growth during the first 24 hours of incubation at room temperature. Although *Candida* proliferates in casein hydrolysate/dextrose PN solutions, the organism does not thrive in crystalline amino acid/dextrose solutions and eventually dies in concentrated dextrose solutions.

Administration of contaminated PN solutions can be a life threatening event. Factors that may help to decrease the possibility of iatrogenic infections are described below.

SOLUTION PREPARATION

Preventing the extrinsic contamination of PN solutions requires the use of strict aseptic technique by pharmacy technicians, pharmacists, nurses, and physicians during every step of the administration process (28). The preparation of all PN solutions by a centralized pharmacy admixture service under a laminar flow hood should reduce the incidence of fluid contamination. Brier and co-workers (29) studied the effect of laminar air flow and clean-room dress on contamination rates of intravenous admixtures. They reported the incidence of contamination of admixtures compounded in laminar air flow conditions as significantly less than those compounded on a clean table top. Clean-room dress did not significantly effect the incidence of admixture contamination and may give the operator a false sense of security.

IN-LINE FILTERS

Many centers with parenteral nutrition programs routinely use in-line membrane filters to decrease the risk of infection from contaminated solutions. The two most commonly used filters are the 0.45 micron and the 0.22 micron filter. Both filters will block the passage of fungi. The 0.45 micron filter will trap most bacteria except some types of *Pseudomonas* species and *Escherichia coli* (28,30). The 0.22 micron filter will block virtually all bacteria, but a pump may be necessary to insure the accurate flow of viscous PN solutions (31). In-line 0.22 micron filters have an added advantage in that they may be employed in testing the sterility of intravenous solutions under actual use conditions (32). Methods for detecting microbial contamination in intravenous fluids that use a total sampling membrane technique are generally superior to those that use an aliquot technique (33). Regardless of the method used, the capability of detecting *Candida* species is essential.

Solution Stability and Component Compatibilities

The literature on PN solution stability and component compatibilities contains many limitations and contradictions. A number of factors influence the stability and compatibility of PN solution components; therefore, absolute statements regarding these problems are often difficult or impossible to make. PN solutions are complex and contain multiple additives. Each of the additives may differ in concentration, preservative content, vehicle, and buffering system. In addition to these differences, the order of mixing, temperature, and storage conditions may effect the compatibility and stability of the final solution.

The two major types of incompatibilities are physical and chemical. Most research that has been conducted to date has evaluated only physical or visual compatibility although chemical decomposition or deterioration may occur even though physical or visual changes are not evident. It is difficult to interpret compatibilities that lack visual changes until data on both the physical and chemical compatibility is known.

TYPES OF INCOMPATIBILITIES

Precipitation, color change, turbidity, and evolution of gas are all examples of visual incompatibilities. This type of incompatibility usually results from a solubility problem or an acid-base reaction producing a poorly soluble, nonionized species or coprecipitate.

Chemical incompatibility usually involves the irreversible degradation of a component, thereby producing inactive, less active, or toxic products. This may or may not be visible. Examples of this type of reaction are oxidation, reduction, photolysis, dextrose catalysis, and hydrolysis.

According to Newton, "There are three bases upon which pharmacists are able to recognize, predict and avoid incompatibilities of parenteral admixture solutions. They are: (1) professional judgment derived from direct experience, (2) a competent understanding of physicochemical principles with particular emphasis on common reactive and labile groups, and (3) reference to pertinent published information" (34).

Sources containing useful information on stability and compatibility of PN solutions and other parenteral medications are listed in Appendix III.

The following are general guidelines for avoiding compatibility problems when preparing PN solutions (34–36)

1. The PN solution should be thoroughly mixed after each additive.
2. Families of drugs or chemical analogues will usually have the same chemical properties and react similarly.
3. PN solutions colored by the addition of vitamins make it difficult to visualize particulate matter.
4. Calcium salts should always be added last to avoid precipitation with phosphate.
5. All final solutions should be visually examined against both white and black backgrounds for particulate matter.

The vast variety of compatibility problems encountered in the use of PN solutions substantiates the need for meaningful compatibility studies. However, due to the complexity of PN solutions, the design of experimentation is extremely difficult.

AMINO ACIDS

Crystalline amino acid (AA) solutions have replaced the protein hydrolysates, which are no longer commercially available, as the intravenous nitrogen source in PN solutions. The assorted commercial products of AA solutions are available in various concentrations, both with and without electrolytes.

Each of the currently available AA solutions (37,38) differ in amino acid content, pH, electrolyte contaminants (Table 1), and osmolality. All of the solutions provide both essential and nonessential amino acids, although clinical superiority of one solution over another has not been established (39). Recent data have suggested that the choice of amino acid product is an important factor in the provision of calcium and phosphorus to neonates (40,41) (see section on calcium and phosphorus in this chapter). A comparison of AA solutions without the added electrolytes is summarized in Table 1.

Stability. Original studies of amino acid/dextrose mixtures without electrolytes, vitamins, or other additives showed stability of the solution for 2 weeks both at room temperature and at 4°C (42). Another study reported that mixed solutions were stable for 12 weeks at 4°C (43). In this study it was noted that increases in temperature enhanced the degradation of the mixed solution; and decomposition,

Table 1. Amino Acid Profiles of Available Solutions Without Added Electrolytes

	Aminosyn 10%	Travasol 10%	FreAmine III 8.5%
Essential amino acids (mg/100 ml)			
Isoleucine	720	480	590
Leucine	940	620	770
Lysine	720	580	620
Methionine	400	580	450
Phenylalanine	440	620	480
Threonine	520	420	340
Tryptophan	160	180	130
Valine	800	460	560
Histidine[a]	300	440	240
Cysteine[a]	—	—	20
Taurine[a]	—	—	—
Nonessential amino acids (mg/100 ml)			
Alanine	1280	2080	600
Arginine	980	1040	810
Proline	860	420	950
Serine	420	—	500
Tyrosine	44	40	—
Glycine	1280	2080	1190
Electrolytes (mEq/L)			
Sodium	—	3	10
Potassium	5.4	—	—
Chloride	—	40	2
Acetate	148	87	74
Phosphate	—	—	20
pH (approximate)	5.3	6.0	6.5

[a]May be essential in infants

due to the Maillard reaction, occurred with time. (The Maillard reaction is an interaction between organonitrogenous agents and dextrose resulting in a darkening of the PN solution [44].) Since microbial contamination may be the limiting factor in solution storage, it is recommended that solutions be stored under refrigeration and administered as soon as possible following admixture (43).

All manufacturers of amino acid preparations recommend that their solutions be protected from light prior to use. Tryptophan decays when exposed to light and also in the presence of sodium bisulfite, a preservative commonly used in parenteral solutions (45). Jurgens et al. (46) studied the stability of a PN solution containing 4.25% crystalline amino acids and 25% dextrose for a period of 2 weeks. The slight decrease in the tryptophan concentration over 2 weeks was more pronounced at room temperature (94.1% ± 1.2 of the initial 100%) than at 4°C (97.5% ± 0 of the initial 100%). The authors concluded that storage of amino acid solutions at 4°C supports tryptophan stability. When tested, changes in concentrations of the other amino acids were within the range of experimental variation.

The stability of amino acids when mixed with hydrochloric acid in PN solutions was addressed by Mirtallo and co-workers (47). Concentrations of proline and histidine had declined at 24 hours after the addition of hydrochloric acid, suggesting a concentration-dependent phenomena. The concentrations of the other amino acids remained unchanged at 24 hours except for that of tryptophan. Tryptophan concentrations decreased over time, independent of the hydrochloric acid concentration. The authors concluded that the available acid, when combined with the PN solutions, may be useful in treating patients receiving PN who have severe metabolic alkalosis.

Phototherapy is commonly used in the neonatal period to enhance the reduction of serum bilirubin and is often used concurrently with PN. Photooxidation may decrease the concentrations of methionine, tryptophan, and histidine in PN solutions (48, 49). Additional studies are necessary to determine the clinical significance of phototherapy during PN.

Compatibility. Compatibility studies involving PN solutions are extremely difficult to design due to the large number of variables—amino acid profile, dextrose concentration, pH, electrolytes, minerals, vitamins, and trace elements (50).

There have been five major studies addressing additive compatibilities in PN solutions, (51-55). Unfortunately, the protein sources used in most of the studies have either been reformulated or are no longer commercially available (e.g., FreAmine, reformulated; FreAmine II, reformulated; protein hydrolysate, discontinued); therefore, interpretation and application of the data to the currently available AA solutions becomes clouded. At present, AA injection solutions are marketed by four companies—Aminosyn, Abbott Laboratories; Travasol, Travenol Laboratories; FreAmine III, American McGaw Laboratories; and Veinamine, Cutter Laboratories. Two of the companies also make renal failure formulas—Aminosyn RF, Abbott Laboratories; and Nephramine, American McGaw Laboratories. None of these solutions is identical and compatability studies to date have not compared all of the available amino acid injection products (56).

DEXTROSE

Concentrations of dextrose injection available for use in PN solutions range between 10% and 70% (57). Dextrose/amino acid solution combinations cannot be stored for prolonged periods of time owing to the Maillard reaction, which occurs slowly at room temperature and results in a darkening or "carmelization" of the mixture.

ELECTROLYTES AND MINERALS

Monovalent inorganic ions, such as sodium, potassium, and chloride, rarely cause solubility problems in PN solutions (44). In general, divalent ions (calcium, phosphates, bicarbonate) form precipitates more readily than do monovalent ions. Whereas magnesium is very soluble in PN solutions (53), other divalent ions, such as calcium, phosphorus, and bicarbonate, have a greater possibility of forming precipitates. Bicarbonate precursors can be given in the form of acetate to avoid the bicarbonate incompatibility problem. Acetate salts are both soluble and stable in PN solutions.

Calcium and Phosphorus. Precipitation of calcium and phosphate in PN solutions and catheter lines has been a continual problem in solution preparation and

Table 2. Composition of Standard Solution[a] per Liter

Sodium	30 mEq
Potassium	20 mEq
Chloride	30 mEq
Acetate	20 mEq
MVI	6.7 ml

[a]Standard solution adapted from Filler RM: *Textbook of Pediatric Nutrition.* New York, Raven Press,1981.

administration (56, 58). The solubility of calcium and phosphorus in PN solutions depends on a number of factors: pH, temperature, amino acid concentration, the amino acid product, the calcium salt, dextrose concentration, the order of calcium and phosphate addition, and contact with intravenous fat emulsion (40, 59). All these factors are important in the preparation of solutions for premature infants who require large quantities of calcium and phosphorus to allow adequate bone mineralization (60).

pH. Phosphate exists simultaneously in both monovalent and divalent forms and, to avoid confusion, should be ordered in millimoles rather than in milliequivalents (61,62). The ratio depends on the pH of the solution and is represented by the following equation:

$$HPO_4^{2-} \underset{[OH^-]}{\overset{[H^+]}{\rightleftharpoons}} H_2PO_4^-$$

Monobasic calcium phosphate (Ca $[H_2PO_4]_2$) is soluble in aqueous solution, but dibasic calcium phosphate ($CaHPO_4$) is much less soluble. Increased concentrations of calcium and phosphorus will be soluble in the monobasic form as the pH of the solution decreases. The pH of a PN solution is determined chiefly by the amino acid product and the dextrose concentration. Therefore, the choice of the amino acid product used in solution preparation may allow more calcium and phosphorus to be administered to premature infants. Each additive may slightly alter the final pH of the solution.

Eggert et al. (40) studied calcium and phosphorus compatibility in PN solutions for neonates and found significant pH differences among two commonly used amino acid products. Aminosyn 2% with dextrose 20% had a pH of 5.1, whereas FreAmine III 2% with dextrose 20% had a pH of 6.4. These differences in pH resulted in distinctly different calcium–phosphate precipitation curves. Thus, more calcium and phosphorus was soluble in Aminosyn than in FreAmine III.

Our own studies have examined the use of calcium and phosphorus in neonatal PN solutions (59). We employed the following procedures: (1) Using concentrations of 10–25% dextrose and 0.5–4.0% of amino acid (Aminosyn) with standard electrolyte and vitamin concentrations (Table 2), calcium and phosphorus additions were made sequentially to determine the critical concentrations at which precipitates formed. (2) The pH of test solutions were determined. (3) Solutions were incubated for 30 hours at room temperature. (4) Following incubation all solutions were observed for calcium–phosphate crystals. (5) Solutions not obviously precipitated were filtered to determine the presence of microprecipitate. Results of the study appear in Figures 1, 2, and 3.

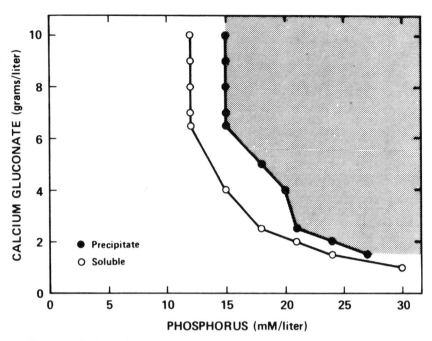

Figure 1 Amino acid (Aminosyn) 0.5%, dextrose 10–25%, pH range 5.7–6.1.

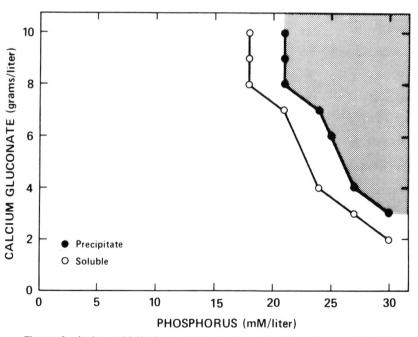

Figure 2 Amino acid (Aminosyn) 2%, dextrose 10–25%, pH range 5.5–5.8.

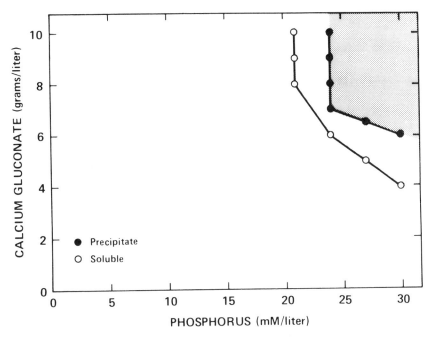

Figure 3 Amino acid (Aminosyn) 4%, dextrose 10–25%, pH range 5.4–5.7.

Temperature.   As the temperature increases, the calcium salt becomes increasingly dissociated, rendering the calcium ion available to complex with phosphate. The warm temperature of an intensive care nursery may alter the solubility of calcium and phosphate in PN solutions.

Amino Acid Concentration.   Increases in the amino acid concentration of PN solutions decreases the pH of the solution, thus increasing the stability of calcium and phosphate (40, 41). This effect is demonstrated in Figure 4. Amino acids in solution exist as ionic species that form soluble complexes with calcium and phosphate. These complexes dissociate to various degrees, depending on the nature of the product formed (63).

Calcium Salt Used.   The data of Henry et al. (63) indicate that a greater concentration of calcium gluconate can be mixed in PN solutions with sodium phosphate than is possible with calcium chloride. This is primarily due to the dissociation characteristics of the two calcium salts. The percent dissociation of calcium gluconate is much less than that of calcium chloride in water (63). Calcium chloride dissociates readily to yield free calcium, making precipitation with phosphates more likely than when the gluconate salt is employed.

Dextrose Concentration.   As dextrose concentrations increase, solution pH decreases slightly. This may contribute to increased stability of calcium and phosphorus; however, our experience has not shown dextrose to be a major factor affecting calcium and phosphorus solubility (41).

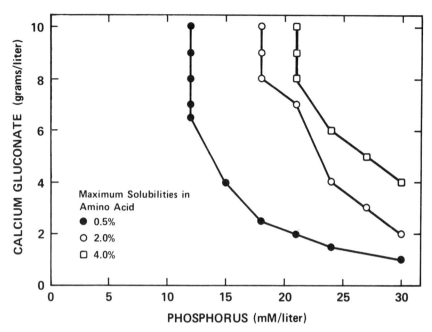

Figure 4 Effect of amino acid on solubility of calcium and phosphorus.

Order of Calcium and Phosphate Addition. Phosphate should be added and diluted as much as possible before adding calcium to PN solutions (40). This tactic avoids high local concentrations of phosphate and immediate precipitation with calcium.

Contact With Intravenous Fat Emulsions. According to Eggert et al. (40), care must be taken not to infuse intravenous fat emulsion into a line containing a PN solution that includes a calcium and phosphate content bordering on the precipitation curve for that solution. As the pH increases, calcium–phosphate crystals may form and be infused into the patient or obstruct the catheter.

VITAMINS

The stability and compatibility of vitamins in PN solutions are subject to a great deal of debate. Data exist reporting multiple vitamin injection to be physically compatible with PN solutions for 24 hours at room temperature (53, 54); however, sorption of the vitamins to plastic or glass, degradation secondary to light exposure, and potential interactions with amino acid/dextrose components are primary concerns. (A comparison of available multiple vitamin injection preparations can be found in Chapter 9.) Available data on vitamin stability and compatibility appear below.

Vitamin A. Several studies have reported vitamin A sorption to plastic containers and administration sets (64–67). This may decrease the amount of vitamin A actually delivered to the patient by 30-65%. Consequently, vitamin A status may require monitoring during prolonged courses of PN (68).

Folic Acid, Vitamin B$_{12}$, and Vitamin K. Some researchers recommend administration of these three vitamins by the intramuscular route rather than as an admixture to the PN solutions, thereby avoiding potential interactions and incompatibilities. However, others have found no physical changes in the PN solutions when these vitamins are included. (53-55). The new intravenous vitamin preparations (MVI-12, MVC 9+3) contain folic acid and vitamin B$_{12}$ for addition to PN solutions just prior to administration. The manufacturers recommend administration of the PN solution within 48 hours following the addition of vitamins. Vitamin K appears to be stable in PN solutions; however, a 10–15% deterioration may be expected over 24 hours when vitamin K is exposed to fluorescent light (69).

Photosensitivity. Vitamins A, D, K, and riboflavin are particularly light sensitive; therefore, exposure to light should be minimized.

Vitamin Interactions With PN Solutions. Multivitamin injection concentrate was tested in PN solutions and found to be physically compatible for 24 hours at 22°C. However, there was a marked alteration of the ultraviolet spectra for both amino acid/dextrose and vitamin components. Whether or not these changes represent an incompatibility is uncertain (54,56).

TRACE ELEMENTS

Trace elements appear as contaminants in amino acid, dextrose, and intravenous fat emulsion preparations (70-73). Since the amount of each trace element varies from lot to lot, the solutions themselves cannot be depended on to deliver fixed amounts of trace elements to the patient.

A number of manufacturers are producing both single entity and multiple trace element solutions for use in PN solutions. Those preparations that are currently available appear in Table 3. Due to the lack of commercially available "pediatric" trace element solutions, we have found it necessary to formulate our own solution to satisfy the needs of our pediatric population. The Stanford University Medical Center pediatric trace element solution is made from zinc sulfate, cupric sulfate, chromium chloride, and manganese sulfate. Each 1 ml of solution contains 100 μg zinc, 20 μg copper, 0.17 μg chromium, 6 μg manganese.

The physical and chemical stability of trace elements added to various PN solutions have been studied over an 8 week period. The researchers concluded that no physical or chemical changes occurred to affect the stability of the solution; no precipitates were formed, no significant pH changes were detected, and the concentrations of the trace elements remained within acceptable ranges (74).

IRON DEXTRAN

The use of intravenous iron dextran in PN solutions has not been extensively studied. Wan and Tsallas (75) reported iron dextran to be stable in PN solutions at room temperature after 18 hours. Their study did not address the potential effects of changes in temperature and pH, sensitivity to light, and prolonged storage time following admixture of the iron dextran and the PN solution. More studies are needed to answer these questions. Halpin has presented an alternate method for administering total dose intravenous iron dextran to patients receiving PN (76).

Table 3. Commercially Available IV Trace Element Preparations

Element	Concentration	Sizes Available (ml)	Manufacturer
Chromium	4 μg/ml	10	USV Laboratories
(chromic		10	Travenol Laboratories
chloride)		10, 30	American Quinine
		10, 30	Abbott Laboratories
Copper	0.4 mg/ml	10	Travenol Laboratories
(sulfate)		10, 30	American Quinine
Copper	0.4 mg/ml	10	USV Laboratories
(cupric		10, 30	Abbott Laboratories
chloride)			
Manganese	0.1 mg/ml	10	Travenol Laboratories
(sulfate)		10, 30	American Quinine
Manganese	0.1 mg/ml	10, 50	Abbott Laboratories
(chloride)		10	USV Laboratories
Zinc	1 mg/ml	10	Travenol Laboratories
(sulfate)		10, 30	American Quinine
Zinc	1 mg/ml	10, 50	Abbott Laboratories
(chloride)		10	USV Laboratories
Selenium	40 μg/ml	10	Lympho-Med,Inc.
(selenious			
acid)			
Multiple trace			
elements			
Zinc	1.0 mg ⎫		
Copper	0.4 mg ⎬ per 10 ml		Travenol Laboratories
Chromium	4.0 μg ⎮		American Quinine
Manganese	0.1 mg ⎭		
Zinc	4.0 mg ⎫		
Copper	1.0 mg ⎬ per 5 ml		Abbott Laboratories
Chromium	10.0 μg ⎮		
Manganese	0.8 mg ⎭		

HEPARIN

Heparin is physically compatible with PN solutions (55), but data on chemical stability and potency are unclear.

INSULIN

The literature on insulin availability from parenteral solutions is both confusing and contradictory. Adsorption of insulin to containers and administration sets ranges between 3% and 80% with an average loss of 40–50% (77–80). Although insulin is rarely administered to pediatric patients receiving PN, the following are guidelines to avoid potential problems:

1. Insulin should be added to the bottle rather than administered subcutaneously; then, if for any reason the PN is discontinued, the insulin will also be discontinued.
2. The insulin addition should be made in a consistent manner just prior to administration of the solution.

ADDITION OF DRUGS TO PN SOLUTIONS

The routine addition of medications such as antibiotics, narcotics, etc. to nutrient solutions is not recommended. Unfortunately, the situation involving a patient with only one venous access site for both PN and medications is common. There are only a few studies addressing drug–nutrient compatibility problems, rendering decisions on compatibility and stability very difficult. Original reference citings are the best method to analyze available data. As previously stated, physical or visual compatibility data are often incomplete and do not give information on chemical stability, activity, and possible toxicity from the combination of drug and PN solution. Quick references for compatibility questions can be found in texts by Trissell (56) and King (81) (see Appendix III).

References

1. Sarubbi FA, Wilson MB, Lee M, et al: Nosocomial meningitis and bacteremia due to contaminated amphotericin B. *J Am Med Assoc* 239:416, 1978.

2. Sanders LH, Mabadeje SA, Avis KE, et l: Evaluation of compounding accuracy and aseptic techniques for intravenous admixtures. *Am J Hosp Pharm* 35:531, 1978.

3. Plouffe JF, Brown DG, Silva J, et al: Nosocomial outbreak of Candida parapsilosis fungemia related to intravenous infusions. *Arch Intern Med* 137:1686, 1977.

4. Zellmer WA: Quality control in admixture services (editorial). *Am J Hosp Pharm* 35:527, 1978.

5. Primary bacteremia. Morbidity and Mortality Weekly Report 25:110, 1976.

6. Stolar MH: Assuring the quality of intravenous admixture programs. *Am J Hosp Pharm* 36:605, 1979.

7. National Coordinating Committee on Large Volume Parenterals: Recommended guidelines for quality assurance in hospital centralized intravenous admixture services. *Am J Hosp Pharm* 37:645, 1980.

8. National Coordinating Committee on Large Volume Parenterals: Recommendations to pharmacists for solving problems with large volume parenterals. *Am J Hosp Pharm* 33:231, 1976.

9. National Coordinating Committee on Large Volume Parenterals: Recommended methods for compounding intravenous admixtures in hospitals. *Am J Hosp Pharm* 32:261, 1975.

10. National Coordinating Committee on Large Volume Parenterals: Recommended procedures for in-use testing of large volume parenterals suspected of contamination producing a reaction in a patient. *Am J Hosp Pharm* 35:678, 1978.

11. National Coordinating Committee on Large Volume Parenterals: Recommended standards of practice, policies, and procedures for intravenous therapy. *Am J Hosp Pharm* 37:660, 1980.

12. National Coordinating Committee on Large Volume Parenterals: Recommendations to pharmacists for solving problems with large-volume parenterals—1979. *Am J Hosp Pharm* 37:663, 1980.

13. Bernick JJ, Brown DG, Bell JE: Adventitious contamination of intravenous admixtures during sterility testing. *Am J Hosp Pharm* 36:1493, 1979.

14. Morris BG, Avis KE: Quality-control plan for intravenous admixture programs. I. Visual inspection of solutions and environmental testing. *Am J Hosp Pharm* 37:189, 1980.

15. Morris BG, Avis KE, Bowles GC: Quality-control plan for intravenous admixture programs. II. Validation of operator technique. *Am J Hosp Pharm* 37:668, 1980.

16. Sanford RL: Cumulative sum control charts for admixture quality control. *Am J Hosp Pharm* 37:655, 1980.

17. Akers MJ, Schrank GD, Russell S: Particulate evaluation of parenteral nutrition solutions by electronic particle counting and scanning electron microscopy. *Am J Hosp Pharm* 38:1304, 1981.

18. Levinson RS, Allen LV, Stanaszek WF, et al: Detection of particles in intravenous fluids using scanning electron microscopy. *Am J Hosp Pharm* 32:1137, 1975.

19. National Coordinating Committee on Large Volume Parenterals: Recommended system for surveillance and reporting of problems with large-volume parenterals in hospitals. *Am J Hosp Pharm* 32:1251, 1975.

20. Rupp, CA Kikugawa CA, Kotabe SE, et al: Quality control of small-volume sterile products. *Am J Hosp Pharm* 34:47, 1977.

21. Sack RA: Epidemic of gram-negative organism septicemia subsequent to elective operation. *Am J Obstet Gynecol* 107:394, 1970.

22. Duma RJ, Warner JF, Dalton HP: Septicemia from intravenous infusions. *N Engl J Med* 284:257, 1971.

23. Maki DG, Rhame FS, Mackel DC, et al: Nationwide epidemic of septicemia caused by contaminated intravenous products. I. Epidemiologic and clinical features. *Am J Med* 60:471, 1976.

24. Maki DG: Sepsis arising from extrinsic contamination of the infusion and measures for control, in Phillips I (ed): *Microbiologic Hazards of Intravenous Therapy.* Lancaster, England, MTP Press Ltd, 1977, p 99.

25. Wilkinson WR, Flores LL, Pagones JN: Growth of microorganisms in parenteral nutritional fluids. *Drug Intell Clin Pharm* 7:515, 1973.

26. Boeckman CR, Krill CE: Bacterial and fungal infections complicating parenteral alimentation in infants and children. *J Pediatr Surg* 5;117, 1970.

27. Deeb EN, Natsios GA: Contamination of intravenous fluids by bacteria and fungi during preparation and administration. *Am J Hosp Pharm* 28:764, 1971.

28. Maki DG, Goldman DA, Rhame FS: Infection control in intravenous therapy. *Ann Intern Med* 79:867, 1973.

29. Brier KL, Latiolais CJ, Schneider PJ, et al: Effect of laminar air flow and clean-room dress on contamination rates of intravenous admixtures. *Am J Hosp Pharm* 38:1144, 1981.

30. Rusmin S, Althauser MB, DeLuca PP: Consequences of microbial contamination during extended intravenous therapy using inline filters. *Am J Hosp Pharm* 32:373, 1975.

31. Butler TH, Pluhar RE: A comparative evaluation of the relative flow rates and the protective capabilities of the 0.22 and the 0.45 micron Millipore filters in preventing mycelial contamination in the course of hyperalimentation therapy in humans. A preliminary study. *Drug Intell Clin Pharm* 7:317, 1973.

32. Lim JC: Technique for microbiological testing of in-use intravenous solutions and administration sets. *Am J Hosp Pharm* 36:1202, 1979.

33. Posey LM, Nutt RE, Thomson PD: Comparison of two methods for detecting microbial contamination in intravenous fluids. *Am J Hosp Pharm* 38:659, 1981.

34. Newton DW: Physicochemical determinants of incompatibility and instability in injectable drug solutions and admixtures, in Trissel LA (ed): *Handbook on Injectable Drugs,* ed 2. Washington, DC, American Society of Hospital Pharmacists, 1980, p 15.

35. Hull RL: Physicochemical considerations in intravenous hyperalimentation. *Am J Hosp Pharm* 31:236, 1974.

36. Rupp CA, Kotabe SE: Common sense guidelines for compatibility. *Drug Intell Clin Pharm* 9:155, 1975.

37. Shatsky F: Substrates available for intravenous nutrition. *Nutritional Support Services* 1:27, 1981.

38. Smith DR: Crystalline amino acids and fat emulsions: Product selection in a pediatric hospital. *Hosp Form* 16:1420, 1981.

39. Mirtallo JM, Schneider PJ, Mauko K, et al: Clinical comparison of two 8.5% amino acid injection products. *Am J Hosp Pharm* 38:83, 1981.

40. Eggert LD, Rusho WJ, MacKay MW, et al: Calcium and phosphorus compatibility in parenteral nutrition solutions for neonates. *Am J Hosp Pharm* 39:49, 1982.

41. Poole RL, Rupp CA, Kerner JA: Calcium and phosphorus in neonatal TPN solutions, *JPEN* (in press).

42. Rowlands DA, Wilkinson WR, Yoshimura N: Storage stability of mixed hyperalimentation solutions. *Am J Hosp Pharm* 30:436, 1973.

43. Laegeler WL, Tio JM, Blake MI: Stability of certain amino acids in a parenteral nutrition solution. *Am J Hosp Pharm* 31:776, 1974.

44. Giovanoni R: The manufacturing pharmacy solutions and incompatibilities, in Fisher JE (ed): *Total Parenteral Nutrition.* Boston, Little, Brown and Company, 1976, p 27.

45. Kleinman LM, Tangrea JA, Gallelli JF, et al: Stability of solutions of essential amino acids. *Am J Hosp Pharm* 30:1054, 1973.

46. Jurgens RW, Henry RS, Welco A: Amino acid stability in a mixed parenteral nutrition solution. *Am J Hosp Pharm* 38:1358, 1981.

47. Mirtallo JM, Rogers KR, Johnson JA, et al: Stability of amino acids and the availability of acid in total parenteral nutrition solutions containing hydrochloric acid. *Am J Hosp Pharm* 38:1729, 1981.

48. Bhatia J, Mims LC, Roesel RA: The effect of phototherapy on amino acid solutions containing multivitamins. *J Pediatr* 96:284, 1980.

49. Moritani D, Lee M, Tung EC: Effect of phototherapy on amino acid solutions, letter. *J Pediatr* 97:600, 1980.

50. Cluxton RJ: Some complexities of making compatibility studies in hyperalimentation solutions. *Drug Intell Clin Pharm* 5:177, 1971.

51. Feigin RD, Moss KS, Shackelford PG: Antibiotic stability in solutions used for intravenous nutrition and fluid therapy. *Pediatrics* 51:1016, 1973.

52. Kaminski MV, Harris DF, Collin CF, et al: Electrolyte compatibility in a synthetic amino acid hyperalimentation solution. *Am J Hosp Pharm* 31:244, 1974.

53. Kobayashi NH, King JC: Compatibility of common additives in protein hydrolysate/dextrose solutions. *Am J Hosp Pharm* 34:589, 1977.

54. Schuetz DH, King JC: Compatibility and stability of electrolytes, vitamins and antibiotics in combination with 8% amino acids in solution. *Am J Hosp Pharm* 35:33, 1978.

55. Athanikar N, Boyer B, Deamer R, et al: Visual compatibility of 30 additives with a parenteral nutrient solution. *Am J Hosp Pharm* 36:511, 1979.

56. Trissel LA (ed): *Handbook on Injectable Drugs,* 2nd ed. Washington, DC, American Society of Hospital Pharmacists, 1980.

57. Chernoff R (ed): *ASPEN Product Resource Manual.* Baltimore, American Society for Parenteral and Enteral Nutrition, Inc, 1981.

58. Pomerance HH, Rader RE: Crystal formation: A new complication of total parenteral nutrition. *Pediatrics* 52:864, 1973.

59. Poole R, Rupp C, Kerner J: Calcium and phosphorus in neonatal TPN solutions, abstract. *JPEN* 5:580, 1981.

60. Knight PJ, Buchanan S, Clatworthy W: Calcium and phosphate requirements of preterm infants who require prolonged hyperalimentation. *JAMA* 243:1244, 1980.

61. Turco SJ, Burke WA: Methods of ordering and use of intravenous phosphate (mEq vs mM). *Hosp Pharm* 10:320, 1975.

62. Hermann JJ: Phosphate: Its valence and methods of quantification in parenteral solutions. *Drug Intell Clin Pharm* 13:579, 1979.

63. Henry RS, Jurgens RW, Sturgeon R, et al: Compatibility of calcium gluconate with sodium phosphate in a mixed TPN solution. *Am J Hosp Pharm* 37:673, 1980.

64. Moorhatch P, Chiou WL: Interactions between drugs and plastic intravenous fluid bags. Part 1. Sorption studies on 17 drugs. *Am J Hosp Pharm* 31:72, 1974.

65. Chiou WL, Moorhatch P: Interaction between vitamin A and plastic intravenous fluid bags. *JAMA* 223:328, 1973.

66. Nedich RL: Vitamin A absorption from plastic I.V. bags. *JAMA* 224:1531, 1973.

67. Hartline JV, Zachman RD: Vitamin A delivery in total parenteral nutrition solution. *Pediatrics* 58:448, 1976.

68. Stromberg P, Shenkin A, Campbell RA, et al: Vitamin status during total parenteral nutrition. *JPEN* 5:295, 1981.

69. Jacobs WC, Lazzara A, Martin DJ: *Parenteral Nutrition in the Neonate.* Chicago, Ill, Abbott Laboratories, 1980, p 21.

70. Bozian R, Sheaver C: Copper, zinc and manganese content of four amino acid and protein hydrolysate preparations. *Am J Clin Nutr* 29:1331, 1976.

71. Haven E, Kaminski M: Trace metal profile of parenteral nutrient solutions. *Am J Clin Nutr* 31:264, 1978.

72. Shearer C, Bozian R: The availability of trace elements in intravenous hyperalimentation solutions. *Drug Intell Clin Pharm* 11:465, 1977.

73. Hoffmann R, Ashby D: Trace element concentrations in commercially available solutions. *Drug Intell Clin Pharm* 10:74, 1976.

74. Tsallas G: The stability and compatibility of trace elements and vitamins in total parenteral nutrition solutions. Presented at the ASPEN 5th Clinical Congress, New Orleans, La, 1981.

75. Wan KK, Tsallas G: Dilute iron dextran formulation for addition to parenteral nutrient solutions. *Am J Hosp Pharm* 37:206, 1980.

76. Halpin TC: Use of intravenous iron dextran in sick patients receiving TPN. *Nutritional Support Services* 2:19, 1982.

77. Weber SS, Wood WA, Jackson EA: Availability of insulin from parenteral nutrient solutions. *Am J Hosp Pharm* 34:353, 1977.

78. Hirsch JI, Fratkin MJ, Wood JH, et al: Clinical significance of insulin adsorption by polyvinyl chloride infusion systems. *Am J Hosp Pharm* 34:583, 1977.

79. Hirsch JI, Wood JH, Thomas RB: Insulin adsorption to polyolefin infusion bottles and polyvinyl chloride administration sets. *Am J Hosp Pharm* 38:995, 1981.

80. Wingert TD, Levin SR: Insulin adsorption to an air-eliminating inline filter. *Am J Hosp Pharm* 38:382, 1981.

81. King JC: *Guide to Parenteral Admixtures.* St Louis, Cutter Laboratories, Inc, 1980.

12
Technical Complications

John A. Kerner, Jr.

The incidence of technical complications due to placement and position of central venous catheters for parenteral nutrition (PN) in infants and children has been reduced significantly in recent years by strict attention to aseptic technique and by documenting the position of the catheter after insertion by obtaining radiographs of the chest. The introduction of nonreactive silicone catheters in place of the less pliable polyvinyl catheters has reduced the incidence of foreign body reaction, thereby reducing the incidence of thrombosis of the subclavian vein or vena cava. Cardiac arrhythmias occur infrequently when the tip of the catheter is placed at the junction of the superior vena cava and right atrium rather than in the heart. Suturing the catheter to the skin at the catheter–cutaneous junction and checking the security of the catheter with each dressing change has also reduced the frequency of catheter displacement (1).

Complications of Central Venous Catheter Insertion

A list of the possible technical complications at the time of catheter insertion is shown in Table 1. The common complications are discussed in detail in Chapter 17 as well as in recent reviews (1–7).

If a catheter breaks and a piece of the material migrates, percutaneous extraction using a snaring wire can be used to remove the foreign body (8,9).

Complications Associated With Ongoing Catheter Use

Complications related to the ongoing use of central catheters are shown in Table 2. Thrombosis of the vein in which the catheter resides may cause venous distention or edema of that part of the body drained by that particular vessel. Most patients

Table 1. Possible Complications at the Time of Catheter Insertion[1-9]

Pneumothorax[a]	Air embolism[a]
Hemothorax	Catheter embolism[a]
Hydromediastinum	Catheter malposition
Subclavian artery injury[a]	Thoracic duct laceration[a]
Subclavian hematoma	Cardiac perforation and
Innominate or subclavian vein	tamponade[a]
laceration	Brachial plexus injury[a]
Carotid artery injury	Horner's syndrome
Arteriovenous fistula	Phrenic nerve paralysis

[a]These complications—including clinical findings and medical and nursing interventions—are described in Table 1 in Chapter 17.

with subclavian vein thrombosis develop edema of the involved arm, neck, and face (6). The *clinical* manifestations of central vein thrombosis are uncommon: Grant's review of the American literature described an incidence of 0.29% (6); Burri and Krischak's review of the European literature was comparable, at 0.24% (10). Burri and Krischak's own experience was 1.4% while Grant's own experience showed a proven incidence of 1.2% and a suspected incidence of 2.9% (6); Valerio and associates' review of five studies revealed a frequency of 2.1% for central vein thrombosis (11).

Cannulation of the subclavian vein may result in microemboli, which are difficult to detect. In addition major pulmonary emboli may occur (6). Firor (12) attributed the death of a neonate to massive pulmonary emboli related to the PN catheter, and Ryan and co-workers reported a similar complication in an adult (13). Awareness that pulmonary embolism can be caused by central venous catheters placed for total parenteral nutrition (TPN) resulted in diagnosis and successful management of pulmonary embolism attributed to a central venous catheter in a neonate (14). Because the tip of the central TPN catheter was located in the right atrium, pulmonary embolism was suspected when this infant had a sudden worsening of respiratory status despite a normal chest film. The diagnosis was confirmed by a technetium 99m lung perfusion scan—a technique useful in the sick neonate (14). The TPN catheter was removed and a thrombus was found adhering to the catheter tip. Heparin therapy was then begun. The authors subsequently found that the addition of one unit of heparin per milliliter of TPN solution does not alter the neonate's partial thromboplastin time, though it might inhibit localized thrombus formation at the catheter tip (14).

Table 2. Possible Complications Related to Use of the Catheter[1,9]

Venous thrombosis
Superior vena cava syndrome
Pulmonary embolus
Catheter dislodgement
Perforation and/or infusion leaks
(pericardial, pleural, mediastinal)

Treatment of subclavian vein thrombosis usually consists of removal of the catheter and treatment with intravenous heparin. Specifics of this treatment are described extremely well by Grant (6). Other suggested treatment regimens include (1) streptokinase therapy followed by heparinization, which resulted in successful clinical resolution of bilateral subclavian, brachiocephalic, and superior vena cava thrombosis associated with central venous catheterization for parenteral nutrition (15); and (2) urokinase instillation, which has saved several occluded catheters from being removed and replaced, (16–19).

Patients receiving PN are at some risk of developing venous thrombosis despite the use of a large caliber vessel with high volume blood flow. Factors contributing to this complication include

1. Local vessel trauma at the time of catheterization
2. Irritation of the vessel intima from the hyperosmolar PN solution, especially when there is a low flow state, resulting in venous stasis secondary to dehydration
3. Hypercoagulable states

Preventive measures might therefore include prompt reversal of dehydration and, when possible, low-dose anticoagulation (6). In Grant's experience duration of subclavian catheterization does not appear to play a significant role, since thrombosis occurred as early as 3 days and as late as 16 days in his series (6).

PN catheters are foreign bodies, no matter what material they are fabricated from or how they are designed (18). As the catheter lies in the blood stream, it becomes surrounded by a layer of fibrin and platelets. The tip of the catheter is the main site of this encrustation. If this accumulation or thrombus reaches an appreciable size, it may occlude the orifice at the catheter tip or become a nidus for infection (18).

Because of the desire to prevent thrombosis many centers use heparin prophylactically in their PN solutions in a concentration of *one unit per milliliter* (1,6). The heparin tends to reduce the formation of a fibrin sheath around the catheter and possibly reduce phlebitis with peripheral PN solutions (1). Grant firmly states that "the addition of 1000 units of heparin per liter of solution completely eliminates catheter clotting (500 units of heparin per liter is inadequate)" (20). Measurement of clotting studies in more than 100 patients showed no anticoagulant effect from the administered heparin (20).

Brismar and associates performed phlebography at the time of catheter insertion and removal (21). In 42 patients, 34 had catheters inserted into the subclavian or external jugular vein with the catheter tip either in the superior vena cava or in the right atrium. Five had insertion through the cubital and three through the femoral veins. Thirty-six of 42 had teflon or polyethylene catheters; only six of 42 had silicone catheters. The frequency of catheter-related thrombosis was 71%, although few had symptoms. In most cases thrombosis, either partial or complete, was detected only through the use of phlebography (21). Valerio and co-workers performed a prospective study of central venous thrombosis associated with the use of polyvinyl chloride catheters in PN (11). They found that although only one of 30 patients had clinical evidence of thrombosis, with superior vena cava syndrome, six of 18 venograms demonstrated a significant clot, which was completely occlusive in three patients. In all these cases, significant venous collaterals developed (11). Both

Valerio and Brismar suggest that prophylactic anticoagulant therapy in long-term catheterization for PN be a standard practice (11,21).

Finally, a phlebographic study in 32 children (22) showed that the infusion of PN solutions caused damage to vessel walls, edema, and disturbances of the venous circulation. The addition of heparin to the solutions greatly reduced the frequency of these complications. In a study evaluating the cheek pouch of the hamster as the biologic tissue, all PN solutions caused some damage to the microcirculation (21). Enger and associates felt that one of the effects of heparin was to reduce the adhesiveness of red blood cells, possibly preventing the initial step of thrombogenesis (22).

Despite the studies previously cited, heparin is *not* routinely used in PN solutions in all medical centers. Centers not using heparin argue that *no controlled* studies have been performed to conclusively demonstrate the benefit of heparin in PN. Our pediatric surgeon uses one unit per milliliter of heparin in PN solutions when PN is given through peripheral vein but does not routinely use heparin for central PN.

Controlled studies of heparin use in PN are needed if we are to make logical decisions about its routine use. If the dose of heparin needed is one unit per milliliter in adults, does the same dose apply for the premature infant? Until these questions are fully answered it is best to consult with your pharmacist and surgeon about heparin use in PN.

Rare Complications With Central Lines

Rare complications have appeared in the literature, including calcification (23), temporary paraplegia from a PN catheter passing into the spinal canal (24), and communicating hydrocephalus (25–28). The last of these complications may result from superior vena cava thrombosis or bilateral internal jugular vein occlusion.

Unusual but major problems with extravasation, beyond those listed in Table 2, have also occurred. A nearly fatal case occurred in an emaciated infant who developed severe ascites after 3 days of TPN (29). Venocavography revealed effusion into the peritoneal cavity due to the catheter having penetrated the wall of the inferior vena cava. Three intrathoracic and two retroperitoneal effusions—one of these producing clinical ascites—due to vein wall perforation have also been reported in infants (30).

Complications With Peripheral PN

Almost all of the technical complications seen with central PN can be avoided by the use of peripheral PN. Phlebitis and superficial skin sloughs are the most common complications in patients receiving peripheral PN (1). Several authors describe this complication in detail with recommendations for treatment (31–33). The incidence of phlebitis is reduced in patients receiving concomitant intravenous fat infusions (1), possibly because the simultaneous infusion of fat lowers the osmolarity of the combined PN solution, since intravenous fat is isotonic. If an infiltrated intravenous site is identified quickly, it is usually benign, and the extravasated fluid is rapidly reabsorbed. Resolution of the extravasation can be aided by moist dressings to the area and by silver sulfadiazine dressings in those few cases in which a skin slough occurs. Very rarely will a skin slough site require skin grafting (1).

References

1. Wesley JR, Saran PA, Khalidi N, et al (eds): *Parenteral and Enteral Nutrition Manual.* Chicago, Abbott Laboratories, 1980, p 37.

2. Fleming CR, Witke DJ, Beart RW Jr: Catheter-related complications in patients receiving home parenteral nutrition. *Ann Surg* 192:593, 1980.

3. Smitherman ML, Balantine TV, Grosfeld JL: Catheter complications with total parenteral nutrition in the first year of life. *J Indiana State Med Assoc* 71:478, 1978.

4. Smitherman ML, Balantine TV, Grosfeld JL: Catheter complications with total parenteral nutrition in the first year of life. Part 2. *J Indiana State Med Assoc* 71:554, 1978.

5. Meszaros WT, Ramulu Y: Complications of indwelling venous catheters. *IMJ* 147:347, 1975.

6. Grant JP: Subclavian catheter insertion and complications. *Handbook of Total Parenteral Nutrition.* Philadelphia, WB Saunders Co, 1980, p 47.

7. Levy JS, Winters RW, Heird WC: Total parenteral nutrition in pediatric patients. *Pediatrics in Review* 2:99, 1980.

8. Chung KJ, Chernoff HL, Leape LL, et al: Transfemoral snaring of broken catheters from the right heart in small infants. *Cathet Cardiovasc Diagn* 6:331, 1980.

9. Fisher RG, Mattox KL: Percutaneous extraction of an embolized hyperalimentation catheter fragment. *South Med J* 71:1438, 1978.

10. Burri C, Krischak G: Techniques and complications of administration of total parenteral nutrition, in Manni C, Magalini SI, and Scrascia E (eds): *Total Parenteral Nutrition.* New York, American Elsevier Scientific Publishing Co, 1976, p 306.

11. Valerio D, Hussey JK, Smith TW: Central vein thrombosis associated with intravenous feeding—A prospective study. *JPEN* 5:240, 1981.

12. Firor HV: Pulmonary embolization complicating total intravenous alimentation. *J Pediatr Surg* 7:81, 1972.

13. Ryan JA, Abel RM, Abbott WM, et al: Catheter complications in total parenteral nutrition: A prospective study in 200 consecutive patients. *N Engl J Med* 290:757, 1974.

14. Wesley JR, Keens TG, Miller SW, et al: Pulmonary embolism in the neonate: Occurrence during the course of total parenteral nutrition. *J Pediatr* 93:113, 1978.

15. Havill JH: Central venous thrombosis following central venous catheterization and parenteral nutrition: Case report. *N Z Med J* 81:420, 1975.

16. Steiger E: Home parenteral nutrition. *Aspen Update* 3(4):1, 1981.

17. Ament ME: Home parenteral nutrition in infants and children. Course in Intravenous nutrition in the pediatric patient, Letterman Army Medical Center, San Francisco, February 13, 1981.

18. Glynn MFX, Langer B, JeeJeebhoy KN: Therapy for thrombotic occlusion of long-term intravenous alimentation catheters. *JPEN* 4:387, 1980.

19. Delaplane D, Scott JP, Riggs TW, et al: Urokinase therapy for a catheter-related right atrial thrombus. *J Pediatr* 100:149, 1982.

20. Grant JP: Administration of parenteral nutrition solutions. *Handbook of Total Parenteral Nutrition.* Philadelphia, WB Saunders Co 1980, p 103.

21. Brismar B, Hardstedt C, Malmborg A-S: Bacteriology and phlebography in catheterization for parenteral nutrition. *Acta Chir Scand* 146:115, 1980.

22. Enger E, Jacobsson B, Sorensen S-E: Tissue toxicity of intravenous solutions: A phlebographic and experimental study. *Acta Paediatr Scand* 65:248, 1976.

23. Al-Salihi FL, Rodriguez EB: Calcification as a complication of hyperalimentation. *J Med Soc NJ* 77:825, 1980.

24. McAlister WH, Keating JP, Shackleford GD: Hyperalimentation catheter passing into the spinal canal causing temporary paraplegia. *Pediatr Radiol* 7:119, 1978.

25. Newman LJ, Heitlinger L, Hiesiger E, et al: Communicating hydrocephalus following total parenteral nutrition. *J Pediatr Surg* 15:215, 1980.

26. Puljic S, Newman LJ, Heitlinger L, et al: Radiography of hydrocephalus after total parenteral nutrition. *Neuroradiology* 16:76, 1978.

27. Stewart DR, Johnson DG, Myers GG: Hydrocephalus as a complication of jugular catheterization during total parenteral nutrition. *J Paediatr Surg* 10:771, 1975.

28. Haar FL, Miller CA: Hydrocephalus resulting from superior vena cava thrombosis in an infant. Case report. *J Neurosurg* 42:597, 1975.

29. Axelsson CK, Knudsen FU: Catheter-induced ascites—An unusual complication of parenteral feeding. *Intensive Care Med* 4:91, 1978.

30. Spriggs DW, Brantley RE: Thoracic and abdominal extravasation: A complication of hyperalimentation in infants. *AJR* 128:419, 1977.

31. Lynch DJ, Key JC, White RR: Management and prevention of infiltration and extravasation injury. *Surg Clin North Am* 59:939, 1979.

32. Brown AS, Hoelzer DJ, Piercy SA: Skin necrosis from extravasation of intravenous fluids in children. *Plast Reconstr Surg* 64:145, 1979.

33. Yosowitz P, Ekland DA, Shaw RC, et al: Peripheral intravenous infiltration necrosis. *Ann Surg* 182:553, 1975.

13
Metabolic Complications

John A. Kerner, Jr.

There are many potential metabolic complications associated with the use of parenteral nutrition (PN) (1–13). Although some complications are unavoidable, most can be controlled or prevented by careful clinical monitoring and by appropriate adjustments of the infusate. Table 1 lists the more common metabolic complications; rarely reported complications of PN are shown in Table 2. This chapter focuses on three common metabolic complications: (1) demineralization of bone and rickets, (2) hepatic dysfunction, and (3) eosinophilia.*

Demineralization of Bone and Rickets

The poor bone mineralization of low birth weight (LBW) infants fed human milk has been recognized for decades but considered inconsequential. As the care provided in intensive care nurseries has improved, there has been a marked increase in the survival of *very* premature infants, and consequently the incidence of rickets, bone demineralization, and fractures has increased (14). In our intensive care nursery these complications are not uncommon in the very LBW infant who is fluid restricted because of underlying pulmonary or cardiac disease. The etiology of the undermineralization of prematurity has been attributed to deficiency of calcium, phosphorus, and vitamin D (15–25), but the precise physiology is not completely understood. The various types of nutritional rickets have also been described in infants and older children (26–30).

INCIDENCE IN ENTERALLY FED INFANTS

Intakes of calcium and phosphorus from human milk as well as from conventional formulas are far below estimated intrauterine accretion values, which are 120–160

---

*The complications listed in Table 1, sections 1–3a, have been discussed previously in the individual chapters on nutrient requirements. Glucose imbalance and electrolyte and mineral disorders are also addressed in Table 1 of Chapter 17. The metabolic monitoring required to prevent or control these complications is depicted in Table 1 of Chapter 15.

Table 1. Potential Metabolic Complications of PN

Complication	Possible Etiology
1. Disorders related to metabolic capacity of the patient	
a. Congestive heart failure and pulmonary edema	Excessively rapid infusion of PN solution
b. Hyperglycemia (with resultant glucosuria, osmotic diuresis, and possible dehydration)	Excessive intake (either excessive dextrose concentration or increased infusion rate)
	Change in metabolic state (e.g., sepsis, surgical stress, use of steroids)
	Common in low birth weight infants if dextrose load exceeds their ability to adapt
c. Hypoglycemia	Sudden cessation of infusate
d. Azotemia	Excessive administration of amino acids or protein hydrolysate (excessive nitrogen intake)
e. Electrolyte disorders	
f. Mineral disorders	Excessive or inadequate intake
g. Vitamin disorders	
h. Trace element disorders	
i. Essential fatty acid deficiency	Inadequate intake
j. Hyperlipidemia (increased triglycerides, cholesterol, and free fatty acids)	Excessive intake of intravenous fat emulsion
2. Disorders related to infusate components	
a. Metabolic acidosis	Use of hydrochloride salts of cationic amino acids
b. Hyperammonemia	Inadequate arginine intake, ? deficiencies of other urea cycle substrates, ? plasma amino acid imbalance, ? hepatic dysfunction
c. Abnormal plasma aminograms	Amino acid pattern of infusate
3. Miscellaneous	
a. Anemia	Failure to replace blood loss; iron deficiency, folic acid and B_{12} deficiency; copper deficiency
b. Demineralization of bone; rickets	Inadequate intake of calcium, inorganic phosphate, and/or vitamin D intake

c. Hepatic disorders
    i. cholestasis
    ii. biochemical and histopathologic abnormalities
	Prematurity; malnutrition; sepsis, ? hepatotoxicity due to amino acid imbalance; exceeding nonnitrogen calorie–nitrogen ratio of 150:1 to 200:1, leading to excessive glycogen and/or fat deposition in the liver; decreased stimulation of bile flow; nonspecific response to refeeding

d. Eosinophilia	Unknown

SOURCE: Modified from Heird WC: Total parenteral nutrition, in Lebenthal E (ed): *Textbook of Gastroenterology and Nutrition in Infancy*. New York, Raven Press, 1981, p 662.

Table 2. Rare Reported Complications of PN

Metabolic bone disease (discussed in Chapter 9)
Hypouricemia[6]
Cholelithiasis in premature infants treated with PN and furosemide[7]
Distended gallbladder (due to lack of oral stimulus to cause contraction)[8]
Nephromegaly[9]
Lactic acidosis in pediatric patients with cancer receiving TPN[10]
Wernicke's encephalopathy[11,12]
Cortical cataracts[13]

---

mg/kg/day of elemental calcium and 75 mg/kg/day of phosphorus (31–32). It is known that calcium and phosphorus supplementation results in improved retention of calcium and phosphorus as well as better bone mineralization (33). In addition, rickets associated with human milk feedings resolves with the provision of supplemental calcium and phosphorus alone (17,34). Thus, regardless of the vitamin D requirements of the LBW infant, it is apparent that many of the reported problems with bone mineralization result from inadequate intake of calcium and phosphorus (14). In response to the above data formulas developed for use in LBW infants have a higher calcium and phosphorus content than standard formulas or human milk (14) (see Table 2 in Chapter 20). The LBW formulas have not been studied in infants who weigh less than 1000 g at birth, in whom the cumulative calcium deficit is likely to be much greater than in heavier LBW infants (14).

The vitamin D content of the new "premature formulas" is higher than that of conventional formulas. Although 400 IU/day of vitamin D may be adequate, rickets has been observed in LBW infants taking this amount of vitamin D (17,25,34).

Although some investigators theorize that the LBW infant has an inability to convert dietary vitamin D to the active 1,25-dihydroxyvitamin D (1,25(OH)$_2$D), plasma levels of the active hormone have been found to be *elevated* in LBW infants with rickets (17,20,25). Steichen and co-workers (20) demonstrated that increased nutritional intake of calcium and phosphorus resulted in healing of rickets, improved bone mineralization, and normalization of serum 1,25(OH)$_2$D concentrations. They speculate that rickets is caused by calcium and phosphorus deficiency rather than by a deficiency in vitamin D metabolism and that the elevation of 1,25(OH)$_2$D may reflect a compensatory mechanism to achieve maximal calcium and phosphorus absorption. They also note that premature infants fed standard proprietary formulas have a maximum calcium absorption of only 50–65 mg/kg/day, which is far below the calculated intrauterine accretion rates (20). Yet, in one case, resolution of rickets was achieved with 1,25(OH)$_2$D supplementation, suggesting that a relative unresponsiveness of the intestine to the action of vitamin D may be an additional factor contributing to rickets of prematurity (25).

INCIDENCE IN PARENTERALLY FED INFANTS

There are few reports of rickets occurring in LBW infants managed on total parenteral nutrition (TPN). Oppenheimer and Snodgrass (35) described neonatal rickets in three preterm infants; each had received prolonged TPN including intravenous vitamin D. Geggel (36) and co-workers described rickets, presenting with fractured ribs, in two premature infants with bronchopulmonary dysplasia and liver disease; both had received TPN. Both patients had received "much less than 400 IU of vitamin D daily" (36). The authors recommended that premature infants be followed for the development of rickets by *monitoring for generalized aminoaciduria* (present in both their patients), which is an early sensitive index of vitamin D deficiency that precedes changes in serum calcium, phosphorus, or alkaline phosphatase values. They felt the etiology of the rickets was multifactorial. Of importance was a rapid rate of growth associated with an insufficient calcium and vitamin D intake; both patients had more than doubled their birth weight prior to the diagnosis of rickets (36).

Leape and Valaes (37) described four cases of rickets in LBW infants receiving TPN. Two have received inadequate vitamin D—20–80 IU/day; two had received apparently adequate vitamin D—600 IU/day. Additionally, the infants were receiving 3 mEq/kg/day of calcium. The authors observed that if TPN in LBW infants is to be effective in achieving intrauterine growth rates, the demand for calcium should, ideally, approximate intrauterine requirements, which have been estimated at approximately 6–8 mEq/kg/day.

A recent retrospective study demonstrated that decreased intake of calcium or phosphate was responsible for the development of rickets in LBW infants, many of whom had been supported on prolonged PN (38). Vitamin D intake, although slightly below the recommended daily dose of 400 IU, was not observed to be related etiologically to rickets in these preterm infants (38).

In the past it was believed to be extremely difficult to provide enough calcium and phosphorus in PN solutions to approach intrauterine accretion rates without encountering precipitation of the two minerals. However, two recent studies have shown that the amounts of calcium and phosphorus needed to approximate intrauterine accretion rates *can* be successfully delivered by PN in all but fluid restricted infants (39,40) (see Chapter 11).

Hepatic Dysfunction

The development of liver disease during TPN was first reported in 1971 in a preterm infant (41). At autopsy the infant's liver revealed cholestasis, bile duct proliferation, and early cirrhosis. Hepatic dysfunction remains one of the most common and most serious complications of TPN. The spectrum of TPN-associated liver complications is depicted in Table 3. A summary of many of the studies documenting hepatic complications in infants and children is shown in Table 4; Table 5 summarizes similar studies in adults. Cholestasis is especially prevalent in very premature infants and in infants on TPN for longer than 2 weeks. The most frequent problem in adults is gradual elevations in transaminases and alkaline phosphatase associated with liver biopsy findings of fatty infiltration within the hepatocytes and some increase in glycogen stores. This last problem appears to result from the infusion of excess carbohydrate calories. The cause of cholestasis is the subject of much debate.

Table 3. TPN-Associated Liver Complications

Hepatomegaly
Hepatic dysfunction
Elevated blood ammonia
Elevated transaminases (SGOT and SGPT)
Cholestasis
Fatty infiltration of the liver
Damage to hepatocytes
Overt liver disease
Fibrosis
Bile duct proliferation
Cirrhosis

CHOLESTASIS

Toulakian and Seashore (42) in a prospective study found that in eight of 19 infants receiving TPN the direct bilirubin increased to greater than 2 mg/dl. Seven of the eight were premature. Beale et al. (43) described intrahepatic cholestasis, which they defined as a direct bilirubin $\geq$ 1.5 mg/dl, in 14 of 62 premature infants who weighed less than 2000 g. The very LBW infants who weight less than 1000 g at birth appear to be at increased risk for cholestasis, with an incidence of 50% compared to 18% for infants 1000–1499 g, and 7% for those 1500–2000 g. Pereira and co-workers (44) also demonstrated a higher incidence of cholestasis in their more immature infants with an inverse correlation between severity of jaundice and the degree of prematurity.

The mean onset of cholestasis was 42 days after initiating TPN (range 5–83 days) in the premature infants studied by Beale et al. (43) After 60 days of TPN, 80% of the premature infants had evidence of cholestasis (43). In the study of Pereira and co-workers (44) infants who developed cholestasis had received TPN for longer periods of time than in infants without cholestasis.

Vileisis and co-workers (45) found that cholestatic jaundice, defined as a direct bilirubin $\geq$ 2 mg/dl, developed in 11 of 33 infants receiving parenteral nutrition for at least 2 weeks. They concluded that the direct bilirubin was the most sensitive and early indicator of cholestasis. Serum glutamic oxaloacetic transaminase (SGOT) and serum glutamic pyruvic transaminase (SGPT) values did not become significantly increased until 2 weeks after the onset of cholestasis. Postuma and co-workers (46) also found in 92 infants that the SGOT elevation occurred significantly later than that of direct bilirubin (after 4.6 weeks for SGOT compared to 2.2 weeks for direct bilirubin).

Serum bile acids, such as cholylglycine and sulfolithocholic acid, may be elevated prior to elevations of direct bilirubin and are more sensitive and specific indicators of cholestasis than standard liver function tests. Sondheimer et al. (47) measured levels of serum conjugates of cholic acid (SCCA) as a sensitive measure of cholestasis. In their infants who weighed less than 2000 g, none had elevations of their SCCA if they had received TPN for less than 2 weeks. In contrast, seven of eight patients of this weight developed increased SCCA values when exposed to TPN for more than 2 weeks; three of these eight patients developed jaundice between the

Table 4. Hepatic Complications of TPN in Infants and Children

Patients	Intravenous Nutrients	Hepatic Dysfunction			Hepatic Pathology							Comments
		↑ Conjugated Bilirubin	↑ SGOT	↑ SAP	Fatty changes	Cholestasis		Portal/Peri-portal Changes	Bile duct Proliferation	Hepatocellular Damage		
						Canalic./duct	Hepato-cyte					
1 infant (1.0 kg)	3.3% P 20% D	—	—	—	—	"Predominantly centrilobular"		—	Prominent	Occasional giant cells		"A definite relationship between the TPN regimen and the development of cholestasis cannot be established" (first reported case). Early cirrhosis.
3 infants (<1.2 kg)	FH 2.6–4 g/kg/day	0/3	0/3	—	Present	"Cholestasis"		—	—	1/3 Hepato-cellular degener-ation		Total: 9 infants. No hepatomegaly.
3 infants (1.2–2.5 kg)	FH and CH 2.2–3.9 g/kg/day	2/3 (>2.0 mg/dl)	2/3	—	1/3	1/3 "Cholestasis"; 2/3 "ascending cholangitis"		—	—	—		Liver biopsies done in 3/7 infants with hyper-ammonemia.
3 infants (0.9–2.8 kg)	5% CH 20% D	3/3 (>2.0 mg/dl)	0/3	3/3	—	—	2/2	—	2/2	2/2 (Minimal)		"Coexistent surgical complications may contribute to the development of cholestasis."
7 children (16 mo–18 yr)	CH FH D	1/3 (> 2.0 mg/dl)	3/3 (Also SGPT)	3/3	—	—	1/3	1/3 Portal triaditis, fibrosis	—	Ballooning of hepatocytes		All 7 patients developed hepatic dysfunction; only 3 reported early rise of transaminases and SAP. Patient with liver biopsy: first biopsy age 16 weeks, last age 6 months, still showing fibrosis and portal triaditis.
5 infants (< 1.5 kg)	4.5% CH 3 g/kg/day 20% D 10% II 3.5 g/kg/day	—	—	—	1/5 (Day 9)	1/5		—	—	—		Total: 23 premature infants, 19 survivors. Supplemental oral feedings. Brown pigment in Kupffer cells.

Group (weight)	TPN regimen	Hyperbilirubinemia					Hepatic histology			Comments
8 infants (1.0–2.6 kg)	2–4% CH 2.6 g/kg/day	8/8 (>2.0 mg/dl)	42%	8/8	5/5	5/5	5/5 / Periportal inflammation	—	5/5 (Minimal)	Total: 19 premature infants. Two infants with abnormal liver histology had conj. bilirubin <2 g/dl; 8/12 infants with hyperammonemia.
9 infants (<1.25 kg)	L-aa 2.5 g/kg/day 10% D 10% II 2–5 g/kg/day	9/9 (>2.0 mg/dl)	—	—	3/9	9/9 / 1/9 "Cholangitis"	5/9 Portal fibrosis	7/9	—	Three infants received supplemental oral feedings, but brief and unsustained. Iron pigment in Kupffer cells.
11 infants (1.1–3.3 kg)	3.3% CH 2.5 g/kg/day 20% D		7/11	4/11	—	11/11 "Cholestasis"	11/11 Portal fibrosis	1/11	Local acute inflammation; 5 with extensive ultrastructural changes	All received supplemental oral feedings. Extensive ultrastructural changes of hepatocytes; persistent hepatic fibrosis in 3.
5 infants (<1.25 kg)	1.7–3.8% L-aa 20% D	11/11 "Elevated"	↑ After 5 weeks	—	1/5	5/5	Portal triaditis	1/5	Minimal	"Elevation of direct reacting bilirubin, earliest clinical manifestation of hepatic dysfunction."
5 infants (1.6–2.2 kg)	5% CH 2.5–3.0 g/kg/day		5/5	—	—	5/5 / 5/5	5/5 Portal triaditis	—	5/5 Ultrastructural changes	Response to cholestyramine in some. Kupffer cell hyperplasia with storage of iron pigment. Mitochondrial changes.
4 infants (1.5–2.9 kg)	Not stated	2/4 (>2.0 mg/dl)	—	—	2/4	2/4	4/4 Portal fibrosis 1/4 Portal triaditis	2/4	Organic crystalline precipitates	Organic crystals containing calcium, phosphate, sulfate (birefringent under polarized light) in bile duct epithelium or hepatocytes, with giant cell transformation.
2 infants (1.0, 1.2 kg)	L-aa 2–4 g/kg/day	?	2/2	2/2	1/2	2/2 / 2/2	1/2 portal triaditis	—	Present	Supplemental oral feedings; treatment with cholestyramine or phenobarbital. Peripheral eosinophilia as early as 2nd week of TPN. Cirrhosis in the smaller infant.

Table 4. (Continued)

Patients	Intravenous Nutrients	Hepatic Dysfunction			Hepatic Pathology			Hepatic Pathology			Comments
						Cholestasis					
		↑Conjugated Bilirubin	↑SGOT	↑SAP	Fatty changes	Canalic./duct.	Hepato-cyte	Portal/Peri-portal Changes	Bile duct Proliferation	Hepatocellular Damage	
62 infants	5% Ch + 8.5% L-aa 2–3 g/kg/day 10–20% D	14/14 (>1.5 mg/dl)	8/14 (SGPT)	—	4/5 Mild to severe	Moderate 7/8	Mild	—	—	7/8 Moderate to severe	"Very low birth weight infants at greater risk to develop cholestasis."
92 infants	FH, CH, and L-aa 2.5 g/kg/day 15% D 10% Il 3 g/kg/day	31/92 (>1.0 mg/dl)	23/83	25/74	Rare, mild	11/14 Centrilobular		Variable portal fibrosis	Uncommon early, more evident with prolonged TPN	—	"Surgical procedure predisposes to earlier and more frequent rise of conjugated bilirubin." Casein hydrolysate: more frequent hepatic dysfunction, earlier rise of bilirubin. PAS-positive (diastase-negative) material in Kupffer cells. Two infants with cirrhosis, 23 or more developed jaundice and liver disease.

SOURCE: Poley JR: Liver and nutrition: Hepatic complications of total parenteral nutrition, in Lebenthal E (ed): *Textbook of Gastroenterology and Nutrition in Infancy.* New York, Raven Press, 1981, pp 744–745. Reprinted with permission.

CH, casein hydrolysate; D, dextrose; FH, fibrin hydrolysate; Il Intralipid; L-aa, L-amino acids; P, protein; SAP, serum alkaline phosphatase; SGPT, serum glutamic pyruvic transaminase; SGOT, serum glutamic oxaloacetic transaminase.

Table 5. Hepatic Complications of TPN in Adults

Patients	Hepatic Dysfunction				Hepatic Pathology					Comments
	Intravenous Nutrients	↑Conjugated Bilirubin	↑SGOT	↑SAP	Fatty Changes	Cholestasis Canalic./Duct.	Cholestasis Hepatocyte	Portal/Periportal Changes	Bile Duct Proliferation	
100 Adults	10% CH L-aa 20–25% D	26% after 8 days (1.4–3.2 mg/dl total bilirubin)	93% > 8 days	56% >20 days	1 Mild 4 Marked	—	—	—	—	↑SGPT in 89% after 10 days of TPN. ↑LDH in 69% after 8 days. Fatty changes early. Toxic effect of tryptophan conversion product suspected.
32 Adults	8.5% L-aa 5% CH 2 g/kg/day 20% D 10% II 3 g/kg/day	19/32 (>2.0 mg/dl)	15/25	24/32 >19 days	—	8/8	—	8/8 Portal triaditis	8/8	Cause of cholestatic jaundice: lipid/dextrose ratios of 3:2 with high protein (>2 mg/kg/day) after 30 days TPN. First abnormality: progressive rise of SAP after 10 days TPN. 8 patients had liver biopsies.
26 Adults (16–80 yr)	—	12/26 (>2.0 mg/dl)	—	After 10–14 days TPN	8/9	Present	Present	2 Fibrosis; portal/periportal triaditis	Present	Progressive rise of SAP: sensitive index of early hepatic dysfunction. Fatty infiltration: early phenomenon.
45 Adults	5% L-aa 25% D	21% (>1.5 mg/dl total bilirubin)	68%	54%	3/4 Marked	1/4 "Mild periportal cholestasis"	—	—	—	Average duration of TPN: 3 weeks. "No evidence that TPN results in chronic liver disease." 4 patients had liver biopsies.

SOURCE: Poley JR: Liver and nutrition: Hepatic complications of total parenteral nutrition, in Lebenthal E (ed): *Textbook of Gastroenterology and Nutrition in Infancy.* New York, Raven Press, 1981, pp 746–747. Reprinted with permission.

fourth and sixth week of TPN. Strikingly, none of the infants above 2000 g had elevations of their SCCA levels after 2 weeks of TPN. Thus, the most immature infants were at the greatest risk for cholestasis. Balistreri and co-workers (48) found measurements of a secondary bile acid, sulfated lithocholate (SL), helpful in monitoring infants on TPN. In patients with cholestasis of any cause there was a marked rise in SL. During serial, prospective monitoring of hepatic function in six patients receiving PN, the concentration of SL was elevated in four patients before routine liver function tests such as bilirubin concentration or transaminases were elevated.

Black and co-workers (49) found in 21 infants randomized into a TPN group and a control (glucose–electrolyte) group that 1 week of TPN resulted in significant elevations of *gamma glutamyl transpeptidase* (GGTP) and *5'-nucleotidase*, whereas SGOT, SGPT, total and direct bilirubin, and serum bile salts were unaffected. Black et al. concluded that the initial effect of TPN appeared to be on the canalicular membrane; the sinusoidal membrane appeared to be unaffected by 1 week of TPN. Thus, the first liver function abnormality seen in infants on TPN is an increase in 5'-nucleotidase and GGTP, usually followed by an increase in bile acids and then an increase in direct bilirubin; serum transaminase levels usually follow direct bilirubin elevations by approximately 2 weeks.

In addition to prematurity and duration of TPN, other factors that may predispose a patient to cholestasis are sepsis (44,50) and the concentration of infused amino acids. Vileisis et al. (51) studied infants receiving 2.3 g/kg/day of protein versus those receiving 3.6 g/kg/day. The incidence of cholestasis was similar in the two groups. However, the high protein intake group developed cholestasis earlier and developed higher levels of direct bilirubin as well.

The majority of patients with cholestasis will have slow resolution of their liver function abnormalities following discontinuation of TPN and initiation of oral feedings. Some will have progression of liver dysfunction for several weeks following discontinuation of TPN with eventual resolution. Less than 10% of patients will develop severe chronic liver disease with cirrhosis, portal hypertension, and death.

The incidence of severe liver disease is highest in patients who have had abdominal surgery (52). Postuma et al. (46) found that the incidence of direct hyperbilirubinemia was 52% in surgical patients compared to 21% in medical patients. Patients with necrotizing enterocolitis (NEC) are at high risk for severe liver disease. Patients with NEC may have inflammatory and fibrosing lesions of the liver, associated with eosinophilic deposits, even without receiving TPN (52). If they survive, they may develop a chronic scarring liver disease (52).

According to Thaler (52), uncomplicated cholestasis associated with TPN is the least serious liver condition; cholestasis associated with sepsis is more serious, and cholestasis associated with gastrointestinal surgical disorders is the most serious. The last two problems predispose to inflammatory and fibrosing lesions of the liver in infants on long-term TPN (52).

Liver biopsies of infants on TPN initially reveal a nonspecific cholestatic hepatitis with bile stasis in canaliculi, Kupffer cells, and hepatocytes. Portal areas often show bile duct proliferation, lymphocyte infiltration, and various degrees of fibrosis. Giant cell transformation is common. In uncomplicated cases follow-up biopsies show resolution of all findings except for mild persistent hepatocellular cholestasis. Electron microscopic findings show persistent canalicular abnormalities months after clinical resolution. A number of recent studies review the spectrum of hepatic disease in infants and children on TPN (53–55).

It should be emphasized that the diagnosis of this syndrome is made on clinical appearance alone, and specific causes of conjugated hyperbilirubinemia must be ruled out. Early sepsis and congenital infections should be considered in all cases. Extrahepatic obstruction due to choledochal cyst or biliary atresia should be evaluated by ultrasound and/or hepatobiliary imaging with Rose Bengal, H-substituted iminodiacetic acid or ^{99m}Tc-para-isopropyl-iminodiacetic acid. Metabolic and genetic disorders such as α_1-antitrypsin deficiency, cystic fibrosis, galactosemia, and tyrosinemia should also be ruled out.

ETIOLOGIC FACTORS

Before the widespread use of lipid infusions, essential fatty acid deficiency was thought to be the cause of hepatic abnormalities. Although intravenous fat has reversed the process in some patients, the routine provision of lipid has not eliminated the problem. Similarly, early protein hydrolysates were thought to contain hepatotoxic levels of ammonia, but the use of crystalline amino acid solutions (with low free ammonia content) has not reduced the degree of hepatic dysfunction. Biliary stasis due to lack of enteral stimulation is still believed to play a role in cholestasis, but many children who now receive a combined enteral and parenteral regimen are still at risk for hepatic dysfunction (56).

Hepatic immaturity apparently puts premature infants at greater risk of permanent liver disease secondary to TPN than adults. Sinatra showed that cholestasis can be readily produced in suckling rats but not in weaned rats, implying that the more immature animals are more susceptible to cholestasis (56a). Impaired bile salt formation and excretion in infants may be one predisposing factor (52). This hypothesis is supported by data previously presented showing that the initial effect of TPN is on the membrane of the bile canaliculi (49).

Direct hepatotoxicity either from specific amino acids or from an imbalance of amino acids is another possible etiology. Amino acid dose has been demonstrated to effect onset and severity of cholestasis (51). Further, an in vitro experiment in which liver slices were incubated with individual amino acids revealed that glycine, leucine, threonine, and isoleucine caused considerable rises in transaminase levels in the liver tissue after 24 hours of incubation (57). When each of the amino acids present in PN solutions were given intraperitoneally to rat pups, *only tryptophan* injection resulted in cholestasis (demonstrated by an increase in serum bile acids) (56a).

Endotoxins, especially from *Escherichia coli*, are another potential source of hepatic dysfunction. Aballi and co-workers (58) administered a single dose of *E. coli* endotoxin to 10 adult male rabbits while six additional rabbits served as controls. SGOT rose and serum albumin fell in all endotoxin-injected animals. Hepatic necrosis was seen in seven out of 10 of the treated animals. The control group demonstrated no abnormalities in liver function or liver histology. In addition, Sonawane and Yaffe (59) demonstrated that hepatic drug metabolism in rat mothers and their neonates is significantly impaired upon exposure to endotoxin. Thus, the human neonate may be at risk for liver dysfunction owing to hepatic immaturity, lack of enteral stimulation, direct hepatotoxicity from amino acids, and gram-negative sepsis. Drugs primarily metabolized by the liver should be used with caution in these situations.

HEPATOMEGALY

Hepatomegaly with mild elevation of serum transaminases in the *absence* of chole-stasis may result from hepatic accumulation of lipid or glycogen secondary to either excess carbohydrate calories or an inappropriate nonnitrogen calorie–nitrogen ratio. Fatty infiltration of the liver due to excessive caloric intake is readily reversible in nearly all instances by reduction of total calories administered and, if necessary, alteration of the nonnitrogen calorie–nitrogen ratio (52).

HEPATIC COMPLICATIONS AFTER INFANCY

Hepatic complications of TPN become less frequent and relatively less severe in patients beyond infancy. However, abnormal liver function tests are not uncommon in patients on PN for long periods of time. Those with chronic intestinal conditions complicated by infection or bacterial overgrowth are particularly susceptible to hepatic complications. In most of these patients, elevated liver enzymes improve with the initiation of partial enteral alimentation (52).

Most adults on TPN develop gradual elevations in alkaline phosphatase, SGOT, and occasionally bilirubin by the second week of therapy. Liver biopsies performed at this time reveal fatty infiltration within the hepatocytes with some increase in glycogen stores; the hepatic architecture is well preserved. The inflammatory and cholestatic changes seen in children are generally absent (56). The fatty liver can be treated by (1) decreasing total carbohydrate load and total calories; (2) decreasing the calorie–nitrogen ratio; (3) substituting lipid for some of the carbohydrate calories ("balanced TPN"—see Chapters 5 and 7); (4) cyclic TPN, allowing a car-bohydrate-free period (see Chapter 22) (60).

In addition to fatty infiltration of the liver, a second type of hepatic lesion is seen in adults on prolonged TPN of greater than 4 weeks duration (60). Up to 30–50% develop a late rise in alkaline phosphatase, bilirubin, and liver enzymes that persists throughout the TPN course and may take months to resolve completely. A liver biopsy at this time shows cholestasis, periportal inflammation, bile duct prolifera-tion, and fibrosis. There is concern that these latter findings may be permanent (60).

Similar to the suspected etiology in children, the etiology of the hepatic injury in adults is not known with certainty but may be due to a toxic effect or deficiency state caused by TPN. The maturity of the adult hepatocyte may simply decrease suscepti-bility and delay the onset of cellular injury. When this hepatic injury occurs, it is wise to discontinue TPN promptly or as soon as the patient's clinical status permits (60).

THERAPY AND PREVENTION

An attempt should be made to reduce the use of TPN in small neonates with functioning gastrointestinal tracts by more persistent efforts at using alternate routes of enteral feeding such as continuous nasogastric or transpyloric feedings. If cholestasis occurs: (1) decrease parenteral and increase enteral feedings, if possible; (2) remove copper and manganese from the TPN solution, since both are normally excreted by the biliary tree and may be hepatotoxic at high concentrations (see Chapter 10).

LIVER MALIGNANCY

Vileisis and co-workers (61) have recently reported an isolated case of liver malignancy in a 26 month-old infant who had previously received PN. The baby was 900 g at birth. Nutritional intake included infusion of dextrose-amino acid solutions into the *portal vein* through an *umbilical venous catheter*. The patient also developed necrotizing enterocolitis in the first few weeks of life. The child went on to require protracted central vein TPN. The authors point out that their description of a heptocellular carcinoma occurring with TPN-related biliary cirrhosis documents the potential for liver malignancy following protracted use of PN (61).

FOLLOW-UP

Marino et al. recently described a two-year follow-up of 10 neonates with PN-induced liver disease. All infants grew at the same rate while on PN. Those infants with chronic active liver disease all had metabolic bone disease and neither height nor weight was normal at 2 years (62).

Eosinophilia

Eosinophilia appears to be a nonspecific finding in sick neonates and is associated with the length of hospitalization, number of days on antibiotic therapy, and the use of PN (63). The incidence of eosinophilia is higher in small preterm infants who have required endotracheal intubation, have received multiple blood transfusions, and have been on PN for prolonged periods of time (64).

Although one report (65) stated that about 80% of the patients on Intralipid develop a peripheral eosinophilia of 5–10%, and occasionally as high as 35%, Kien and Chusid (66) could not demonstrate an association of eosinophilia with Intralipid. In the latter study, 14 of 21 patients, aged five days to 17 years receiving PN developed eosinophilia. Of the 14 only seven had received Intralipid. There was no difference in the prevalence of eosinophilia between PN patients with or without liver dysfunction. The authors concluded that eosinophilia is often encountered in children receiving PN but is not directly attributed to PN. The complication seems to be benign and transient and, therefore, probably does not require further work-up.

Practical Guidelines

1. Table 1 in Chapter 15 outlines specifics of the metabolic monitoring necessary to prevent or manage complications listed in Table 1 of this chapter.
2. Calcium, phosphorus, and alkaline phosphatase should be obtained weekly in premature infants at risk for osteopenia or rickets. Chest x-ray films should be assessed carefully for evidence of osteopenia. If possible, immature infants should be periodically screened for early rickets with urinary amino acid screens, since generalized amino aciduria is an early sensitive

index of vitamin D deficiency and precedes changes in calcium, phosphorus, and alkaline phosphatase (36).

3. If the SGOT or SGPT rise in association with a normal or near normal direct bilirubin and alkaline phosphatase, check the total caloric intake and the calorie–nitrogen ratio. Reduce the caloric intake and/or decrease the non-nitrogen calorie–nitrogen ratio, which ideally should be approximately 150–200:1.

4. Monitor for early evidence of cholestasis.
   a. Use either the GGTP, 5'-nucleotidase, or serum bile acids.
   b. If the above tests are not easily obtainable measure the *direct* bilirubin on a weekly basis.

5. For an excellent current reference on cholestasis, please see Sinatra FR: Cholestasis in infancy and childhood. *Curr Prob in Pediatr* 12(12):6, 1982.

References

1. Heird WC: Total parenteral nutrition, in Lebenthal E (ed): *Textbook of Gastroenterology and Nutrition in Infancy.* New York, Raven Press, 1981, p 662.

2. Seashore JH: Metabolic complications of parenteral nutrition in infants and children. *Surg Clin North Am* 60:1239, 1980.

3. Wesley JR, Saran PA, Khalidi N, et al (eds): *Parenteral and Enteral Nutrition Manual.* Chicago, Abbott Laboratories, 1980, p 38.

4. Levy JS, Winters RW, Heird WC: Total parenteral nutrition in pediatric patients. *Pediatrics in Review* 2:99, 1980.

5. Filler RM: Parenteral support of the surgically ill child, in Suskind RM (ed): *Textbook of Pediatric Nutrition.* New York, Raven Press, 1981, p 350.

6. Al-Jurf A, Steiger E: Hypouricemia in total parenteral nutrition. *Am J Clin Nutr* 33:2630, 1980.

7. Whitington PF, Black DD: Cholelithiasis in premature infants treated with parenteral nutrition and furosemide. *J Pediatr* 97:647, 1980.

8. Barth RA, Brasch RC, Filly RA: Abdominal pseudotumor in childhood: Distended gallbladder with parenteral alimentation. *AJR* 136:341, 1981.

9. Cochran ST, Pagani JJ, Barbaric ZL: Nephromegaly in hyperalimentation. *Radiology* 130:603, 1979.

10. Merritt RJ, Ennis CE, Thomas DW, et al: Lactic acidosis in pediatric patients with cancer receiving total parenteral nutrition. *J Pediatr* 99:247, 1981.

11. Meyers CC, Schochet SS Jr, McCormick WF: Wernicke's encephalopathy in infancy: Development during parenteral nutrition. *Acta Neuropathol (Berl)* 43:267, 1978.

12. Blennow G: Wernicke's encephalopathy following prolonged artificial nutrition. *Am J Dis Child* 129:1456, 1975.

13. Catalano JD, Monteleone JA: Cortical cataracts following total parenteral nutrition. *Birth Defects* 12(5):39, 1976.

14. Okamoto E, Heird WC: Feeding the low-birth-weight infant. *Pediatric Annals* 10(11):37, 1981.

15. Lewin PK, Reid M, Reilly BJ, et al: Iatrogenic rickets in low-birth-weight infants. *J Pediatr* 78:207, 1971.

16. Koon SW, Fraser D, Reilly BJ, et al: Rickets due to calcium deficiency. *N Engl J Med* 297:1264, 1977.

17. Rowe JC, Wood DH, Rowe DW, et al: Nutritional hypophosphatemic rickets in a premature infant fed breast milk. *N Engl J Med* 300:293, 1979.

18. Hoff N, Haddad J, Teitelbaum S, et al: Serum concentrations of 25-hydroxyvitamin D in rickets of extremely premature infants. *J Pediatr* 94:460, 1979.

19. Callenbach JC, Sheehan MB, Abramson SJ, et al: Etiologic factors in rickets of very-low-birth-weight infants. *J Pediatr* 98:800, 1981.

20. Steichen JJ, Tsang RC, Greer FR: Elevated serum 1,25 dihydroxyvitamin D concentrations in rickets of very-low-birth-weight infants. *J Pediatr* 99:293, 1981.

21. Kulkarni PB, Hall RT, Rhodes RG, et al: Rickets in very-low-birth-weight infants. *J Pediatr* 96:249, 1980.

22. Steichen JJ, Gratton TL, Tsang RC: Osteopenia of prematurity: The cause and possible treatment. *J Pediatr* 96:528, 1980.

23. Glasgow JFT, Thomas PS: Rachitic respiratory distress in small preterm infants. *Arch Dis Child* 52:268, 1977.

24. Seino Y, Ishii T, Shimotsuji T, et al: Plasma active vitamin D concentration in low birthweight infants with rickets and its response to vitamin D treatment. *Arch Dis Child* 56:628, 1981.

25. Chesney RW, Hamstra AJ, DeLuca HF: Rickets of prematurity: Supranormal levels of serum 1,25 dihydroxyvitamin D. *Am J Dis Child* 135:34, 1981.

26. Lapatsanis P, Makaronis G, Vretos C, et al: Two types of nutritional rickets in infants. *Am J Clin Nutr* 29:1222, 1976.

27. Maltz HE, Fish MB, Holliday MA: Calcium deficiency rickets and the renal response to calcium infusion. *Pediatrics* 46:865, 1970.

28. Glorieux FH, Marie PJ, Pettifor JM, et al: Bone response to phosphate salts, ergo calciferol, and calcitriol in hypophosphatemic vitamin D-resistant rickets. *N Engl J Med* 303:1023, 1980.

29. Rudolf M, Arulanantham K, Greenstein RM: Unsuspected nutritional rickets. *Pediatrics* 66:72, 1980.

30. Kooh SW, Jones G, Reilly T, et al: Pathogenesis of rickets in chronic hepatobiliary disease in children. *J Pediatr* 94:870, 1979.

31. Ziegler EE, O'Donnell AM, Nelson SE, et al: Body composition of the reference fetus. *Growth* 40:329, 1976.

32. Fomon SJ: *Infant Nutrition.* Philadelphia, WB Saunders Co, 1974.

33. Day GM, Chance GW, Radde IC, et al: Growth and mineral metabolism in very-low-birth-weight infants. II. Effects of calcium supplementation on growth and divalent cations. *Pediatr Res* 9:568, 1975.

34. Sagy M, Birenbaum E, Balin A, et al: Phosphate-depletion syndrome in a premature infant fed human milk. *J Pediatr* 96:683, 1980.

35. Oppenheimer SJ, Snodgrass GJAI: Neonatal rickets: Histopathology and quantitative bone changes. *Arch Dis Child* 55:945, 1980.

36. Geggel RL, Pereira GR, Spackman TJ: Fractured ribs: Unusual presentation of rickets in premature infants. *J Pediatr* 93:680, 1978.

37. Leape LL, Valaes T: Rickets in low birth weight infants receiving total parenteral nutrition. *J Pediatr Surg* 11:665, 1976.

38. Winslow C, Morriss F, Conley S, et al: Rickets in very low birth weight infants: Growth exceeding mineral intake. *Clinical Research* 28:897A, 1980.

39. Eggert LD, Rusho WJ, MacKay MW, et al: Calcium and phosphorus compatibility in parenteral nutrition solutions for neonates. *Am J Hosp Pharm* 39:49, 1982.

40. Poole R, Rupp C, Kerner J: Calcium and phosphorus in neonatal TPN solutions. *JPEN* 5:580, 1981.

41. Peden VH, Witzleben DL, Skelton MA: Total parenteral nutrition. *J Pediatr* 78:180, 1971.

42. Touloukian RJ, Seashore JH: Hepatic secretory obstruction with total parenteral nutrition in the infant. *J Pediatr Surg* 10:353, 1975.

43. Beale EF, Nelson RM, Bucciarelli RL, et al: Intrahepatic cholestasis associated with parenteral nutrition in premature infants. *Pediatrics* 64:342, 1979.

44. Pereira GR, Sherman MS, DiGiacomo J, et al: Hyperalimentation-induced cholestasis: Increased incidence and severity in premature infants. *Am J Dis Child* 135:842, 1981.

45. Vileisis RA, Inwood RJ, Hunt CE: Laboratory monitoring of parenteral nutrition-associated hepatic dysfunction in infants. *JPEN* 5:67, 1981.

46. Postuma R, Trevenen CL: Liver disease in infants receiving total parenteral nutrition. *Pediatrics* 63:110, 1979.

47. Sondheimer JM, Bryan H, Andrews W, et al: Cholestatic tendencies in premature infants on and off parenteral nutrition. *Pediatrics* 62:984, 1978.

48. Balistreri WF, Suchy FJ, Farrell MK, et al: Pathologic versus physiologic cholestasis: Elevated serum concentation of a secondary bile acid in the presence of hepatobiliary disease. *J Pediatr* 98:399, 1981.

49. Black DD, Suttle EA, Whitington PF, et al: The effect of short-term total parenteral nutrition on hepatic function in the human neonate: A prospective randomized study demonstrating alteration of hepatic canalicular function. *J Pediatr* 99:445, 1981.

50. Manginello FP, Javitt NB: Parenteral nutrition and neonatal cholestasis. *J Pediatr* 94:296, 1979.

51. Vileisis RA, Inwood RJ, Hunt CE: Prospective controlled study of parenteral nutrition-associated cholestatic jaundice: Effect of protein intake. *J Pediatr* 96:893, 1980.

52. Thaler MM: Liver dysfunction and disease associated with total parenteral alimentation. *ASPEN 6th Clinical Congress*, San Francisco, 1982, p 67.

53. Cohen C, Olsen MM: Pediatric total parenteral nutrition: Liver histopathology. *Arch Pathol Lab Med* 105:152, 1981.

54. Dahms BB, Halpin TC Jr: Serial liver biopsies in parenteral nutrition-associated cholestasis of early infancy. *Gastroenterology* 81:136, 1981.

55. Benjamin DR: Hepatobiliary dysfunction in infants and children associated with long-term total parenteral nutrition: A clinico-pathologic study. *Am J Clin Path* 76:276, 1981.

56. Boraas M: Hepatic complications of total parenteral nutrition. Part 1. Description and etiology. *Clinical Nutrition Newsletter*. Philadelphia, Hospital of the University of Pennsylvania, August issue: 1, 1981.

56a. Merritt RJ, Sinatra FR, Henton DH: Cholestatic effect of tryptophan and its metabolites in suckling rat pups. *Pediatr Res* 16:171 A, 1982.

57. Cohen M: Changes in hepatic function, In Winters R, Hasselmeyer E (eds): *Intravenous Nutrition in the High Risk Infant*. New York, John Wiley & Sons, 1975, p 293.

58. Aballi AJ, Karayalcin G, Costales F, et al: Liver damage in rabbits from administration of a single dose of gram-negative endotoxin. *Pediatr Res* 12:646, 1978.

59. Sonawane BR, Yaffee SJ: Gram-negative endotoxin administration decreases hepatic drug-metabolizing enzymes during development of rats. *Pediatr Res* 14:939, 1980.

60. Boraas M: Hepatic complications of total parenteral nutrition. Part II. *Clinical Nutrition Newsletter*. Philadelphia, Hospital of the University of Pennsylvania, October issue: 1, 1981.

61. Vileisis RA, Sorensen K, Gonzalez-Crussi F, et al: Liver malignancy after parenteral nutrition. *J Pediatr* 100:88, 1982.

62. Marino L, Hack M, Dahms B, et al: Two-year follow-up: Growth and neonatal PN-associated liver disease. *JPEN* 5:569, 1981.

63. Lawrence R Jr, Church JA, Richards W, et al: Eosinophilia in the hospitalized neonate. *Ann Allergy* 44:349, 1980.

64. Bhat AM, Scanlon JW: The pattern of eosinophilia in premature neonates. A prospective study in premature infants using the absolute eosinophil count. *J Pediatr* 98:612, 1981.

65. Filler RM: Parenteral support of the surgically ill child, in Suskind RM (ed): *Textbook of Pediatric Nutrition*. New York, Raven Press, 1981, p 341.

66. Kien CL, Chusid MJ: Eosinophilia in children receiving parenteral nutrition support. *JPEN* 3:468, 1979.

14
Septic Complications

Amy S. Andolina

Over the past decade, investigators have demonstrated an association of systemic infection with the delivery of parenteral nutrition (PN) through a central venous catheter (1,2). Sepsis continues to be a major complication of centrally infused PN in pediatrics. An infection may originate from preparation of the solution, catheter insertion, catheter site care, the administration set, the solution container, or any manipulation of the system.

Almost all patients who are candidates for PN are in some way compromised hosts. The newborn infant is immunologically impaired in his defense against microorganisms (3,4). A child with cancer, hepatic dysfunction, burns, fistulas, or gastrointestinal malfunction is predisposed to infectious complications. Antibiotics, chemotherapy, steroids, and radiation therapy may further depress the host's defense mechanisms.

In the early use of PN, the incidence of bacterial and fungal septicemia was unacceptably high, with rates of 14–37% (5–10). The realization that PN related infections were iatrogenic spurred steps to reduce this complication. The development of written protocols (11) covering every aspect of solution preparation and handling (12) and patient care (13,14), along with the evolution of PN teams (2,15–17) has greatly reduced the incidence of infection. Over the last 5 years it has been demonstrated that in hospitals where teams practice strict asepsis, rates of PN related sepsis are very low—0–2% (18). However, the incidence of sepsis remains higher in children—approximately 15% (19).

Sources of PN Related Infections

SOLUTION

In 1981, the Center for Disease Control reported that fluids used for PN, including protein hydrolysates and fat emulsions, can support the growth of a wide variety of organisms (Table 1) (20). Intrinsic contamination of intravenous solutions has been documented (21–24). However, this type of contamination of PN components leading to demonstrated clinical sepsis has not been widely described (2). Extrinsic contamination can occur during admixture and administration (2). Fortunately,

Table 1. Micro-organisms Frequently Found in PN Solutions[2,21,22]

Amino Acid/ Dextrose	Protein Hydrolysate/ Dextrose	Fat Emulsion
C. albicans	C. albicans	C. albicans
Pseudomonas aeruginosa	Torulopsis glabrata	Pseudomonas aeruginosa
Enterobacter aerogenes	S. aureus	S. aureus
	Escherichia coli	Escherichia coli
	Proteus mirabilis	Klebsiella species
	Klebsiella species	
	Enterobacter cloacae	

delivery of contaminated PN solutions has not been known to be correlated with bacterial or fungal septicemia in the patient (25–29). Although the PN solutions are usually not the source of significant clinical infection, the potential for infection is always possible. Therefore, meticulous compounding of the PN solution by a pharmacist under a laminar flow hood (2) and the use of final in-line filters (discussed in Chapter 17) are recommended.

As stated by the National Coordinating Committee on Large Volume Parenterals, the PN solution should be kept refrigerated until use and administered within 48 hours after pharmacy admixture. Fat emulsion and PN solution bottles should not hang for more than 24 hours (30). Fischer et al. report that Intralipid may enhance the risk of bacterial sepsis in certain patients (31).

CATHETER

The most common source of sepsis in the patient receiving central line PN is the catheter (1) (see Table 2 for most common organisms). Several mechanisms have been postulated. It is thought that organisms from an infection site may colonize the central catheter and lead to sustained septicemia because of ongoing seeding. A fibrin sleeve that forms at the tip of the catheter may also be a trap for microorganisms (32). Another probable cause of catheter-related sepsis is growth of organisms along the exterior of the catheter from skin flora around the insertion site, or growth of organisms down the interior of the catheter due to a break in the closed system (32).

The location of the catheter may also play a role in catheter-induced sepsis. In children receiving PN the incidence of infection in peripheral vein infusion was 0% compared to a 10.5% incidence related to central vein delivery (33).

The likelihood of sepsis can be related to the duration of therapy. A review of the experience at the Toronto Children's Hospital with PN using central venous catheters indicated that 16% of the patients had one or more systemic complications. For each week of therapy after the first week, the risk of sepsis increased by approximately 5% (34). Some investigators believe that a central PN catheter that is inserted and maintained properly may be left in place for weeks to months without increased risk of septicemia (32,35,36).

The incidence of sepsis may also be linked to catheter composition. With the trend toward using silicone rubber catheters there has been a corresponding decrease in the incidence of sepsis (37,38). Sepsis is rarely associated with steel nee-

Table 2. Microbial Pathogens Most Frequently Associated With PN Catheters[18]

Candida species (30–50%)
Torulopsis glabrata
Staphylococcus aureus
Klebsiella species—*Enterobacter* species
Enterococci

dles; therefore, they are recommended for peripheral vein infusions, with site rotation every 48–72 hours (20).

Tunneling of the central venous catheter to a distant exit site has also been shown to decrease infection (5,7), although Von Meyenfedt et al. (39) relate no significant difference in tunnelling of polyvinyl chloride catheters on sepsis rate. The Hickman and Broviac catheters, when used for home parenteral nutrition, are associated with a relatively low infection rate (40–42). The use of strict aseptic technique during catheter placement, line maintenance, and catheter insertion site care are the most important measures in preventing septicemia (see Chapter 17).

INTRAVENOUS ADMINISTRATION SET

The infusion administration sets can become contaminated from a variety of sources. Laboratory and epidemiologic studies have demonstrated that infusion of contaminated fluid even for a short period of time can result in persistent contamination of the administration set (24,43,44). Retrograde contamination of administration sets from a contaminated intravenous catheter can more than likely occur (1) since microorganisms can migrate against a steady flow of fluid (45). However, extrinsic contamination of administration sets results from manipulation of the system, for example, administration of medication and blood or blood products, flushing clotted catheters, or withdrawing blood (1,9,44,46). It is therefore recommended that administration sets be changed every 24 hours and that the catheter be used for the administration of PN *only* (20,46).

Types of Infectious Organisms

Microbial pathogens causing PN-associated sepsis have been identified (2,9,17,18, 25,35,46,47). Gram-positive cocci accounted for the majority of septic episodes with *Staphylococcus epidermidis* and *S. aureus* isolated most often. Gram-negative bacteria are isolated less frequently (2,17,18,25,35,46). Fungi are also responsible for an important percentage of the PN-associated infections. Candida species are most frequently found, especially *C. albicans* (2,9,17,18,25,45,47). The catheter is the most frequent source of PN-associated infection (18).

CANDIDA

Since *Candida* is the most difficult organism to treat, it will be discussed in detail. The most common points of entry for *Candida* are intravenous sites, the gastrointestinal tract, and open wounds. Candidal septicemia is usually seen in the compromised host. *Candida* is cleared by the reticuloendothelial system in various organs, particularly the kidney. Venous blood cultures are frequently negative despite existing septicemia and the presence of *Candida*. Arterial blood cultures, therefore, may be more helpful in identifying the organism. The diagnosis of candidal septicemia is made by positive blood cultures, fundoscopic examination, and a Wright's stain of a blood smear (32). Physical examination at the onset of fungemia may reveal no characteristic signs beyond signs of sepsis. A few patients have been noted to have inflammation of the intravenous catheter entry site from which a white cheesy exudate could be expressed (48). Occlusive dressings, which are used often for PN catheter care, have come under suspicion as fostering *Candida* growth (2).

Complications Associated with *Candida*.   By the time a blood culture is positive for *Candida*, disseminated candidiasis could have already occurred. When tissue invasion occurs, the kidney, heart, and retina are commonly involved (32).

Candidal endophthalmitis is a diagnostic sign of systemic dissemination and may occur as a complication of candidal septicemia even though the fungemia may be transient (48). Thus, all patients with a positive blood culture for fungus should have routine ophthalmologic examinations. Although spontaneous resolution of candidal endophthalmitis has been reported, present knowledge suggests a progressive disease that results in scarring and loss of visual acuity. Other complications of candidal septicemia that have occurred during PN in infants are candidal osteomyelitis (49), meningitis (50), arthritis and osteitis (51), and thrombophlebitis (52).

Diagnosis of Sepsis

Determining the cause of fever in a child with a clinical picture of sepsis is made difficult because many patients receiving PN have other sources for infection besides the catheter itself. The following are points of emphasis (2,17,32,34,35, 46,53,54).

1. Patients receiving PN may have the following signs of sepsis:
   a. Persistent temperature spikes from 38.9°C (102°F) to 40°C (104°F) every 12–24 hours
   b. Chills
   c. Sudden glucose intolerance (glucosuria, elevated serum glucose)
   d. Leukocytosis
   e. Failure to gain weight
   f. Deteriorating clinical or mental status
   g. Hypotension
   h. Oliguria
2. It is important to look for potential sources of infection through:
   a. History and physical examination
   b. Complete blood count with differential and sedimentation rate
   c. Inspection of peripheral and central venous insertion sites

   d. Throat, urine, sputum, stool, skin, and wound cultures

   e. Urinalysis

   f. Peripheral blood cultures (for aerobes, anaerobes, fungi)

   g. Lumbar puncture for cell count, chemistries, Gram stain, and culture (if indicated)

   h. Work-up for abscess or pneumonia (if indicated)

3. If the PN solution or intravenous tubing is suspected:

   a. Remove PN solution and tubing and send for culture (for aerobes, anaerobes, fungi)

   b. Replace with new tubing and PN or dextrose solution

   c. If fat emulsion is infusing, discontinue it and send for culture

4. If a source of infection is found, treat appropriately.

5. If no other source of infection is found in 24–48 hours, most authorities recommend removal of the catheter (exceptions will occur—Pollack and co-workers (42) described antibiotic therapy *without* catheter removal in an infant and in a 64 year-old man with terminal cancer because of the continuous need for venous access and the lack of further insertion sites).

6. Removal of the catheter:

   a. Before removing the catheter, obtain blood cultures from the catheter as well as from a peripheral vein

   b. Culture the catheter insertion site if it is suspicious

   c. The catheter insertion site should be cleansed with normal saline or sterile water

   d. The catheter sutures should be removed

   e. The catheter should be removed in a sterile manner

   f. The catheter tip should be sent for bacterial and fungal studies (8,50–52) Snip the catheter tip using sterile scissors; then drop the tip into a sterile container

   g. A new infusion of IV dextrose must be started to avoid hypoglycemia

7. Absolute indications for catheter removal include:

   a. Septic shock (prior to culture results)

   b. Embolic phenomena

   c. Laboratory proven bacteremia or fungemia

   d. Persistent fever with no other source of infection or underlying disease

Many investigators recommend that 24–48 hours elapse after removing a catheter and instituting antibiotic therapy before reinserting a new catheter (17,46). This recommendation is reasonable, since it is possible that the hiatus will prevent seeding organisms on the new catheter (46).

Management

Prompt removal of the catheter alone may effectively treat bacterial or fungal catheter-related sepsis (2,8,17,25,46). Some investigators suggest treating a bacterial septicemia with antibiotics immediately (35). If tissue invasion with fungus has occurred or if bacterial foci are identified, treatment with intravenous antibiotics or antifungal agents is indicated, as well as catheter removal (2).

It has been reported that only 15–25% of the catheters removed on the basis of suspected bacterial colonization were, in fact, found to be contaminated (15,46,55). An aseptic technique to replace central venous catheters using the *same* insertion site has been described by Padberg et al. The procedure involves inserting a guide-wire along the course of the catheter, then withdrawing the "contaminated" cathe-ter, leaving the guidewire in place. The guidewire serves as a track over which a new catheter can then be threaded. Lastly, the guidewire is withdrawn (15,56).

Glynn et al. (57) have described using urokinase, with and without antibiotics, for thrombosis and associated infection occurring in implanted silastic catheters. As the infected thrombotic clot is dissolved by the urokinase, antibiotics are able to reach the "hiding organisms." Prophylactic use of systemic antibiotics (32,36) to prevent bacteremia and routine flushing of the PN catheter with amphotericin B to prevent fungemia, is not generally recommended (2,32,35,46).

Conclusion

Infectious complications have presented a challenge in caring for the child receiv-ing PN. The importance of establishing and adhering to protocols in the areas of pharmacy technique, catheter placement, PN delivery, and catheter care cannot be overemphasized. Individuals or a team well versed in these methods will enhance the efficacy of PN therapy.

References

1. Maki DG: Sepsis arising from extrinsic contamination of the infusion and measures for control, in Phillips I, Meers PD, D'Arch PF (eds): *Microbiologic Hazards of Intravenous Therapy.* Lancaster, England, MTP Press Ltd, 1977, p 99.
2. Allen JR: The incidence of nosocomial infection in patients receiving total parenteral nutrition, in Johnston IDA (ed): *Advances in Parenteral Nutrition, Proceedings of an International Symposium, Bermuda, May 16–19, 1977.* Lancaster, England, MTP Press, Ltd, 1977, p 339.
3. Wilfert CM: The neonate and gram negative bacterial infections, in Krugman S, Ger-shon AA (eds): *Infections of the Fetus and the Newborn Infant.* New York, Liss, 1975, p 167.
4. Quero J, Omenaca F, Garcia FE, et al: Parenteral nutrition in management of sick low birthweight infants. *An Esp Pediatr* 10:141, 1977.
5. Dudrick SJ, Groff DB, Wilmore DW: Long term venous catheterization in infants. *Surg Gynecol Obstet* 129:805, 1969.
6. Groff DB: Complications of intravenous hyperalimentation in newborns and infants. *J Pediatr Surg* 4:460, 1969.
7. Filler RM, Eraklis AJ: Care of the critically ill child: Intravenous alimentation. *Pediatrics* 46:456, 1970.
8. Ashcraft KW, Leape LL: Candida sepsis complicating parenteral feeding. *JAMA* 212:454, 1970.
9. Cury CR, Quie PG: Fungal septicemia in patients receiving parenteral alimentation. *N Engl J Med* 285:1221, 1971.

10. Heird WC, Driscoll JM, Schullinger JN, et al: Intravenous alimentation in pediatric patients. *J Pediatr* 80:351, 1972.

11. Sorg JL: Protocol for hyperalimentation in a community hospital. *Am Surg* 42:716, 1976.

12. Vidt DG: Use and abuse of intravenous solutions. *JAMA* 232:533, 1975.

13. Colley R, Wilson JM, Wilhem MP: Intravenous nutrition—Nursing considerations. *Issues in Comprehensive Pediatric Nursing.* 1:5, 1977.

14. Phillips KJ: Nursing care in parenteral nutrition, in Fischer JE (ed): *Total Parenteral Nutrition.* Boston, Little Brown & Co, 1976, p 101.

15. Padberg FT, Ruggiero J, Blackburn GL: Central venous catheterization for parenteral nutrition. *Ann Surg* 193:264, 1981.

16. Nehme AE: Nutritional support of the hospitalized patient: The team concept. *JAMA* 243:1906, 1980.

17. Sanders RA, Sheldon GF: Septic complications of total parenteral nutrition. *Am J Surg* 132:214, 1976.

18. Maki DG: Nosocomial bacteremia: An epidemiologic overview. *Am J Med* 70:727, 1981.

19. Ward J: TPN infection: Prevention in sick children. *ASPEN 6th Clinical Congress, San Francisco, 1982.*

20. Methods of prevention and control of nosocomial infections. Guidelines for the prevention and control of nosocomial infections. Center for Disease Control. U.S. Department of Health and Human Services/Public Health Service. March, 1981.

21. Holmes CJ, Allwood MC: The growth of micro-organisms in parenteral nutrition solutions containing amino-acids and sugars. *International Journal of Pharmacology* 2:325, 1979.

22. Melly MA, Meng HC, Schaffner W: Microbial growth in lipid emulsions used in parenteral nutrition. *Arch Surg* 110:1479, 1975.

23. Mackel DC, Maki DG, Anderson RL, et al: Nationwide epidemic of septicemia caused by contaminated intravenous products: Mechanisms of intrinsic contamination. *J Clin Microbiol* 2:486, 1975.

24. Maki DG, Rhame FS, Mackel DC: Nationwide epidemic of septicemia caused by contaminated intravenous products. I. Epidemiologic and clinical features. *Am J Med* 60:471, 1976.

25. Sanderson I, Deitel M: Intravenous hyperalimentation without sepsis. *Surg Gynecol Obstet* 136:577, 1973.

26. Debb EN, Natsios GA: Contamination of intravenous fluids by bacteria and fungi during preparation and administration. *Am J Hosp Pharm* 28:764, 1971.

27. Miller RC, Grogan JB: Incidence and source of contamination of intravenous nutritional infusion systems. *J Pediatr Surg* 8:185, 1973.

28. Miller RC, Grogan JB: Efficacy of inline bacterial filters in reducing contamination of intravenous nutritional solutions. *Am J Surg* 130:585, 1975.

29. Maki DG, Anderson RL, Shulman JA: In-use contamination of intravenous fluid. *Appl Environ Microbiol* 28:778, 1974.

30. National Coordinating Committee on Large Volume Parenterals. Recommended methods for compounding intravenous admixtures in hospitals. *Am J Hosp Pharm* 32:261, 1975.

31. Fischer GW, Hunter KW, Wilson SR, et al: Diminished bacterial defenses with Intralipid. *Lancet* 2:819, 1980.

32. Ryan JA: Complications of total parenteral nutrition, in Fischer JE (ed): *Total Parenteral Nutrition.* Boston, Little Brown & Co, 1976, p 55.

33. Ziegler M, Jakobowski D, Hoelzer D, et al: Route of pediatric parenteral nutrition: Proposed criteria revision. *J Pediatr Surg* 15:472, 1980.

34. Filler RM: Parenteral support of the surgically ill child, in Suskind RM (ed): *Textbook of Pediatric Nutrition.* New York, Raven Press, 1981, p 341.

35. Copeland EM, MacFayden BV, McGown, et al: The use of hyperalimentation in patients with potential sepsis. *Surg Gynecol Obstet* 137:377, 1974.

36. Sinatra A, Giannalia L: Septic complications, due to the catheter, in parenteral nutrition and continuous peridural anesthetic block. Cases from an intensive care center. *Minerva Anestesiol* 46:1117, 1980.

37. Filler RM, Coran AG: Total parenteral nutrition in infants and children: Central and peripheral approaches. *Surg Clin North Am* 56:395, 1976.

38. Parsa MH, Habif DV, Ferrer JM, et al: Intravenous hyperalimentation: Indications, technique, and complications. *Bull NY Acad Med* 48:920, 1972.

39. Von Meyenfeldt MM, Stapert J, De Jong PC, et al: TPN sepsis: Lack of effect of subcutaneous tunnelling of PVC catheters on sepsis rate. *JPEN* 4:514, 1980.

40. Fleming CR, Witzke DJ, Beart RW: Catheter-related complications in patients receiving home parenteral nutrition. *Ann Surg* 192:593, 1980.

41. Gatti JE, Reichek N, Mullen JL: Endocarditis complicating home hyperalimentation. *Arch Surg* 116:933, 1981.

42. Pollak PF, Kadden M, Byrne W, et al: 100 Patient years' experience with the Broviac silastic catheter for central venous nutrition. *JPEN* 5:32, 1981.

43. Michaels L, Ruebner B: Growth of bacteria in intravenous fluids. *Lancet* 1:772, 1953.

44. Maki DG, Goldman DA, Rhame FS: Infection control in intravenous therapy. *Ann Intern Med* 79:867, 1973.

45. Weyrauch HM, Bassett JB: Ascending infection in an artificial urinary tract. An experimental study. *Stanford Med Bull* 9:25, 1951.

46. Ryan JA, Abel RM, Abbott WM, et al: Catheter complications in total parenteral nutrition. A prospective study of 200 consecutive patients. *N Engl J Med* 290:757, 1974.

47. Boekman CR, Krill CE: Bacterial and fungal infections complicating parenteral alimentation in infants and children. *J Pediatr Surg* 5:117, 1970.

48. Klein JJ, Watanakunakorn C: Hospital acquired fungemia: Its natural course and clinical significance. *American Journal of Medicine* 67:51, 1979.

49. Berant M, Kristal C, Wagner Y: Candida osteomyelitis as a complication of parenteral nutrition in an infant. Successful treatment with flucytosine. *Helv Pediatr Acta* 34:155, 1979.

50. Mercer HP, Gupta JM: Candida meningitis causing aqueductal stenosis following parenteral nutrition in an infant with meconium peritonitis. *Aust Pediatr J* 14:286, 1978.

51. Businco L, Iannaccone G, Del Principe D, et al: Disseminated arthritis and osteitis by Candida albicans in a two-month-old infant receiving parenteral nutrition. *Acta Pediatr Scand* 6:393, 1977.

52. Wiley EL, Hutchins GM: Superior vena cava syndrome secondary to candida thrombophlebitis complicating parenteral alimentation. *J Pediatr* 91:977, 1977.

53. Wesley JR, Saran PA, Khalidi N, et al: *Parenteral and Enteral Nutrition Manual.* Chicago, Abbott Laboratories, 1980, p 40.

54. Forlaw L: Parenteral nutrition in the critically ill child. *Critical Care Quarterly* 3:7, 1981.

55. Grant JR: Septic and metabolic complications: Recognition and management, in Grant JR (ed): *Handbook of Total Parenteral Nutrition.* Philadelphia, WB Saunders Co, 1980, p 128.

56. Hopkins BS: Diagnosing bacterial complications of temporary central venous catheters. *Clinical Consultations.* 2:14, 1982.

57. Glynn MFX, Langer B, Jeejeebhoy KN: Therapy for thrombotic occlusion of long term intravenous alimentation catheters. *JPEN* 4:387, 1980.

Part IV
Practical Aspects

15
Monitoring the Patient on Parenteral Nutrition

John A. Kerner, Jr.

Meticulous monitoring of pediatric patients receiving parenteral nutrition (PN) is necessary to (1) detect and frequently prevent complications; (2) determine if proper and adequate nutritional ingredients are being infused; and (3) to document positive clinical benefits. To insure maximal success of this monitoring, a "team" approach utilizing the skills of a physician, pharmacist, nurse, and nutritionist is essential.

The nurse will be involved in gathering, assessing, and interpreting essential bedside data (see Chapter 17). Skilled nursing care is imperative to facilitate the maintenance of PN therapy whether delivered by central or peripheral vein. Catheter-related complications are most likely to be detected by the primary care provider, the nurse. The responses of an aware nurse can be critical in maintaining safe long-term PN.

Most metabolic complications can be prevented or detected before they cause serious consequences if an adequate biochemical monitoring regimen is rigidly followed. At many centers the pharmacy actively monitors patients receiving PN. This method has been shown to improve the patient's clinical response to PN, reduce the pharmacy's costs, and reduce patient charges for PN (1).

The monitoring approach recommended by our nutritional support service is shown in Table 1 (2). To carry out such monitoring, your clinical laboratory must be able to perform microchemistries (i.e., blood tests that can be performed on blood volumes small enough that they can be obtained by heelstick or fingerstick). Judicious ordering of blood tests is very important in infants and children because of their small blood volume. Although the monitoring listed in Table 1 is "ideal," compromises must frequently be made, especially for low birth weight infants. For example, one or two liver functions tests can be done, instead of measuring an entire panel. SGOT and direct bilirubin can be measured instead of SGOT, SGPT, alkaline phosphatase, and direct bilirubin—this will still give you a measure of hepatocyte inflammation (with the SGOT) and biliary function (with the direct

Table 1. Metabolic Monitoring During Peripheral or Central Parenteral Nutrition

Variables to be Monitored	Initial Period[a]	Later Period[b]
Growth		
Weight	daily	daily
Height	weekly	weekly
Head circumference	weekly	weekly
Skin fold thickness/mid-upper arm circumference[c]	every 2 weeks	every 2 weeks
Laboratory		
Plasma electrolytes (Na, K, Cl, CO_2)	weekly	3×/week
BUN	3×/week	2×/week
Plasma calcium, magnesium, phosphorus	2×/week	weekly
Acid-base status	3–4×/week	weekly
Albumin	2×/week	weekly
Transferrin	weekly	weekly
Nitrogen balance studies	weekly	weekly
Urine glucose[d]	2–6×/day	2×/day
Liver function tests	weekly	weekly
Hgb or Hct	2×/week	weekly
Platelet count	weekly	weekly
Fe, TIBC, retic count	as indicated	as indicated
Serum folate and vitamin B_{12}	monthly	monthly
Serum copper and zinc	monthly	monthly
Serum turbidity[e] (or nephelometry level)	daily	daily
Serum triglyceride, cholesterol and free fatty acids (or FA/SA)[e]	2×/week	weekly
Blood NH_3	2×/week	weekly
Screening for Signs of Infection		
WBC and differential	as indicated	as indicated
Cultures	as indicated	as indicated
Clinical observations (activity, vital signs, etc.)	daily	daily

SOURCE: Adapted from Levy JS, Winters RW, Heird WC: Total parenteral nutrition in pediatric patients. *Pediatrics in Review* 2:99, 1980.

[a]The period before maximum doses of glucose, amino acids, or intravenous fat are achieved, or any period of metabolic stability.

[b]The period during which the patient is in a metabolic steady state.

[c]If you have access to a trained nutritionist.

[d]If urine glucose is negative, it is safe to assume that serum glucose is not high enough to cause problems; although Dextrostix determinations are not sufficiently accurate to determine worrisome degrees of hyperglycemia, they are useful in monitoring for hypoglycemia (e.g., in the case of an infiltrated IV, or sudden cessation of a deep line, until a new line can be started).

[e]When patient is receiving intravenous fat.

bilirubin). Measurement of *direct bilirubin alone* may be an adequate liver function screen *early* in PN, since cholestasis has been shown to occur before the elevation of transaminases (3,4). It is extremely helpful to check with your hospital's clinical laboratory to find out blood volumes necessary for various blood chemistries. Minimums required at Stanford University Hospital's clinical laboratory to run various studies are shown in Table 2.

Calculations of caloric intake and total fluid intake can be performed either by the pharmacist, nutritionist, physician, or even by computer (see Chapter 25). Tangible evidence for clinical benefits from PN can best be demonstrated by improvement in nutritional assessment parameters (see Chapter 2). Flow sheets can also be devised to summarize all important monitoring data; such sheets are worthwhile for efficient decision making (Fig. 1).

Practical Guidelines

1. Before intitiating either peripheral or central PN, obtain the following baseline lab work. Follow Table 1 for monitoring frequency.
   a. CBC with platelets
   b. Urinalysis
   c. Total protein, albumin, and transferrin
   d. Calcium, phosphorus, magnesium, electrolytes, and glucose
   e. BUN
   f. SGOT, SGPT, alkaline phosphatase, total and direct bilirubin
   g. Blood ammonia
   h. Serum triglycerides, cholesterol, and free fatty acids (or FA/SA level)
   i. Serum zinc, copper, vitamin B_{12}, and folate (if you expect the patient to be on *TPN* for at least 1 month)
   j. 24 hr urine for urea nitrogen (UUN—used to help determine *nitrogen balance* (see below)
2. Keep strict intake and output records. In addition to recording volume and concentration of PN solutions infused, any enteral intake must receive equal importance—record total volumes infused, name, and concentration (i.e., 1/2 strength, 3/4 strength, etc.) of the enteral product. In this way both total fluid volume and accurate caloric intake can be properly calculated.
3. Anthropometric measurements such as triceps skinfold thickness and mid-upper arm circumference should be performed at least every 2 weeks.
4. If urinary reducing substances are present in concentrations of mg/dl, or mg% (2+ or greater), monitor Dextrostix (if Dextrostix is elevated, confirm with a blood glucose). The dextrose content of the solution may need to be decreased to prevent osmotic diuresis. A systematic review of all possible etiologies for glucosuria includes
   a. Use of steroids
   b. Use of other medications
   c. Dietary indiscretions

Table 2. Clinical Lab Pediatric Specimen Requirements[a]

Chemistry Test	Minimum Amount of Whole Blood per Test	
CHEMISTRY I SLIP		
Individual tests		
Na	0.2 ml	*or* 0.2 ml
K	0.2 ml	for both
Cl	0.2 ml	
CO$_2$	0.2 ml	
Creatinine	0.2 ml	
Glucose	0.2 ml	*or* 0.2 ml
BUN	0.2 ml	for both
Bilirubin (total)	0.2 ml	if ≤ 1 yr
Bilirubin (direct)	0.2 ml	*or* 0.2 ml for both
Albumin	0.2 ml	
Mg	0.2 ml	
P	0.2 ml	
Ca	0.3 ml	
Gamma GPT	0.4 ml	
Protein (total)	0.4 ml	if child is ≤ 1 yr
CPK	0.5 ml	
Alkaline phosphatase	0.6 ml	
Bilirubin (total)	1.2 ml	1.2 ml if child
Bilirubin (direct)	1.2 ml	≥ 1 yr for
Protein (total)	1.2 ml	any or all tests
SGOT	1.2 ml	
SGPT	1.2 ml	1.2 ml for any
Uric acid	1.2 ml	*or* all tests
LDH	1.2 ml	
Surveys		
Renal I panel	0.3 ml	*or* 0.5 ml
Electrolyte panel	0.4 ml	for both
	If child ≤ 1 yr	
Fasting metabolic	1.2 ml	If more than one
Renal II panel	1.6 ml	survey ordered,
General survey	1.8 ml	draw only the
Hepatic panel	2.0 ml	*larger* amount
	If child ≥ 1 yr	
Fasting metabolic	1.2 ml	
Renal II panel	1.2 ml	1.2 ml for any
General survey	1.2 ml	*or* all tests
Hepatic panel	1.2 ml	
HEMATOLOGY III SLIP		
Serum osmolality	0.7 ml	

[a]These are *minimum microtainer whole blood* volumes. If less blood is drawn, the test cannot be run.

	Baseline	1	2	3	4	5	6	7
Date								

Intake
ml/kg/24 hr _____
cal/kg/24 hr _____
Protein/kg/24 hr _____
Non-nitrogen cal/
  nitrogen grams _____

Nutritional Assessment
Weight _____
Length/head circumference _____
Triceps skinfold thickness _____
Mid-upper arm circumference/arm
  muscle circumference _____
Skin testing (+/−) _____
Transferrin _____
Nitrogen balance _____
Absolute lymphocyte count _____

Lab Assessment
Na/K _____
Cl/CO_2 _____
BUN/creat _____
Mg/glucose _____
Ca/P _____
Folate/B_{12} _____
Zn/Cu _____
TGL/chol _____
FFA (FA/SA) _____
WBC _____
Poly/band/eos _____
Hgb/Hct _____
MCV/retic _____
Fe/TIBC _____
SGOT/SGPT _____
Alk phos/GGTP _____
T. bili/D. bili _____

Figure 1 Monitoring sheet for peripheral or central parenteral nutrition.

   d. Error in PN delivery rate
   e. *Possible sepsis*
5. If a PN line infiltrates, an alternate source of dextrose and fluids must be provided immediately PO or IV to avoid hypoglycemia.
6. When the decision is made to discontinue PN on an elective basis, PN should be tapered over at least 1–2 days. The patient's enteral intake at the time of cessation should ideally provide at least maintenance fluids and at least three fourths of the daily caloric needs.
7. Following each increase in the dose of intravenous fat (IVF) a serum triglyc-

eride level should be obtained to document tolerance. After tolerance has been established, the IVF dose can be increased again.

8. A 24 hr urine collection for UUN is necessary to determine nitrogen balance. UUN is measured in mg/100 ml.

9. Nitrogen balance is determined in the following manner (5):

$$\text{N}_2 \text{ balance} = \frac{\text{grams of protein (intake)}}{6.25} - (\text{UUN} + 3)$$

Protein intake should include grams of protein provided by oral or enteral feeds *plus* those provided by IV amino acids.

   a. Dividing by 6.25 converts the protein intake into grams of nitrogen.

   b. UUN in this equation is expressed in grams (e.g., if UUN = 500 mg/100 ml or 5000 mg/liter and patient's 24 hr urine is 2 liters, UUN = 10,000 mg or 10 g/24 hr).

   c. The constant of 3 in the equation corrects for non-urea nitrogen losses (~2 g/day), fecal losses (~1 g/day), and skin, hair, and nail losses (~0.2 g/day). This constant has been established in adult balance studies. *It is not clear that the same constant can be used for premature infants or young children* (please see Chapter 2 for further discussion).

References

1. Mutchie KD, Smith KA, MacKay MW, et al: Pharmacist monitoring of parenteral nutrition: Clinical and cost effectiveness. *Am J Hosp Pharm* 36:785, 1979.

2. Levy JS, Winters RW, Heird WC: Total parenteral nutrition in pediatric patients, *Pediatrics in Review* 2:99, 1980.

3. Inwood R, Vileisis R, Hunt CE: Hepatic cholestasis associated with parenteral nutrition in infancy: Incidence and clinical utility of liver function tests. *J Pediatr* 96:158, 1980.

4. Postuma R, Trevenen CL: Liver disease in infants receiving total parenteral nutrition. *Pediatrics* 63:110, 1979.

5. Grant A: *Nutritional assessment guidelines.* Berkeley, Calif, Cutter Laboratories, 1979, p 40.

16
Writing Parenteral Nutrition Orders

Robert L. Poole

Parenteral nutrition (PN) solutions can be ordered using either of two basic formats, tailored or standardized. Tailored solutions are formulated specifically to meet the daily nutritional requirements of the individual patient, whereas standardized solutions are designed to provide a formulation that meets the majority of the nutritional needs of those patients with stable biochemical and metabolic parameters. Both of these order methods have advantages and disadvantages associated with their use.

Standardized Solutions

A standardized PN solution contains fixed amounts of each component per unit volume. Filler et al. (1) pioneered the use of this type of solution in pediatric patients. More recently, Filler's group (2) has modified their formulations, employing primarily six standard solutions: two premature infant formulas, central and peripheral solutions for infants and young children aged 0–7 years, and central and peripheral solutions for children and adolescents aged 7–18 years. Standardized solutions have been used quite successfully in the older pediatric and adult patients (3,4). There are several advantages associated with standardized solutions. (1) They are easy for the physician to order; that is, the type of solution, either peripheral or central, and the infusion rate are the only two items that need to be ordered. (2) All essential nutrients are included in fixed amounts in the solution, thus eliminating the chance for inadvertent omissions. (3) The pharmacist spends less time labeling and calculating formulation worksheets through the use of preprinted labels and a standard formulation worksheet for the actual compounding of the solution. This also reduces the potential for pharmacy errors in labeling and compounding. The major disadvantage of standardized solutions is their lack of patient specificity. Therefore, they may not meet the nutritional needs of the critically ill patient whose metabolic capacity is impaired or whose electrolyte status is in a state of flux.

Tailored Solutions

Tailored PN solutions are patient-specific formulations designed to meet the nutritional requirements peculiar to each patient. In support of tailored parenteral nutrient regimens, Dudrick stated,"No single parenteral regimen could be ideal for all patients with a wide variety of pathological processes, nor for all age groups, nor for the same patient during all aspects of a particular disorder" (5). With advances in nutrition research on the requirements of patients with various diseases, Wood concluded that patient-specific formulas are likely to be necessary in order to provide optimal nutritional support (6). The Committee on Nutrition of the Mother and Preschool Child recently stated,"An absolute requirement for successful parenteral nutrition is a flexible system for mixing the nutrient infusates" (7). The primary advantage of tailored parenteral nutrition solutions is flexibility. Each solution is specially formulated for an individual patient and can be altered as that patient's nutritional needs and metabolic, electrolyte, or clinical status changes.

The use of tailored PN solutions assumes the physician is knowledgeable in all aspects of the nutritional support of their patient. The individual ordering of each component, which is necessary with patient-specific solutions, may be viewed as a potential disadvantage to the use of this format. The time involved in calculations and label preparation by the pharmacy service is an additional disadvantage; however, computer programs are available to expedite these pharmacy functions and to help eliminate this costly time factor (see Chapter 25).

Orders for PN solutions must be written clearly to avoid confusion in their interpretation and errors in their compounding. The order for a tailored parenteral nutrition solution requires the careful analysis of biochemical parameters and of fluid, electrolyte, and nutrient requirements. Table 1 contains the components of PN solutions that we currently believe are essential for growth, repair, and normal metabolic functions. Reference to a detailed PN protocol (8) and the use of a standardized daily PN order sheet can facilitate the ordering of these complex solutions.

The purpose of the detailed PN order sheet we employ (Fig. 1) is to aid the clinician in producing a complete order that avoids omissions that could lead to serious electrolyte abnormalities and nutrient deficiency states. This order sheet also assists the pharmacy in the accurate preparation of PN solutions by providing the physician with a standard outline. Thus, all orders generated by the physician will have the same format for the pharmacist's interpretation. An additional function of the PN order sheet is to familiarize housestaff physicians with the essential components of PN solutions and to provide them with protocol recommendations based on current literature.

The following is a step-by-step approach for the writing of tailored PN orders utilizing the order sheet illustrated in Figure 1.

1. Enter the patient's most recent body weight in kilograms.
2. Determine the patient's 24-hour fluid requirements in ml/kg/day.
3. Calculate the daily carbohydrate, protein, electrolyte, mineral, vitamin, and trace element requirements based on the patient's clinical status, current laboratory parameters, and protocol recommendations.
4. Once appropriate quantities of each nutrient component have been calculated,

Table 1. Essential Components of PN Solutions

Carbohydrate
Dextrose
Protein
Crystalline amino acids
Electrolytes
Sodium
Potassium
Chloride
Calcium
Magnesium
Phosphorus
Vitamins
Multivitamins
Vitamin K
Vitamin B_{12}
Folate
Trace Elements
Zinc
Copper
Chromium
Manganese
Fat emulsion[a]

[a]Fat emulsions must be ordered in a separate bottle from dextrose–amino acid solution

enter the amounts in the corresponding areas of the order sheet. When phosphorus is added to PN solutions, it must be ordered in millimoles to avoid any possible confusion in compounding (9,10). Special attention must be given to the increased calcium and phosphorus requirements of the preterm infant. Calcium and phosphorus may form an insoluble precipitate when mixed in PN solutions in the amounts exceeding critical concentrations (for further discussion see Chapter 11).

5. Intravenous fat emulsion is available in either 10% or 20% solutions. Fat emulsion should be added to the PN regimen when indicated (see Chapter 7).

6. To calculate the total caloric intake, the following factors should be used: dextrose, 3.4 cal/g; fat emulsion—10% solution contains 1.1 cal/ml; 20% solution contains 2.0 cal/ml. Protein contains 4 cal/g but is intended for protein synthesis and not considered to be broken down as a source of calories.

Standardized and tailored solutions each have their place in the provision of nutritional support for pediatric patients. Advances in the area of parenteral nutrition may demonstrate the need for exclusive use of tailored solutions. Dice et al. (11) employing tailored PN solutions in neonates, reported that "close monitoring provided a greater mean daily weight gain, allowed a greater amount of nutrients to be provided, and was cost effective when compared with the use of a standardized solution."

The writing of patient-specific PN orders can be facilitated through the use of a standardized order sheet. The stepwise approach to writing orders presented above

Patient Name:
Medical Record Number:

STANFORD UNIVERSITY HOSPITAL
STANFORD UNIVERSITY MEDICAL CENTER
Stanford, California 94305
PHYSICIAN'S ORDERS
FOR
PEDIATRIC PARENTERAL NUTRITION
—

addressograph stamp

A. Please send TPN orders to the Pharmacy before 11:00 A.M. DAILY.
B. Orders cannot be processed without the patient's current weight.
C. Order all additives on a 24-hour basis; i.e., mEq/Kg/day, mM/Kg/day,
   ml/day, ml/Kg/day, etc.

PERIPHERAL___or CENTRAL___TPN LINE(check one)   Today's WEIGHT____Kg
DATE ORDERED___/____/___(month/day/year)   Next Bottle #_____
DUE DATE___/___/___(month/day/year)   TIME DUE_____(AM PM)
TOTAL FLUID INTAKE (ml/Kg/day)_____
AMOUNT OF FAT EMULSION (gm/Kg/day)_____
CONCENTRATION OF FAT EMULSION_____10%_____20%(check one)

How many IV lines exist which will not be used for TPN?_____
Enter their flow rates (ml/hr):
(1) Arterial line ☐ 0.45%NaCl ☐ 0.9%NaCl(check one) _____
(2)_____(3)_____(4)_____
If taking enteral feeds, complete the following section: Check one
____1. Total fluids administered as: parenteral and advancing
        enteral. (Additives are calculated as if total fluids were
        given parenterally)
____2. Total fluids administered as: parenteral and fixed enteral.
        (Additives are distributed in parenteral fluids only;
        ignores electrolyte content of enteral fluids)
____3. Total fluids ordered will be administered parenterally.
        (Enteral feeds will be given in addition to the total
        parenteral fluids)
Enter Amount_____(mls), Frequency:q_____hrs, & Calories/Ounce_____

Enter AMINO ACID (gm/Kg/day)_____   Enter DEXTROSE CONCENTRATION_____

TODAY'S ADDITIVES   PROTOCOL RECOMMENDATION

TRACE ELEMENTS AND VITAMINS:
1. PEDIATRIC TRACE
    ELEMENTS*   ____ml/Kg   1.0 ml/Kg/day (weight <20 Kg)
2. ADULT TRACE ELEMENTS* ____ml/day 5.0 ml/Kg/day (weight >20 Kg)
3. MULTIPLE VITAMIN   1.0 ml/day – infants
    INJECTION   ____ml/day   2.0 ml/day – older children
4. FOLIC ACID   ____mcg/day   50 mcg/day – infants
                                    1 mg/day – older children
5. ZINC (additional) ____mcg/Kg/day 200 mcg/Kg/day – Premies
6. VITAMIN K   ____mg/day   0.5 mg/day
7. VITAMIN B-12   ____mcg/day   5.0 mcg/day
    ELECTROLYTES, HEPARIN AND INSULIN:
1. PHOSPHORUS*   ____mM/Kg/day 1-2 mM/Kg/day
2. SODIUM   ____mEq/Kg/day 2-3 mEq/Kg/day

3. POTASSIUM   ____mEq/Kg/day 2-3 mEq/Kg/day
4. ACETATE   ____mEq/Kg/day 2-3 mEq/Kg/day
5. MAGNESIUM   ____mEq/Kg/day 0.25 – 0.5 mEq/Kg/day
6. CALCIUM GLUCONATE* ____mg/Kg/day 200 – 500 mg/Kg/day
7. HEPARIN   ____Units/ml   0.5 - 1.0 Units/ml
8. INSULIN   ____Units/ml   ---------------------------
9. OTHER (specify)   ____   ---------------------------

---

*DO NOT EXCEED: Pediatric Trace Elements   20 ml/day
                 Adult Trace Elements   5 ml/day
                 Calcium Gluconate 400 mg and P 2 mM per 100 ml

_____MD

_____RN

Figure 1 Physician order sheet for pediatric parenteral nutrition.

236

should provide the patient with a solution that contains total nutritional support. Once the final PN formulation has been ordered, a computer can expedite the calculation, preparation, and labeling required in the pharmacy (12) (see Chapter 25).

References

1. Filler RM, Eraklis AJ, Rubin VG, et al: Long-term total parenteral nutrition in infants. *N Engl J Med* 281:589, 1969.

2. Filler RM: Parenteral support of the surgically ill child, in Suskind R (ed): *Textbook of Pediatric Nutrition.* New York, Raven Press, 1981, p 341.

3. Sceppa JM, Barza M, Leape LL, et al: Metabolic abnormalities associated with a standardized TPN formulation. *JPEN* 1:31A, 1977.

4. Seltzer MH, Asaadi M, Coco A, et al: The use of a simplified standardized hyperalimentation formula. *JPEN* 2:28, 1978.

5. Dudrick SJ: Presidential address: The common denominator and the bottom line. *JPEN* 2:13, 1978.

6. Wood WA: Patient-specific total parenteral nutrient formulas. *Am J Hosp Pharm* 35:1068, 1978.

7. Committee on Nutrition of the Mother and Preschool Child, National Research Council: Nutritional requirements of newborn infants. *Nutrition Services in Perinatal Care.* Washington, DC, National Academy Press, 1981, p 48.

8. Kerner JA, Sunshine P: Parenteral alimentation. *Semin Perinatol* 3:417, 1979.

9. Turco SJ, Burke WA: Methods of ordering and use of intravenous phosphate. *Hosp Pharm* 10:320, 1975.

10. Hermann JJ: Phosphate: Its valence and methods of quantification in parenteral solutions. *Drug Intelligence and Clinical Pharmacy* 13:579, 1979.

11. Dice JE, Burckart GJ, Woo JT, et al: Standardized versus pharmacist-monitored individualized parenteral nutrition in low-birth-weight infants. *Am J Hosp Pharm* 38:1487, 1981.

12. Giacoia GP, Warden LK, Canfield BG: Computerized total parenteral nutrition formulas for newborn infants. *Am J Hosp Pharm* 37:22, 1980.

17
Nursing Care of the Pediatric Patient on Parenteral Nutrition

Alice I. Morrow
Louise Poirier-Kerner
Amy S. Andolina
M. Eileen Walsh

Successful delivery of pediatric parenteral nutrition (PN) is directly dependent on the quality of nursing care. Nursing responsibilities begin once the medical decision for PN has been made. Both the family and the child will require education and support: therefore, the nurse should have a thorough understanding of PN. This chapter describes basic nursing care standards for PN that are applicable for nurses working in a variety of institutional settings. Nursing responsibilities to be discussed include

1. Intravenous (IV) catheters for PN
2. Central venous catheter placement
3. IV infusion devices
4. Equipment needed for PN
5. Monitoring a pediatric patient on PN
6. Dressing changes and catheter care during PN
7. Approach to complications of PN
8. Associated aspects of nursing care
9. Transition from parenteral to enteral feedings
10. Central venous catheter removal

Intravenous Catheters Used for Parenteral Nutrition

Many types of IV catheters are used to administer PN to pediatric patients. Both the selection of the catheter and the site of insertion (i.e., central venous versus peripheral) should be based on the following:

1. The nature of the infusate (i.e., concentrations of greater than 12.5% dextrose in water must be administered through a central vein)
2. The age and size of the patient
3. The estimated length of time PN will be required
4. The level of expertise of the individual performing the catheter insertion

Institutional experience and familiarity with infusion catheters also play an important role in catheter type and insertion site selection.

PERIPHERAL PN

Peripheral PN can be administered by either a stainless steel needle with plastic wings ("butterfly" $\frac{1}{2}$–$1\frac{1}{4}$ inch length with 17–25 gauge inner diameter) or a polyethylene over-the-needle catheter (Intracath 1–$5\frac{1}{2}$ inch length with 12–22 gauge inner diameter). The polyethylene catheters tend to be more stable and reliable; however, they can be more difficult to insert in the patient with poor venous access. The venipuncture site should be prepared with an iodophor solution and allowed to dry for 2 minutes. Once the catheter is inserted, it should be taped, while allowing for easy inspection of the site. At the insertion site, an iodophor ointment should be applied and covered with a gauze dressing. The site should be examined and redressed daily.

Peripheral PN catheters are valuable because they are less frequently implicated in the septic and thrombotic complications associated with central venous catheters. However, the logistics of locating viable IV sites, constantly restarting peripheral IVs, and dealing with the inherent problems of a peripheral IV can be prohibitive on busy pediatric units. One possible solution for long-term peripheral PN access in neonates has been described by Tanswell (1). Using a 19-gauge scalp needle with the tubing removed, a 10 cm silicone rubber tubing (0.0635 cm outer diameter) is threaded 3 cm into a peripheral vein. The distal tip of the catheter is identified by palpation and marked with a grease pencil. Redness or swelling are indications for immediate catheter removal. After 250 catheterizations over 3 years on infants as small as 900 g, Tanswell's technique caused no local or systemic catheter-related complications. The catheters were in place for up to 37 days, with a mean of 9 days (1).

Central Venous PN

To achieve a high caloric intake, a hyperosmolar infusate should be delivered through a central, large-bore vein with high volume blood flow to minimize the risk of venous thrombosis and phlebitis. There are polyvinyl, polyethylene, and silastic catheters available for central venous PN administration. The polyvinyl or polyethylene inside-the-needle catheters (INCs) are available in 14–19 gauge with a needle length of $1\frac{1}{2}$–2 inches and a catheter length of 8–36 inches. These catheters are the most likely to cause catheter embolism if pulled back over the needle. Silastic catheters have been used effectively in pediatric central venous PN for many years. They are adapted to the IV infusion system with a blunt needle. Complications with this method are leakage or perforation of the catheter. Silastic catheters are preferred to polyvinyl or polyethylene catheters; they have a high degree of flexibility,

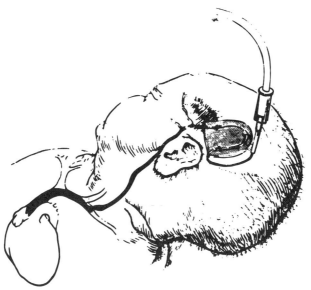

Figure 1 Percutaneous catheter placement. (Riordan TP: Placement of central venous lines in the premature infant. *JPEN* 3:381, 1979. Copyright © 1979, Williams Wilkins Co. Reproduced with permission.)

a soft nonwetting surface that works to resist clotting, durability, and decreased association with catheter-related sepsis and thrombophlebitis (2). Two unique types of silastic catheters available are the Hickman and Broviac catheters, which are discussed later in the chapter.

Placement of the central venous PN catheters is by either a percutaneous or a venous cutdown technique. The choice of sites for insertion includes the scalp, common facial, internal jugular, external jugular, cephalic, and subclavian veins.

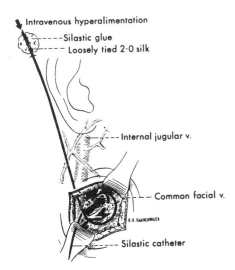

Figure 2 Common facial vein catheterization. (Vain NE, Georgeson KE, Cha CC, Swarner OW: Central parenteral alimentation in newborn infants: A new technique for catheter placement. *J Pediatr* 93:865, 1978. Copyright © 1978, CV Mosby Co. Reproduction with permission.)

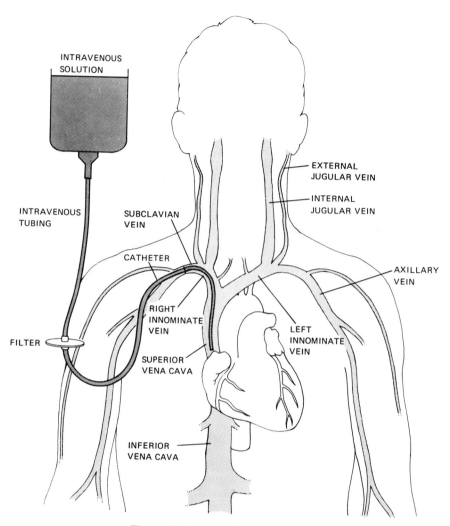

Figure 3 Anatomy of venous access.

Examples of both a percutaneous and a cutdown technique for infants follow. Riordan (3) described a percutaneous technique by which a 19-gauge "butterfly" needle is inserted into a scalp vein and a silastic catheter (0.030 × 0.060 mm) is threaded through the needle into the superior vena cava (Fig. 1). Vain et al. (4) reported a cutdown technique for catheter placement in neonates that appears to lower the frequency of superior vena cava obstruction, a frequent complication of central PN. In Vain and co-workers' technique, a catheter is inserted by a cutdown into the common facial vein, and a portion of the catheter is looped into place in the subcutaneous neck tissue before advancement of both ends of the catheter (Fig. 2). The loop of the catheter allows free movement of an infant's head, thereby preventing "pistoning" of the end of the catheter in the superior vena cava and possible thrombosis.

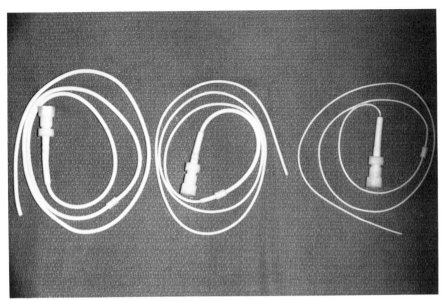

Figure 4 Central venous catheters. Left to right: Hickman, Adult Broviac, and Pediatric Broviac catheters. (Courtesy of Dr. Stephen Shochat.)

Once the central venous catheter is inserted, it is advanced into the superior vena cava to its junction with the right atrium (Fig. 3). It is desirable for the catheter to float in the superior vena cava instead of in the right atrium. Placement of the catheter in the atrium can stimulate cardiac arrythmias or cause the catheter to incorporate itself in the endocardium. It is possible to provide better catheter stability and to decrease the risk of infection by subcutaneously tunneling the catheter of choice to a distant exit site.

Two specially designed catheters for long term PN are the Hickman and Broviac catheters. The catheter may be placed by either a cutdown incision or a percutaneous method (5). After the catheter is placed, a separate incision is made on the chest or abdomen so that the distal end of the catheter can be directed through a subcutaneous tunnel between the two incisions. The catheter is then trimmed to an appropriate estimated length so it will terminate in the superior vena cava. The Hickman and Broviac catheters differ from the traditional silastic catheter in the following ways: (1) The portion of the catheter extending from the patient as well as the catheter neck is reinforced with Teflon in order to reduce the risk of cracking and breakage. (2) The distal end of the catheter has a Luer-Lok connector to enable snug insertion of IV tubing and to allow secure screw-capping of the catheter when not in use. (3) A Dacron cuff attached to the midportion of the catheter is placed subcutaneously at the catheter exit site; this stimulates the formation of dense fibrous adhesions that anchor the catheter securely and create a barrier for ascending bacteria. This process takes approximately two weeks, at which time the cutaneous sutures at the exit site can be removed. (4) The catheter is constructed so that it may be spliced if the external portion becomes cracked or cut, or if the adapter piece disconnects. The manufacturers provide a special repair kit (6) which is essential to have on hand.

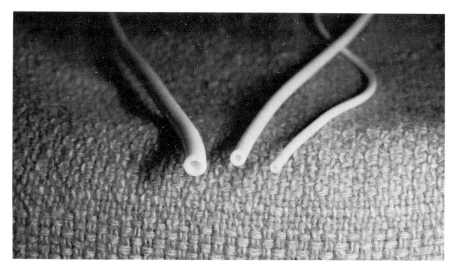

Figure 5 Catheter lumens. Left to right: Hickman, Adult Broviac, and Pediatric Broviac catheters. (Courtesy of Dr. Stephen Shochat.)

The Hickman and Broviac catheters are similarly constructed, differing mainly in internal diameter. The Hickman catheter has a 1.6 mm internal diameter; the Broviac catheter is available in pediatric and adult sizes of 0.7 mm and 1.0 mm, (Figs. 4 and 5). The larger lumen of the Hickman catheter does facilitate collection of blood samples and infusion of multiple parenteral therapies. (This practice is not recommended if the catheter is being used to deliver PN.) Patient size and therapy needs are determining factors in the choice of catheter.

After the insertion of any type of central venous catheter, chest films are mandatory to confirm proper placement and to rule out mechanical complications secondary to catheter placement. Each catheter type is radiopaque; catheter visualization can be made more distinct after injection with renografin-60. Infusion of hypertonic PN solutions or fat emulsions should not be initiated until the film has been interpreted. During the interim, an isotonic solution should be infused slowly.

Central Venous Catheter Placement

Depending on institutional protocol, central venous catheterization is performed either in the operating room or on the patient care unit. The placement of a central venous catheter to deliver PN can be facilitated by a nurse familiar with the procedure. The nurse will be expected to explain the procedure to the patient, to assemble the equipment, to assist the physician, to lend support to the patient, and to recognize and assist with any associated immediate complications (Table 1).

Due to the risk of septic complications, the catheter placement should be treated as an aseptic surgical procedure, requiring masks, gowns, and gloves. Complications can be minimized or prevented with strict sterile technique, proper equipment

Table 1. Complications of Pediatric Parenteral Nutrition

Complications	Clinical Findings	Medical and Nursing Interventions
CENTRAL CATHETER RELATED: INSERTION COMPLICATIONS		Observance of strict aseptic technique; insertion by a skilled physician; selection of the most appropriate insertion site. Proper patient positioning and preparation will help to minimize insertion complications.
Pneumothorax	Sudden tachypnea and respiratory distress, decreased breath sounds, cyanosis, pain, decreased cardiac output, and shift in location of heart sounds. Rarely, a slow-leaking pneumothorax may present at a later stage with similar findings.	STAT chest film; discontinue infusion; closed-tube thoracostomy after needle thoracentesis; symptomatic treatment with oxygen; place patient in high-Fowler's position; provide emotional support. Follow-up films within 24–48 hr may be needed to assess an insidious pneumothorax.
Hydrothorax	Tachypnea, pain, cyanosis, dyspnea, decreased cardiac output.	STAT chest films; discontinue infusion; closed-tube thoracostomy after needle thoracentesis; symptomatic treatment. Morbidity from hydrothorax can be minimized by slow infusion of an isotonic solution after catheter insertion until placement is verified by chest x-ray films.
Arterial puncture	Rapid hematoma formation, internal or external bleeding at insertion site, pallor, weak pulse, tachycardia, hypotension, upper airway impingement if trachea is compressed.	Remove catheter; direct firm pressure for 15 min or until hemostasis is achieved; Hct assessment is indicated if blood loss appears significant; prepare for vascular volume replacement.
Thoracic duct injury	Lymphous drainage from the insertion site. Chylothorax resembles hydrothorax in symptoms	Remove catheter; perform needle thoracentesis and closed-tube thoracostomy for chylothorax. The

Table 1. (Continued)

Complications	Clinical Findings	Medical and Nursing Interventions
	except drainage is milky white on aspiration.	patient with hepatic disease has an enlarged thoracic duct due to lymphatic flow alteration; therefore, subclavian insertion should not be attempted on the left side.[a]
Embolism Air	Sudden respiratory difficulty, tachypnea, cyanosis, chest pain, apnea, hypotension, cardiac arrest, aphasia, seizures, hemiplegia, coma; "mill-wheel churning" found over anterior precordium on auscultation.	Immediately clamp the catheter; place patient in a left lateral Trendelenburg position to raise the right side of the heart.[b] Prompt syringe aspiration of the air through the catheter; administer oxygen; resume infusion once line is clear. To avoid this complication, instruct the child to perform the Valsalva maneuver when vein is cannulated and each time the catheter is open to air.[a] Tape and/or Luer-Lok all connections securely; use an air eliminating IV filter.
Embolism Catheter	Chest pain, cardiac arrhythmias.	Chest films; transvenous retrieval of broken piece of catheter with guidewire snare. Prevent by withdrawing the needle simultaneously with the catheter to avoid the needle cutting off the catheter tip.[a]
Cardiac perforation with tamponade	Tachycardia, gallop rhythm, muffled heart sounds, neck vein distention, decreased cardiac output with hypotension.	Remove catheter; perform pericardial tap if patient is critically symptomatic; may require surgical intervention for performance of pericardial window and mediastinal drainage tube placement.

Table 1. (Continued)

Complications	Clinical Findings	Medical and Nursing Interventions
Brachial plexus injury	Tingling of fingers, pain shooting down arm, paralysis.	Remove catheter. Prevent with skilled insertion technique.
CENTRAL CATHETER (CC) OR PERIPHERAL LINE (PL): MAINTENANCE COMPLICATIONS		When catheter removal is indicated during maintenance PN therapy, an alternate source of intravenous or oral fluids and dextrose must immediately be provided.

Thrombosis/thrombophlebitis and phlebitis
  Central vein
    Thrombosis
	Frequently patients are asymptomatic; may develop edema of the involved arm, neck, and face (superior vena cava syndrome); may rarely present with signs and symptoms of pulmonary embolism (shortness of breath, chest pain, cyanosis, tachycardia, rales with or without pleural friction rub).	Notify physician; remove catheter, culture catheter tip, and begin treatment with intravenous heparin (some centers will instill urokinase to dissolve the thrombus, avoiding catheter removal, in selected cases). (See discussion in Chapter 12.) May decrease incidence of this complication with: use of nonreactive silicone catheters; maintenance of adequate hydration; prophylactic use of heparin in PN solution (Standard: 1 unit heparin/ml PN solution).

Thrombophlebitis (partial or complete occlusion of a vein by a thrombus with secondary inflammation of the vein wall) —may also occur with PL use.	Patient may be febrile and may have symptoms of central vein thrombosis; insertion site may show signs of inflammation.	Decrease incidence of this complication as described above. Incidence of phlebitis is reduced in PL use in patients receiving concomitant IV fat emulsion. For treatment, consult your surgeon.
Peripheral vein Phlebitis	Pain, tenderness, inflammation, skin discoloration, redness, heat and burning along the course of vein.	Remove IV; initiate comfort measures, e.g., local cold then heat application. Restart IV using stainless steel needle.

Table 1. (Continued)

Complications	Clinical Findings	Medical and Nursing Interventions
Bacteremia and Septicemia (seen almost exclusively with CC use)	Glucosuria, fever, leukocytosis with a shift to the left; possible lethargy, abdominal distention, vomiting, hypothermia.	Thoroughly examine the patient; obtain cultures of peripheral blood, urine, stool, and throat for bacteria and fungus; obtain cultures of tracheal aspirate and CSF, and chest film when appropriate; culture infusate and infusion tubing. If after 24–48 hr the catheter seems the most likely source, obtain blood culture from the line, remove the catheter, and send the tip for culture. The suspicion of sepsis usually requires broad-spectrum IV antibiotic coverage until sepsis has been ruled out or proven by culture. The Center for Disease Control found that 54% of TPN septicemias are fungal, usually *Candida*. Gram-positive and to a lesser extent, gram-negative bacteria may cause PN related septicemia.
Fungemia (seen almost exclusively with CC use)	Fever, lethargy, failure to gain weight; positive blood culture and/or positive site culture; unusual symptoms of pain in the eye, veils and spots in front of the eye, loss of vision, eyes may be red and tender. *Note*: Visual symptoms may be a latent finding related to PN fungemia.	Remove catheter; begin course of IV amphotericin B depending on clinical course; oral course of nystatin is indicated if *Candida* is isolated from the stool or mouth.
Catheter insertion site inflammation (seen with both CC and PL)	Local erythema, drainage, pain, cellulitis.	Culture and sensitivity of exudate. If patient is not septic, catheter removal is not mandatory but the situation should be followed closely to rule out progression of the infection. Broad spectrum

Table 1. (Continued)

Complications	Clinical Findings	Medical and Nursing Interventions
		antibiotic coverage may be indicated until culture results are available. Vigorous skin care of the cellulitis site.
Perforation of central veins	Rapidly developing evidence of hypovolemic shock secondary to blood loss (pallor, thirst, restlessness, weak pulse, tachycardia, hypotension); possible visible hematoma formation at infusion site.	STAT chest films; apply firm local pressure over neck veins if hematoma formation is visible; remove catheter. Surgical evacuation of hematoma may be indicated for vascular repair. Prepare for vascular volume replacement; type and crossmatch for blood and transfuse as necessary.
Air embolism (see insertion complications and interventions) seen almost exclusively with CC use		Great care should be exercised in maintaining integrity of connections in the PN administration system to prevent this complication (e.g., taping connections lengthwise, Luer-Lok connections, etc.). Always use Valsalva maneuver when appropriate; if air emboli are suspected, place in the left Lateral Trendelenburg position.
Extravasation of the infusate (seen with both CC and PL)	Swelling, edema, pain, and coolness over catheter site or of head, neck, face; possible vesicles; discoloration and/or sloughing of skin at the infusion site.	Discontinue infusion; remove catheter; symptomatic management of skin as per institutional protocol (e.g., steroid creams, Silvadene, split-thickness skin grafting after debridement if skin damage is severe).
METABOLIC COMPLICATIONS (Similar in both central and peripheral PN with the exception of problems of		The metabolic complications outlined below include only the most common relating to glucose and electrolyte imbal-

Table 1. (Continued)

Complications	Clinical Findings	Medical and Nursing Interventions
marked hyperglycemia associated with hypertonic dextrose given by central lines.)		ances. These complications can be avoided or detected early by routine monitoring (as described in Chapter 15); more extensive descriptions of various metabolic complications of PN are present in each of the chapters on the PN nutrients.
Glucose Hyperglycemia	Glucosuria ≥ 2+ using Clinitest tabs; polyuria; polydipsia; clinical evidence of dehydration (dry, hot, flushed skin, fatigue).	Identify the etiology of the hyperglycemia. May reflect the development of infection, increased stress, too great a dextrose load, alterations in rate of infusion of the dextrose–amino acid solution, or the use of glucocorticoids. Therapy is dependent on the cause and should include evaluation for presence of sepsis, decrease in either rate or concentration of dextrose infusion, assessment of level of hydration and possible infusion of isotonic solution to rehydrate if indicated. Generally, insulin is not required in pediatric patients in the management of hyperglycemia. An appropriate decrease in the dextrose load is effective. Constant nursing monitoring of the infusion rate is critical in avoiding hyperglycemia. Search carefully for other signs and symptoms of infection.
Hyperosmolar nonketotic dehydration	Persistent glucosuria without ketosis, hyperglycemia, serum osmolality > 350 mg%, confusion, dehydration, seizures, coma.	The syndrome should be recognized and treated before neurologic findings are present. Treatment: discontinuation of the dextrose—amino acid solution; rehydration with 5%

Table 1. (Continued)

Complications	Clinical Findings	Medical and Nursing Interventions
		dextrose and hypotonic saline; insulin in small doses to gradually reduce blood sugar (rapid reduction in blood glucose can precipitate cerebral edema); monitoring of serum glucose, osmolality, sodium and potassium, and urine glucose, ketones, specific gravity, and volume.
Hypoglycemia	Serum glucose < 50 mg%, muscle weakness, diaphoresis, nervous instability, trembling, faintness, headache, hunger, palpitations, diplopia, confusion.	Hypoglycemia usually occurs secondary to a sudden drop in the concentration or rate of the dextrose infusion. Can be caused by interrupted or too rapid weaning of the dextrose infusion. Prevention of this problem: meticulous monitoring of the infusion system; careful tapering of the concentration and rate of the dextrose infusion. Clinical suspicion of hypoglycemia should be validated with an immediate Dextrostix test followed, if necessary, by a serum glucose test. Treat hypoglycemia with a bolus of a 25% glucose solution IV or oral glucose (if possible). Hypoglycemic episodes may cause permanent neurologic deficits when prolonged, unrecognized, or untreated. Whenever a hypertonic PN infusion is disrupted, an alternate source of dextrose must be provided immediately, either orally (if possible) or IV as $D_{10}W$.

Table 1. (Continued)

Complications	Clinical Findings	Medical and Nursing Interventions
Electrolyte and mineral imbalance		Corrections of an electrolyte imbalance may require concomitant correction of another electrolyte because of their interdependence. Use of IV, IM, or oral route is determined by the patient's condition and the acuteness of the situation.
Hypokalemia	Vomiting, paralytic ileus, mental clouding, lethargy, weak pulse, faint heartsounds, hypotension, generalized weakness, diminished reflexes. ECG reveals U waves, low voltage T waves, and prolonged QT interval. A urine K^+ concentration of ≤ 10 mEq/liter suggests severe K^+ depletion.	Obtain laboratory confirmation. Institute IV or oral replacement therapy. If IV bolus used, monitor ECG pattern for arrhythmias. Reevaluate maintenance therapy. Obtain lab determinations prn.
Hyperkalemia	Diarrhea, colic, nausea (all reflect GI hyperactivity), dizziness, paresthesia, muscle weakness, cramps, pain. ECG reveals high peaked T waves, increased PR interval and widened QRS, depressed ST segment, atrioventricular or intraventricular heart block. If serum K^+ is ≥ 7.5 mEq/liter, there is a danger of heart block, ventricular flutter, and ventricular fibrillation.	Obtain laboratory confirmation. Eliminate sources of K^+ intake. Patient may need: Kayexalate enemas; IV insulin plus dextrose administration; extrarenal dialysis. Monitor ECG pattern. Obtain lab determinations prn.
Hypocalcemia	Abdominal cramps, paresthesias, carpopedal spasm, positive Trousseau's sign, positive Chvostek's sign, hyperactive reflexes, tetany, twitching; ECG reveals prolonged QT interval relative to rate.	Obtain laboratory confirmation. Institute replacement therapy IV or orally. If IV bolus used, monitor ECG pattern for arrhythmias. May need to correct another electrolyte imbalance concomitantly. Obtain lab determinations prn.

Table 1. (Continued)

Complications	Clinical Findings	Medical and Nursing Interventions
Hypercalcemia	Muscle hypertonicity, decreased DTRs, deep bony pain, flank pain secondary to renal calculi, polydipsia, polyuria, azotemia, thirst, nausea, vomiting, anorexia, constipation, dehydration, mental confusion, lethargy, coma, arrhythmias, extraskeletal calcification.	Obtain laboratory confirmation. Eliminate sources of Ca^{2+} intake; consider use of steroids. Obtain lab determinations prn.
Hypomagnesemia	Disorientation, agitation, depression, CNS irritability, tremors, ataxia, convulsions, muscle cramps, paresthesias, tetany, positive Chvostek's sign, tachycardia, hypotension. Note: may be associated with hypocalcemia.	Obtain laboratory confirmation. IM or IV administration of Mg^{2+} in the form of $MgSO_4$; or oral replacement. Obtain lab determinations prn.
Hypermagnesemia	Lethargy, hypotension, loss of DTRs, respiratory depression. ECG reveals prolonged QT interval, atrioventricular block; cardiac arrest with extreme elevations.	Obtain laboratory confirmation. Eliminate sources of Mg^{2+} intake. Obtain lab determinations prn.
Hypophosphatemia	Muscular hypotonia, paresthesias, hyperventilation, respiratory distress, thickened tongue, lethargy, mental confusion, coma, decreased erythrocyte 2,3-diphosphoglycerate.	Obtain laboratory confirmation. Administer IV or oral phosphate. Obtain lab determinations prn.
Hyperphosphatemia	Same as hypocalcemia but less severe.	Obtain lab confirmation. Eliminate sources of phosphate intake.

[a]Salmond SW: Monitoring for potential complications of total parenteral nutrition administration. *Critical Care Quarterly* 3:23, 1981.
[b]Ostrow LS: Air embolism and central venous lines. *AJN* 81:2036, 1981.

and lighting, appropriate patient preparation and positioning, and a nurse's assistance.

The patient should undergo "preoperative" assessment to determine the need for general anesthesia, with its attendant risks. The patient may require a sedative, tranquilizer, or an analgesic to tolerate the procedure. Coagulation studies should be performed and an allergy history (e.g., to anesthetics and contrast drugs) should be obtained. A signed consent may be needed prior to the procedure, depending on the hospital policy.

Explanation of the procedure to the patient and family will reduce anxiety, increase understanding, and ultimately enhance cooperation. The child's age, level of understanding, and questions will be a guide to how much information and detail should be offered. The patient and/or parent should be told that a preoperative medication may be administered for the child's comfort, and that a nurse will always be at the bedside for emotional support and observation. The appearance of people in masks and gowns may be frightening to a child. The child should be prepared for the sight of masks, gowns, gloves, and in general, the sterile technique. A graphic description of the catheter may be helpful. Just prior to the local skin preparation, the child should be forewarned of the uncomfortable sting of the local anesthetic. To prevent the possible complications of air entry into the catheter, the child should be taught the Valsalva maneuver before catheter placement. The child should be instructed to, "take a deep breath; hold it; and bear down with your mouth closed." The Valsalva maneuver will be used at several strategic moments during the catheterization; therefore, the patient should be allowed to practice it several times. The child should also be informed that he will be placed in a Trendelenburg position during the procedure; this position can be easily demonstrated at the bedside to further dispel fears and mystery surrounding the upcoming procedure.

The following is a general guide, with rationale, for the nurse assisting during the central line placement through a cutdown incision:

1. Perform "preoperative" teaching.
2. Check the signed consent form.
3. Assemble the equipment for easy access.
4. Give premedication, if ordered.
5. Auscultate breath sounds as a baseline.
6. Assemble an IV administration set with an isotonic solution, needed to infuse at a keep-open-rate until the catheter placement is confirmed by x-ray films.
7. Shave area, if necessary.
8. Perform a friction scrub over the area with an iodophor solution; allow it to set for its antibacterial–antifungal effect.
9. Place the patient in Trendelenburg position to promote filling and distention of the subclavian vein. Also, place a rolled towel under and along the thoracic spine to drop the shoulders and head back for better localization of the vein.
10. Turn the patient's head away. Drape around the selected site with sterile towels to provide a sterile working field.
11. The physician will administer a local anesthetic of 1–2% lidocaine hydrochloride to the subcutaneous tissue. The cutdown is then performed to locate the vein.

12. Instruct the patient in the Valsalva maneuver as the needle is inserted into the vein to prevent air embolism.
13. Observe the patient for symptoms indicating complications; continue to monitor for strict observance of sterile technique; continue to provide emotional support.
14. There should be blood return as the needle is withdrawn. Instruct the patient in the Valsalva maneuver as the needle is completely withdrawn, than attach the IV to the end of the catheter hub and infuse at a keep-open-rate. All connections should be securely taped or Luer-locked.
15. The catheter will be sutured in place followed by closure of the cutdown incision.
16. An iodophor ointment should then be applied to the catheter insertion and cutdown site.
17. Apply a sterile dressing. Tape securely.
18. Make the patient comfortable. Auscultate breath sounds.
19. A chest film should be taken.
20. Continue to observe the patient for signs and symptoms indicating complications.
21. Chart the procedure in the nurses' notes, including: physician's name, time, placement site, catheter size and type, IV solution hung, patient's condition, any complications, preprocedure and postprocedure descriptions of the patient's breath sounds, and chest film confirmation of placement.
22. The first bottle of PN can be hung upon receiving radiologic confirmation that the catheter terminates in the superior vena cava.

If the central venous catheter is to be inserted at the bedside or in a treatment room, the nurse will be responsible for assembling the necessary equipment. The equipment should be checked for proper functioning and sterility. Sterile duplicates should also be readily available during the procedure for replacement of contaminated items. One or more of the following should be assembled:

1. Isotonic solution with a primed IV administration set
2. Sterile gloves
3. Sterile masks and gowns
4. Sterile drapes and clips
5. Vials of 1% and 2% lidocaine
6. 3 ml syringes with needles
7. Sterile scalpels
8. Sterile scissors
9. Sterile hemostats
10. 3-0 silk thread with straight needle
11. Sterile forceps
12. Sterile gauze sponges
13. Good light source
14. Sterile catheters in various sizes (duplicates)

15. Iodophor solution
16. Iodophor ointment
17. Sterile 4 inch × 4 inch gauze pads
18. Sterile 2 inch × 2 inch gauze pads
19. Adhesive tape—various widths
20. Hypoallergenic tape—various widths
21. Towel for the patient to lie on

IV Infusion Devices

The pediatric PN patient is administered small volumes of fluid. Severe complications may occur as a result of inappropriate rate of administration. It is, therefore, essential to use an IV infusion pump or controller to regulate the infusates. There are different types of infusion devices available. Among these are the syringe pump, volumetric pump, peristaltic pump, and the IV controller (7).

Infusion pumps automatically deliver IV fluids at a preselected flow rate by exerting positive pressure on the IV tubing (peristaltic pumps) or by pushing the IV fluid through a cylinder (piston or cylinder pumps). The pumps deliver the rate either in drops per minute or in milliliters per hour (volumetric). The volumetric pump is preferred because milliliters are more precise than drops. Drop size can vary with temperature, fluid viscosity, weight, and the type and make of administration set used. Volumetric pumps generally require a special tubing cassette that peristaltic pumps do not. Infusion pumps have both audible and visible alarm systems. The alarm system should alert the nurse to air in the line, occlusion, infusion complete, low battery, or whether or not the pump is operating. The pumps vary in their sensitivity to detect a change in flow resistance. One type of occlusion alarm may react immediately to the change in resistance of a freshly infiltrated peripheral IV whereas another type may not give an alarm until the IV line is completely kinked. An IV controller, like a pump, delivers a fluid amount accurately but works by "gravitational" force, requiring that the IV container be at least 30 inches above the infusion site. It is *essential* that the nurse fully understands the type of pump used, its operation, alarm system, and limitations.

Equipment Needed for PN

The arrangement of the PN administration system varies among institutions and between pediatrics and adults. Basic concerns related to all administration set-ups are safety, effectiveness, and simplicity. The ideal administration set for pediatric PN patients would be a preassembled, packaged, closed system. Components of a standard pediatric administration system with rationale are described below:

Components	Rationale and Points of Emphasis
1. Volume control fluid chamber with disc valve between volume chamber and drip chamber (note if vented or nonvented administration set is needed).	1. Facilitates accurate delivery of small volumes of fluid; disc valve reduces risk of introducing air into the system if volume chamber empties.

1a. Micro (pediatric) drip burette (60 gtts = 1 ml).

1a. Simplifies rate calculation (gtts/min = ml/hr); facilitates accurate delivery of small fluid volumes; useful if not using a pump or controller.

2. 0.22 micron bacterial particulate, and air-eliminating IV filter.

2. Decreases risk of sepsis, thrombophlebitis, air emboli, and particulate contamination.

3. Y-connector

3. Provides access for fat emulsion administration.

4. IV controller or infusion pump with accompanying adapter or administration set, e.g., cassette.

4. Flow-rate may be preselected. Alarm system includes some or all of the following: occlusion, air in the line, infusion complete, not operating, battery low; alerts nurse to unexpected occurrences between routine IV checks.

5. Luer-Lok extension tubing.

5. Provides for increased mobility of patient; decreases the risk of disconnection.

6. Smooth, rubber-tipped clamp.

6. Facilitates tubing changes; should be with patient and attached to infusion pump at all times, readily available for accidental disconnection of the line.

Once the administration equipment has been assembled, but before the PN solutions are hung, the PN solution should be systematically checked. The PN formula and fat emulsion should be validated against the physician's orders to insure accuracy in amount, additives, and administration rate. The pharmacist's expiration date on the dextrose–amino acid and fat emulsion solutions should also be noted. The dextrose-amino acid solution should be refrigerated up until the time of use to reduce the risk of bacterial or fungal growth. The refrigerated dextrose–amino acid solution can be used immediately from the refrigerator because it will be warmed by room environment as it passes through the infusion set. The fat emulsion bottle does not require refrigeration. The PN containers should be examined for defects. The dextrose–amino acid solution should be scrutinized for cloudiness and particulate matter, while the fat emulsion should be checked for separation ("oiling out") of the emulsion. All additives to the PN solution should be added in the pharmacy under the laminar flow hood. The need to shield specific PN additives (MVI, vitamin K, etc.) is controversial (for further discussion, see Chapter 11). However, when the additives are in the PN solution bottle, the bottle may need to be protected from light to preserve the integrity of the additive by covering with a brown paper bag.

Assembly of the PN administration system should be performed in a clean, nonturbulent area with adequate counterspace to permit aseptic assembly. The components of the administration system should be assembled as diagrammed (Fig. 6). Once the materials are properly assembled, the rubber stopper of the PN solution bottle should be swabbed with an iodophor solution; after allowing it to stand for 2 minutes, the top should be rewiped with alcohol. The IV tubing can then be introduced into the PN solution, and the administration system can be primed. Although it is best for fat emulsion to be infused in a separate IV site, it may be piggybacked into a PN solution line. When fat emulsion is given in combination with any IV solution, it must be given as close to the port of entry as possible by a Y-connector. The fat emulsion line must always be located distal to *any* IV solution

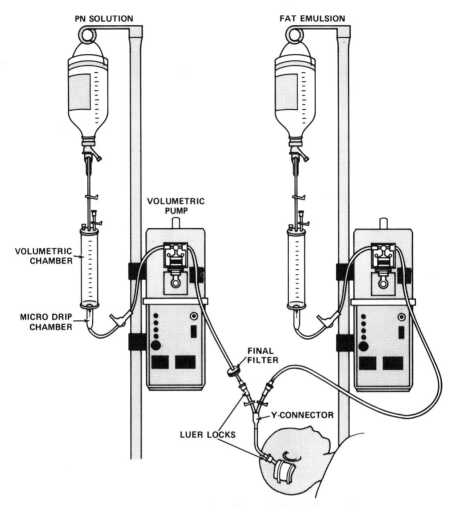

Figure 6 The parenteral nutrition administration system.

and/or filter because (1) mixing with any dextrose solution may "crack" and separate the fat emulsion, and (2) lipid particles are too large to filter. Inadvertent disconnection of the line could result in an air embolism, and increase the risk of infection; therefore, all connections should be securely taped or Luer-locked.

Final filters with dextrose-amino acid infusates have been controversial (8). In-line filters were designed to remove particulate matter, prevent phlebitis, and prevent sepsis. The National Coordinating Committee on Large Volume Parenterals' (NCCLVP) recommendation for the "ideal" filter is one that will remove and retain bacteria, fungi, and particulate matter and will eliminate air. It should offer uniform, sufficiently high, gravity flow-rates, and maintain the prescribed flow-rate throughout its use. It should also be designed to protect the patient from the bolus presentation of collected contaminants (9). From the research currently available, the best all-purpose filter is a 0.22 micron in-line final filter (10–12).

The described administration system is well suited for either central or peripheral PN. Additional stopcocks should not be placed in the system since this encourages use of the line for administration of medications, blood, and blood products, withdrawal of specimens for lab analysis, or obtaining CVP measurements. Particularly in central administration, it is important to use the line only for the administration of PN components. Use of the central PN line for purposes other than PN administration is strongly discouraged, since it is believed to increase the risk of sepsis. Blood should not be withdrawn from or given through the catheter, since this increases formation of a fibrin sleeve and clotting of the catheter. In an emergency, the PN solution may be discontinued, and the line may be used for blood drawing and drug administration. When the patient is stable, the PN infusion can be resumed after the insertion of a new catheter (13).

Merritt et al. (14) described a year of experience with Hickman catheters in 18 pediatric oncology patients. The Hickman catheters were used for the delivery of routine IV fluids and PN solutions, as well as for blood and blood products. Blood specimens were routinely drawn from the catheters for laboratory analysis. They reported a 19% incidence of serious complications requiring catheter removal, which they thought was not ideal, but not prohibitive, for such a high-risk group of patients. Their report reflects experience with a small number of cancer patients cared for by a limited number of personnel. These findings should not be interpreted to indicate that previous infection-control guidelines for central PN patients can be disregarded. There are no controlled studies comparing use of the Hickman or Broviac catheters for exclusive administration of PN versus the multi-purpose use described by Merritt and co-workers. Further research is needed to determine the relative incidence of complications such as clotting of the catheter and sepsis.

Monitoring the Pediatric Patient on PN

Careful monitoring of the pediatric patient receiving PN is a major nursing function (see Table 1). It is generally the nurse's responsibility to assure that blood and urine specimens required for metabolic monitoring are obtained in an appropriate and timely manner. Abnormal results should be promptly reported to the physician.

Recording of accurate patient weights on a routine basis is essential for the pediatric patient. In an unstable infant, the weight may be checked every 8 hours. In a more stable child, daily weights may be adequate. It is vital that the same scale be used and that the patient be consistently clothed or unclothed. If arm-boards or sandbags are used to stabilize IV sites, they should be weighed, labeled, and their weights should be subtracted from the total weight. The patient should be weighed at the same time daily. Significant weight gains or losses should be double checked, and reported.

Strict intake and output records are essential to prevent or correct fluid imbalances. In the pediatric, incontinent patient, preweighed plastic diapers permit accurate measurment of urine output. After subtracting the weight of the dry diaper, the number of grams of the urine weight equals the volume of urine in cubic centimeters.

Urine testing for sugar, acetone, pH, blood, protein, and specific gravity should be performed every 2–8 hours depending upon the stability of the patient. Glucosuria can indicate PN intolerance; *sudden* glucosuria may indicate a response to stress or may herald a septic episode. Prolonged glucosuria will lead to osmotic diuresis and dehydration. If glucosuria is 2+ or greater, a Dextrostix reading should be obtained. The Dextrostix is a bedside tool that permits a gross estimate of the serum glucose level; an unusually high reading should be followed by laboratory determination.

Vital signs are also important parameters for the nurse to measure and record every 2–8 hours, depending on the stability of the patient. Fever in the pediatric patient receiving PN is always of concern. A persistent rise in temperature or a fever preceded by an isolated temperature elevation several days earlier may be related to catheter sepsis. Significant changes in pulse, respiration, or blood pressure may indicate additional complications as well as fluid imbalance. Routine physical assessment of the child receiving PN should particularly focus on (1) changes in behavioral and mental status (indicating metabolic versus psychological problems), (2) dependent or generalized edema (indicating low serum albumin versus fluid overload), and (3) skin turgor (indicating hydration).

It is critical that the nurse examine the administration system and infusion site every 30–60 minutes to assess infusate delivery and integrity of the system and site. The initial infusion of PN solution should be increased only in gradual, systematic increments to help avoid glucose intolerance. The routine discontinuation of PN solution involves a gradual and systematic decrease in volume to minimize the risk of rebound hypoglycemia. Occasionally there are indications for more rapid weaning. However, this increases the risk of hypoglycemia. When the PN infusion has been abruptly discontinued, the nurse should reassess the patient's acute and short-term needs for alternative carbohydrate delivery (15). PN solutions should infuse at a constant rate. No attempt should be made to catch up or slow down the solution. The infusion rate must be delivered as ordered and alterations of ±10% from the prescribed rate must be reported to the physician. It is helpful to carefully "time-tape" the PN solution bottles (Fig. 7). This is a convenient method for the nurse to quickly assess whether the appropriate infusion rate is being maintained by comparing the fluid level line with the hour on the tape. Early recognition of infusion site or system complications can reduce morbidity.

Fat emulsion should be infused continuously over 24 hours whenever possible to provide the fat in the safest and most physiologic manner. The initial rate of fat infusion in pediatric patients should not be greater than 0.1 ml/min over the first 10–15 minutes; if no allergic reaction, respiratory distress, or fever occurs, the rate may be increased to the prescribed maintenance rate.

All patients receiving fat emulsion infusion require a serum turbidity check every 24 hours. This is only a gross indicator of fat clearance but can alert the nutritional support team to impaired fat tolerance. Fat clearance can be further evaluated through lab analysis of free fatty acids and serum triglycerides. To perform a serum turbidity test, the nurse must perform a capillary stick of either the heel or fingertip and fill one capillary tube with blood. After the specimen is centrifuged, the serum should be examined under bright light for evidence of turbidity (cloudiness). Any evidence of turbidity should be reported to the physician for further evaluation.

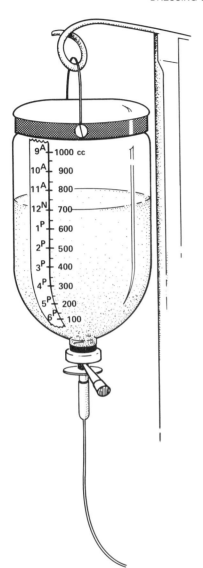

Figure 7 Time-taping of the intravenous bottle.

Dressing Changes and Catheter Care During PN

Septicemia is one of the most common complications associated with PN. The incidence of reported catheter-related sepsis ranges from 0–27% (16). The skin around the catheter insertion site is frequently implicated in septic complications. Most institutions have established protocols for catheter care, with infection rates

Table 2. Dressing Change Procedure

EQUIPMENT
Face masks
Paper bag for refuse
PN dressing kit including the following sterile items:
1 pair gloves
3 alcohol swabs (70%)
1 package of 3 iodophor swab sticks
1 package iodophor ointment
1 cotton-tipped applicator
1 3 inch × 3 inch pre-cut gauze sponge
1 roll 2 inch × 3 inch durapore tape

PROCEDURE	RATIONALE AND POINTS OF EMPHASIS
1. Explain procedure to patient and/or parent. Check for allergies to iodophor or tape.	Promote family's understanding of care.
2. Wash hands.	
3. Gather all supplies and bring to patient's bedside.	
4. Clean work area with antiseptic solution and dry thoroughly.	
5. Wash hands.	
6. Instruct all persons at the head of the bed (nurse, patient, parents) to don masks.	Prevents respiratory organisms from contaminating the insertion site. If a patient is unable to wear a mask, he can turn his head away from the catheter.
7. Open kit or assemble equipment on sterile field.	
8. Carefully remove old dressing and discard into paper refuse bag.	Remove dressing carefully to prevent catheter dislodgement.
9. Inspect the catheter insertion site and surrounding skin for any signs of erythema, swelling, tenderness, drainage, or extravasation of fluid. Document in the patient's chart and notify physician.	Catheter insertion site should be changed when signs of persistent inflammation occur to minimize the potential for infection.
10. Observe the catheter for	
a. Stabilizing sutures; notify physician if not intact.	
b. Dislodgement; note edema of the neck or oozing of solution from catheter site and notify physician.	Catheter position should be confirmed.
c. Position of the needle guard.	If necessary, it should be repositioned or replaced to ensure catheter protection.
d. Leakage; if present, notify physician.	Closely inspect the area for actual site of leakage—reduce rate.
e. Kinking	Reposition catheter. Note: sterile gloves should be worn if the catheter is manipulated.

Table 2. (Continued)

PROCEDURE	RATIONALE AND POINTS OF EMPHASIS
11. Monitor skin integrity	
a. Allergic reaction to cleansing solutions or tape.	Any allergic reactions should be evaluated and the dressing procedure should be altered as needed. A skin protection agent (e.g., Skin Prep or tincture of benzoin) may be indicated.
b. Shaving preparation of dressing site.	The adolescent male may need a dressing site shaved to remove potential bacteria-harboring hair and to facilitate occlusiveness.
12. Put on sterile gloves and open packages inside kit.	
13. Using an alcohol swab, surgically scrub the skin in a clean-to-dirty fashion. Beginning at the catheter insertion site and including the catheter, scrub in increasingly larger circles and move out to the periphery.	To remove debris acetone should not be used; it is irritating to the skin, and is not a proven antibacterial agent. (Acetone use may also be corrosive to the catheter.)
14. Clean site with three iodophor swabsticks in the same surgical fashion.	
15. Allow iodophor to set for 2 minutes. Do not wipe off.	To maximize antibacterial and antifungal action.
16. Apply iodophor ointment to catheter insertion site with applicator.	To prevent bacterial and fungal growth at catheter site.
17. Slide precut, sterile 3 inch × 3 inch gauze sponge under catheter to cover insertion site and hub only; fold sponge over catheter.	Consider everything under the gauze sponge as sterile.
18. Optional: Paint the skin area around the gauze dressing with tincture of benzoin. *Allow to dry.*	Benzoin has two purposes: It enhances sticking of tape; when dried well, benzoin adds a protective layer to the skin. If it is not allowed to dry, it can cause maceration of the skin. When dry, benzoin feels "tacky."
19. Secure gauze sponge with porous tape.	Waterproof tape is not used routinely since it prevents air circulation (altering skin flora) and early detection of leakage. *Exception:* Use waterproof tape if tracheostomy or draining wound is adjacent to the site.
20. Tape looped tubing to the skin.	To prevent tension on catheter.
21. Remove masks.	
22. Label dressing with date, time, and initials. Also note if catheter is not sutured.	Informs unit staff of day of dressing change.
23. Document in the patient's chart the dressing change, appearance of catheter site, and any problems encountered.	Provides information for unit staff and maintenance of the medical record.

263

from 2–7%. Generally, institutions assign the responsibility for dressing changes to a small group of individuals who are well acquainted with the technique. Dressing changes may be delegated to PN nurse specialists, house officers, or staff nurses. In situations where there will be a need for home PN, patients and parents may be taught to perform the dressing changes. The dressing change should be performed every 24–72 hours, and immediately whenever the dressing becomes wet, soiled, or loose. Jarrad et al. (17) lowered the incidence of positive skin cultures from 3.5% to 0% with daily dressing changes and recommend this for patients at high risk for septic complications. For practical purposes, to allow for maximum nursing staff coverage, Colley et al. (18) suggested a Monday-Wednesday-Friday schedule for dressing changes. Most institutions have adopted a standard dressing change technique for control of catheter-related sepsis (see Table 2).

An alternative to the gauze-and-tape dressing is the transparent dressing. Transparent dressings currently available are Op-site (Acme United Corporation) (19–22), Ensure (Deseret), Bioclusive (Johnson & Johnson), and Tegaderm (3M Corporation) (23). The transparent dressing is a clear, permeable, adhesive dressing that permits easy inspection of the catheter site and, therefore, less frequent dressing changes. Whenever the catheter site appears dirty, moist, or infected, a dressing change is mandatory. Each transparent dressing should be applied as recommended by the manufacturer. The following guide to applying Op-site is an example:

1. Before applying Op-site, cleanse the catheter insertion site (as described in Table 2, 13–16) with 70% alcohol, an iodophor, then apply a small amount of an iodophor ointment. Note: Some neonatal units apply a very small gauze dressing before applying Op-site.
2. Choose a dressing size that will allow a 1–2 inch margin.
3. Pull off only a small portion of the backing on the Op-site dressing and anchor it to the skin on one side of the catheter.
4. Holding the anchored side with one hand, pull the Op-site over the catheter. While maintaining enough pull to prevent wrinkling, it is important to allow the dressing to "relax" slightly before smoothing it down. If Op-site is applied under tension, it can cause skin irritation and patient discomfort.
5. Smooth Op-site carefully across the catheter surface with a gauze sponge, and seal the dressing to the surrounding skin. The green handles can be left on or removed by cutting the corners with scissors and pulling them off.
6. Op-site removal: Carefully use an alcohol swab, or *sterile* gauze sponges, water, and an iodophor soap to release the Op-site from around the sides of the catheter. Never pull the Op-site directly across the catheter surface since the catheter may become dislodged.

The IV tubing and filter should be changed and dated every 24 hours, preferably to coincide with dressing and bottle changes. The PN solution bottle should be changed every 24 hours to reduce the incidence of bacterial and fungal growth. The tubing junctions should be secured with tape or Luer-locked to prevent disconnection. Use of only minimal amounts of tape will facilitate easy removal. When changing the PN IV tubing or when heparin-locking a central line, instruct the patient to perform the Valsalva maneuver.

Care of the Hickman and Broviac Catheters

Hickman and Broviac catheter care is essentially the same as that described for any central venous catheter. The design of the catheter is such that they can remain patent for prolonged periods of time when not being used for IV solution infusions. The process by which this is accomplished is called *heparin-locking*. A heparin-lock is performed by filling the catheter with a heparin solution and sealing the end of the catheter with a Luer-Lok injectable cap. The purpose of the heparin-lock is to prevent clotting of the catheter while an IV solution is not infusing, thereby increasing patient mobility and independence. The flushing technique and heparin-locking procedure requires the following equipment:

1. Smooth, rubber-tipped clamp
2. 10 ml syringe filled with sterile normal saline
3. 3 ml syringe with needle
4. 1 vial heparin solution (100 U heparin/ml normal saline)
5. Iodophor solution
6. Sterile gauze to apply iodophor
7. 3 alcohol swabs
8. ¼-inch adhesive tape
9. 1 Luer-Lok injection cap

To perform the flushing technique and heparin-locking procedure:

1. Wash hands thoroughly.
2. Arrange supplies.
3. Wipe top of heparin solution vial with iodophor solution; wait 2 minutes.
4. Wipe top of vial with an alcohol swab.
5. Draw up 3 ml heparin solution in 3 ml syringe, removing all air bubbles. Cap needle and set aside.
6. Remove tape at the junction of the catheter and the IV tubing.
7. Wipe junction with an iodophor solution; wait 2 minutes. Wipe with an alcohol swab.
8. Clamp the catheter and turn off the IV flow.
9. Disconnect IV tubing.
10. Attach 10 ml syringe with normal saline and flush to clear the viscous PN solution.
11. Clamp the catheter.
12. Attach Luer-Lok injectable cap.
13. Unclamp the catheter.
14. Wipe the injection cap; using iodophor then alcohol as before.
15. Inject 2.5 ml of heparin solution through the injection cap into the catheter, withdrawing the needle as the final 0.5 ml is delivered to ensure a positive pressure within the catheter to prevent backflow at the catheter tip.
16. Securely tape the cap to the catheter.

A patent Hickman or Broviac catheter can be maintained for prolonged periods of time even without the infusion of an IV solution. To accomplish this the catheter must be flushed every 12–24 hours (through the injectable cap) with a heparin solution.

The injectable cap should be changed every 1–4 days, as described previously. The procedures for changing the cap and heparin injection should coincide (24).

In conclusion, although a variety of techniques have been effective in different institutions, the most critical factor in any institution is the adoption of a standardized nursing care practice.

Approach to Complications of PN

As a primary care provider, the nurse is in a key position to prevent complications and to recognize early any problems in PN therapy. The nurse needs to be aware of potential complications, their signs and symptoms, and the appropriate nursing response. Early recognition of complications can significantly reduce morbidity and mortality. Complications of PN may be classified into two categories: catheter-related (mechanical and infectious) and metabolic. Table 1 summarizes these complications and the appropriate nursing and medical interventions.

Associated Aspects of Nursing Care

Children receiving PN can experience musculoskeletal problems due to prolonged immobility, muscle mass wasting from long-term malnourishment, and disturbances in calcium and phosphorus levels. Nursing care related to musculoskeletal function should include a level of physical activity that the child can tolerate without excessive caloric expenditure. Exercise also helps promote better incorporation of protein into muscle. An exercise program can range from passive range of motion with frequent position changes to walks to the playroom where therapeutic and developmentally stimulating activities are offered.

Maintenance of skin integrity is another concern. Children receiving PN are predisposed to skin breakdown if they have (1) excessive diarrhea secondary to their primary disease process, (2) bony prominences due to long-standing malnutrition, (3) skin rashes due to lack of trace elements, (4) dry skin secondary to essential fatty acid deficiency, (5) activity level restrictions intended to reduce caloric expenditure, and (6) critical illness that prohibits physical activity. Nursing care for the child with potential or actual skin breakdown should aim at keeping the skin meticulously clean, dry, and lubricated. Useful pressure-relieving modalities include frequent position changes, sheep skins, egg-crate mattresses, and waterbeds. Massage, exposure to air, and dry heat are additional methods that can increase blood supply to pressure areas and either prevent breakdown or enhance healing. Prevention is the primary goal, since an alteration in skin integrity increases the risk of infection. Skin complications that result from extravasation of peripheral dextrose-amino acid solutions can be severe and may necessitate debridement and split-thickness skin grafting; therefore, IV sites should be carefully monitored.

Oral hygiene also needs attention because of the problems associated with prolonged fasting, possible oral trauma from the presence of tubes, reactions from chemotherapy or radiation therapy, and infections from bacterial, viral, or fungal organisms. Reidun Daeffler, an oncology clinical nurse specialist, summarizes five goals for oral hygiene (25):

1. Keep the oral mucosa clean, soft, moist, and intact to prevent infection in the oral cavity.
2. Keep the lips clean, soft, moist, and intact.
3. Remove tooth debris and plaque without damaging the oral mucosa to prevent caries and periodontal disease.
4. Alleviate oral pain and discomfort to enhance oral intake.
5. Prevent halitosis; a fresh feeling in the mouth promotes patient comfort.

Her survey of current oral hygiene practice reveals a great amount of discrepancy and little current research. Her recommendations for oral care include:

Frequency—Oral care should be evaluated on an individual basis, but performed around the clock in the acutely ill patient, especially if the patient is NPO, mouth-breathing, or receiving oxygen.

Cleansing—Mouthwash removes crusts and mucous, moistens and softens oral mucosa, and flushes away loose debris. Commercial mouthwashes as well as full strength hydrogen peroxide are often too irritating. Normal saline (1 teaspoon sodium chloride per liter of water) is an effective mouthwash but will not remove crusting. Mechanical cleansing with nonwaxed dental floss and a soft, small tooth brush is important, and should be performed unless contraindicated by pain and bleeding. Lemon-glycerine swabs may be irritating if stomatitis is present. Foam sticks are helpful in stimulating gum circulation. An effective mouthwash regime, used at Children's Hospital at Stanford, is a half-strength hydrogen peroxide wash, followed by a salt-and-soda wash. The half strength hydrogen peroxide wash is one part water to one part hydrogen peroxide. The salt and soda solution is 2 heaping teaspoonfuls of baking soda plus 1 heaping teaspoonful of salt in 1 liter of water.

Moistening—Research is needed in this area to find an effective agent. Daeffler (25) recommends a water-soluble lubricant for lips and gums.

Support of the Patient During Transition From Parenteral to Enteral Feedings

As gastrointestinal function returns, the patient can be weaned from PN with the gradual introduction of enteral nutrition. During this transition, several concerns should be incorporated into the child's nursing care plan.

To prevent rebound hypoglycemia during the transition from parenteral to enteral feeding, the dextrose–amino acid solution concentration and rate should be tapered gradually over 1–2 days. During the tapering, Dextrostix assessment of glucose metabolism should be performed when any sign or symptom of hypoglycemia is evident. Laboratory glucose determinations should be performed on a routine basis if the Dextrostix finding is abnormal.

The initiation of enteral feedings is dependent on the child's age, disease process, return of gastrointestinal function, and toleration of the feedings. Typically, feedings will be introduced in small amounts of low concentrations of formula or clear liquids. Nursing care during this transition involves administration of the appropriate amount and type of feeding and observations for signs of enteral intolerance, e.g., abdominal distention, discomfort, nausea, vomiting, and excessive stooling. The developmental feeding needs of each child should be taken into consideration. The infant may need a soft nipple and support of his jaw to regain a strong suck. The older child may be anorectic or afraid to eat. Thus, support and creativity in the feeding situation are also important.

Central Venous Catheter Removal

The PN catheter should not be removed until the child has demonstrated tolerance of at least three fourths of his or her daily enteral requirement. Some weight loss—due to diuresis—is expected during this transition period; however, it should not exceed 3% of the total body weight and should level off before the catheter is removed. Depending on hospital policy, either the nurse or the physician will remove the central venous catheter. At the time of catheter removal, the child should be instructed to perform the Valsalva maneuver to prevent air from entering the catheter. After removal, the entire catheter should be examined for size and smoothness to assure intactness. The catheter tip should be kept sterile and sent to the laboratory for culture. Once the catheter is removed, firm pressure to the exit site should be applied for 5–10 minutes to prevent local hemorrhage or hematoma formation. Before applying a sterile dressing, a small amount of iodophor ointment should be applied to the exit site. The site should be examined, cleansed, and redressed daily until healed.

The removal of the Hickman or Broviac catheter should be performed by the physician or the PN nurse specialist. The exit site should be cleaned with an iodophor solution. The catheter is wrapped firmly around the hand and steadily pulled for approximately 2–3 minutes until the fibrous tissue around the Dacron cuff loosens and the catheter slides free; the steady pull can then be released. Again, the catheter should be wrapped around the hand and the catheter pulled with a firm, steady pressure to remove the entire catheter. After the Hickman or Broviac catheter is removed, an iodophor ointment and a sterile pressure dressing should be applied to the exit site. This will be done at the patient's bedside unless there is a problem. The Dacron cuff will remain under the skin and eventually dissolve or it may be surgically removed. Jerking pulls on a stubborn catheter should be avoided to prevent breaking. If the catheter breaks or is difficult to remove, the catheter should be cleansed and a pressure dressing applied; the patient will need to be prepared for surgical removal of the catheter.

Conclusion

Nursing care for the child receiving PN is complex and requires a skilled, knowledgeable, and alert practitioner. Adopting standardized nursing procedures can promote the effectiveness of PN and minimize the potential for complications. PN is a therapy in evolution. Keeping pace with new findings remains a continuous challenge for the nurse.

References

1. Tanswell AK: Long-term peripheral intravenous access in the neonate. *J Pediatr* 94:480, 1979.

2. Welch GW, McKeel DW, Silverstein P, et al: The role of catheter composition in the development of thrombophlebitis. *Surg Gynecol Obstet* 138:424, 1974.

3. Riordan TP: Placement of central venous lines in the premature infant. *JPEN* 3:381, 1979.

4. Vain NW, Georgeson KE, Cha CC, et al: Central parenteral alimentation in newborn infants: A new technique for catheter placement. *J Pediatr* 93:5, 1978.

5. Rubenstein R, Michalak J, Stegman R, et al: Hickman catheter insertion via the percutaneous subclavian route. *Nutritional Support Services* 2(6):9, 1982.

6. Pollack PF, Kadden M, Byrne WG, et al: 100 patient years' experience with the Broviac silastic catheter for central venous nutrition. *JPEN* 5:34, 1981.

7. Labry J: Infusion monitoring devices. *NITA* 4:5, 1981.

8. Millan DA: Final inline filters. *AJN* 79:1272, 1979.

9. National Coordinating Committee on Large Volume Parenterals. Recommendations to pharmacists for solving problems with large-volume parenterals–1979. *Am J Hosp Pharm* 37:663, 1980.

10. Bivins BA, Rapp RP, DeLuca PP, et al: Final inline filtration: A means of decreasing the incidence of infusion phlebitis. *Surgery* 85:4, 1979.

11. Holmes CJ, Kundsin RB, Ausman RK, et al: Potential hazards associated with microbial therapy. *J Clin Microbiol* 12:6, 1980.

12. Turco S, Davis NM: Clinical significance of particulate matter: A review of the literature. *Hosp Pharm* 8:137, 1973.

13. Forlaw L: Parenteral nutrition in the critically ill child. *Critical Care Quarterly* 3:7, 1981.

14. Merritt RJ, Ennis CE, Andrassy RJ, et al: Use of Hickman right atrial catheter in pediatric oncology patients. *JPEN* 5:85, 1981.

15. Hyperalimentation nursing standards of practice. *NITA* 4:2, 1981.

16. Goldman DA, Maki DG: Infection control in TPN. *JAMA* 223:1360, 1973.

17. Jarrad MM, Olson CM, Freeman JB: Daily dressing change effects on skin flora beneath-subclavian catheter dressings during total parenteral nutrition. *JPEN* 4:392, 1980.

18. Colley R, Wilson JM, Wilhem MP: Intravenous nutrition—Nursing considerations. *Issues in Comprehensive Pediatric Nursing.* 1:5, 1977.

19. Curtas S, Grant J: Evaluation of Op-site as a total parenteral nutrition dressing. *NITA* 4:414, 1981.

20. Schwartz-Fulton J, Colley R, Valanis B, et al: Hyperalimentation dressings and skin flora. *NITA* 4:355, 1981.

21. Palidar P, Simonowitz D, Oreskovich M: Use of Op-site as an occlusive dressing for total parenteral nutrition catheters. *JPEN* 6:150, 1982.

22. Freeman P, Boyer J: How to get the most out of Op-site. *RN* 45:32, 1982.

23. Tegaderm technical support information. 3M Corporation. St. Paul, MN, 1982.

24. Hospital and home care of the Hickman catheter. Children's Hospital at Stanford nursing guidelines, 1980.

25. Daeffler R: Oral hygiene measures for patients with cancer. *Canc Nurs* 4:33, 1981.

18
Psychosocial Aspects of Pediatric Parenteral Nutrition

M. Eileen Walsh

A spectrum of psychological and social problems has emerged as parenteral nutrition (PN) therapy has advanced (1). As research with respirator-dependent polio victims (2,3) and hemodialysis-dependent (4) patients has shown, dependence on life-support systems creates emotional and social turmoil. Research on adult patients receiving PN confirms these findings (5–11).

The variability and intensity of adult psychosocial reactions to PN therapy depend primarily on the duration of PN. Patient response to PN therapy evolves from denial to acceptance. During the first week of PN therapy, patients are generally depressed, anxious, and paranoid, refusing to acknowledge their dependence on an external life support system. Gradually, their attitudes change. Patients become introspective as they attempt to cope with PN. They become hopeless and angry because they feel they no longer control their own lives. PN patients also grieve over the loss of their normal digestive functions. PN patients resent being deprived of the important social function of eating. People rely on meals for social interactions, to demarcate the day, to satisfy hunger, and to relieve tedium. Patients suffering from pre-PN therapy induced malnutrition may also feel unattractive. This negative body image may continue throughout long-term PN therapy. Patients who receive PN therapy beyond 3 months may also continue to feel hopeless and depressed. Unresolved depression may result in suicidal ideation and acts. By simply neglecting their PN care, some patients passively commit suicide. Many long-term patients overcome this depression, however, and achieve a new sense of equilibrium, enjoying a state of good health and nutrition not felt in a long time.

Other concerns—the expense of treatment, limitations on activity, employment possibilities, and detrimental effects on their marriage—also affect an adult's psychosocial response to PN therapy. It appears the adult's reaction stages are dependent on one or more of the following factors:

1. The duration of PN therapy
2. The patient's diagnosis and prognosis for recovery from the primary pathology

3. The hope of the return of normal ingestion and gastrointestinal function
4. The patient's personality (i.e., ego strength and determination)
5. The personality of the patient's family (i.e., quality of support)
6. For home PN patients, the family's receptivity to a home program, and the patient's and/or family's mastery of the PN technique

These findings are derived solely from PN studies of adults because there is a paucity of studies concerning children. The following five cases reflect the experiences of children who received hospital or home PN from Stanford University Hospital or the Children's Hospital at Stanford during the past five years.

Clinical Examples

CASE 1

M.J. was an 11-year-old girl with newly diagnosed Crohn's disease. She received total parenteral nutrition (TPN) and nothing by mouth (NPO) for 1 week. She was interviewed in the hospital after being weaned from TPN. She noted that while NPO, everything—all television shows, magazine advertisements, and books—seemed to be about food. Yet, she denied any reaction to being NPO: "I just ignored it." She had no conscious complaints about hunger. Her sole, but frequent, complaint was the discomfort and "burning" of the peripheral PN catheter insertion site.

It is difficult to ascertain whether TPN and /or being NPO caused any psychological upset in 1 week. Another event during that week, however, may have obscured her reaction to receiving TPN and being NPO; she was told that she had a chronic illness, Crohn's disease.

CASE 2

M.L. was a 12-year-old girl with Crohn's disease. She received TPN and was placed NPO for 6 weeks. Two months after her discharge, she wrote a letter describing her TPN experience. She explains that at first, "I resented it because I couldn't eat and everyone else in my room could." Later she said, "It didn't bother me much . . . but, I very much looked forward to the day I could eat again." Notations in her hospital chart showed that she frequently cried at mealtimes, saying she was "depressed and hungry." After 2 weeks of TPN and being NPO, her parents informed her that she would remain NPO for an additional month. She began to cry hysterically and pulled the IV tubing apart. Her conversations continued to focus on food; she would question the staff and patients on the ward concerning the foods they ate at mealtimes. Summarizing her experience, M.L. wrote, "For all the money in the world, I wouldn't want to relive the summer of 1981."

It is difficult to determine the causes of M.L.'s reactions to TPN. M.L.'s parents were filing for divorce during her hospitalization. The child may have worried about who was going to provide her emotional nurturance. The entire family received psychiatric consultation during the child's hospitalization. From a psychiatric viewpoint, deprivation of food both symbolized and exacerbated her concern over the family situation. This case demonstrates that TPN and being NPO can become intertwined with preexisting psychological difficulties.

CASE 3

C.S. was a 16-year-old girl with ulcerative colitis. For 6 weeks she was NPO and received TPN. In the final week of TPN therapy she was weaned from continuous (24 hours/day) to cyclic (18-16-14-12 hours/day) TPN. Six weeks after her hospital discharge, she wrote a letter describing her reactions to TPN. She complained that the TPN apparatus made "using the bathroom very hard because of having to unplug everytime" and made it difficult for her to change clothes. The infusion pump's very sensitive buzzers annoyed her, especially "at night when trying to rest." Another complaint was "trying to keep the line dry" during baths and showers. Sleeping was unpleasant because her arms were always entangled in the lines.

In response to being NPO she was very disappointed the first few days and "wanted to *taste, smell,* even *see* food." She coped by "talking to others about it all the time." She found that "being with my family" and other patients was an important diversion. When food was reintroduced, she was initially "very scared to eat again . . . eager but cautious." She was weaned from continuous to cyclic TPN and felt very happy and relieved when the line was removed. Her final statement was, "If someone told me I had to be on machines to live, it would be like having a 500 pound lead ball chained to me . . . no freedom!"

C.S. appeared to compensate successfully for her need to eat. It is difficult to assess her psychosocial response because there are so many unknowns. Was talking with others an adequate substitute for eating? Her statement of being "very scared to eat again" when food was reintroduced raises many questions. Did she wonder if her body was still working? Did she fear that the ulcerative colitis would become exacerbated? Or was she frightened that eating would cause strange abdominal sensations? These questions must be answered before definitive psychosocial statements can be made. Children need assistance to explore and understand their feelings.

CASE 4

S.C. was a 7-year-old girl who had repeated lengthy hospitalizations for TPN therapy during the year following her diagnosis of intractable diarrhea of unknown etiology. During her final 6 months of hospitalization, the health care team was concerned that her chronic illness could cause her psychological disability. She received psychological evaluations and support daily. Throughout most of the hospitalization, S.C. was NPO, although in the final month she was allowed to eat a few items. Chart review of 4 months of a psychologist's notes reveals the following:

S.C. described herself as "having stomach problems" and being "unable to eat." Her play sessions, both with and without the psychologist, revolved around food. She drew pictures of fruits, vegetables, hamburgers, and hot dogs that were personified with hats and feet that would dance. Her alphabet letters were all represented by pieces of food. Once she showed the psychologist a Jack-in-the-box that she described as "crying because he's hungry." She would play a guessing game: "You can tell what type of food a person likes by looking at their face" (i.e., salami face, pretzel face, etc.). If she were not pretending to be preparing food, she would take the psychologist on walks to show her all the eating locations in the building. Her favorite toys were a punchbowl, dishes, and toy boxes of food. She liked talking about her favorite foods. She frequently asked the psychologist to eat her (S.C.'s) favorite foods and then spontaneously verbalized her own refusal to eat. Sometimes she pretended that her dolls stole food from the table settings and would punish them for it.

S.C.'s growth was stunted and she appeared malnourished on her hospital admission. Her drawings and Silly Putty play revealed her concern about her body image. She once drew pictures of two houses, one narrow and one wide, and then rejected the wide house, saying it was ugly. One day she stretched Silly Putty into a fat man figure until he snapped, while she chanted, "He got fatter and fatter and fatter and then he burst."

Her choice of books also demonstrated her concern about eating and her body image:

Archie comics—Her favorite character was Jughead, an adolescent boy with an insatiable appetite

Dr. Seuss's *Green Eggs and Ham*

Hansel and Gretel—She was awed by an edible house!

A story about a rodent named Uncle Skinny

Babar the Elephant

Also, a Walt Disney cartoon exposé on the consequences of overeating would put her in good humor.

S.C. was preoccupied with her loss of eating and body image. She did in play what she would have liked to have been able to do in reality. She also identified with the forces oppressing her (being NPO), since she punished the doll and "reminded" herself not to eat. She clearly craved food and its associated pleasures.

At the end of this final hospitalization, TPN was discontinued and S.C. was discharged. All medical therapy failed and no further treatment could help her. Home TPN was apparently not an option. S.C. died shortly after her discharge.

CASE 5

S.A. was a 14-year-old boy with an underlying immune deficiency complicated by *Cryptosporidium*-induced secretory diarrhea. He had received 11 weeks of in-hospital TPN 3 years earlier and has received home PN for the past year. He was interviewed in his home about both TPN experiences.

During the 11 weeks of peripheral TPN, S.A. was also NPO. Receiving nothing by mouth was the most difficult aspect of TPN for him. Watching the other children eat at mealtimes could bring tears to his eyes.

S.A. craved gum, particularly the imaginary Willy Wonka Gum that promised a complete seven-course meal upon mastication. Later, he was allowed Life-Savers—only one pack per day. Each morning he would ceremoniously line up the 20 varieties of Life-Savers and make a selection. He would then smash the pack into tiny pieces and savor each sliver one by one throughout the day. While NPO he also craved hot drinks. When allowed one cup of ice per day, S.A. would save the entire cup for dinner time.

During the past year while receiving 12-hour cyclic PN at home, S.A. was allowed to eat. Although his oral nutrients were not absorbed and exacerbated his diarrhea, S.A. enjoyed eating. He ate only one meal a day, usually dinner with his family. Instead of eating during school lunchtime, S.A. played basketball. He participated in all sports except body contact ones. He was also allowed to swim, providing he could redress his central catheter insertion site within 20 minutes of emerging from the pool. S.A. felt wonderful about the 4 inches he grew in 1 year since being on home PN, his first height gain in 6 years. S.A.'s mother noted that S.A. developed self-esteem and pride in the independent management of his PN (i.e., dressing changes, setting up and taking down infusions). His mother attributed some of his pride to the peer support he received and to the doctor who taught him about home PN (this doctor managed her own home PN care for 5 years). S.A.'s most difficult problem with PN was enuresis caused by the high PN infusion flow-rate during the night. He slept so soundly that the urge to void would not awaken him, and he would find wet bed sheets every morning. S.A. viewed enuresis as an inconvenience without a solution. Home PN in children is so recent that this problem has not been described before, although adult TPN patients have complained of having to wake every 2 hours to void.

At present, S.A. has achieved a new state of equilibrium on long-term PN therapy. A contributing factor is his supportive, intact family. He hopes that a cure will be found for his *Cryptosporidium*-induced diarrhea and that normal gastrointestinal function will return. Meanwhile, home PN is a way of life. Nocturnal cyclic PN affords him the freedom to participate in an average adolescent's daily living activities with only a few restrictions.

In summary, all five children had chronic gastrointestinal illnesses. Therapy with TPN was not only necessary to improve their nutritional status, but also to allow their gastrointestinal tracts to rest and heal. In the final two cases, long-term PN was the only means of survival since intractable diarrhea prohibited adequate gastrointestinal nutrient absorption.

Any lengthy illness or therapy during childhood tends to interfere with the normal, healthy course of a child's physical and psychosocial development. Not only does the child grieve over the loss of a "normal," healthy self, but parents and brothers or sisters must adapt to not having a "normal" child or sibling. Further discussion on the needs of the family of the chronically ill child are beyond the constraints of this chapter. Suffice it to say that many variables should be taken into consideration when attempting to understand and to attend to a child's psychosocial reactions to PN.

Adapting to PN Therapy

From this pilot survey of children treated with PN, certain themes hallmark children's psychosocial reactions. Similar to adults in the early stages of therapy, children on PN experience denial, negative body image, and grief over the loss of eating and its concomitant social pleasures. Children appear to become preoccupied with food. They focus on food items in magazines, on television, and in their environment, and they are jealous of others' ability to eat. Children should be allowed to express their interest in food. Talking and seeing food is apparently a means of dealing with its deprivation. Although avoiding food-oriented situations would seem wise and kind, when a child expresses the need to talk about food, it should be recognized as necessary and therapeutic and should not be discouraged. Children receiving PN have unique adaptive mechanisms for vicarious gratification of their desire to eat. Young children find satisfaction in their real and pretend play, in reading books about food, and in talking to and watching others eating their favorite foods. Older children use diversionary activities to sublimate the social function of mealtimes (e.g., playing sports and visiting with friends and family). Once some food is allowed, PN is less traumatic for children of all ages.

Adaptation to long-term pediatric PN is not easy to define since so few children receive long-term PN. Case five exemplifies one child's healthy adaptation to a year of home PN therapy.

Similar to those for adults, contributing factors to a child's reaction to any form of PN therapy include

1. The duration of PN
2. The child's diagnosis and prognosis for recovery from the primary pathology
3. The hope for the return of normal ingestion and gastrointestinal function
4. The personality of the child
5. The personalities of the child's parents and siblings
6. For children receiving home PN, the family's receptivity to a home program and mastery of the PN technique

If long-term PN is necessary, home PN is the ideal option. Because home PN has extensive ramifications for an entire family, it is mandatory that an assessment be made of the family's suitability for the home program. Parfitt and Thompson (12) suggest the following guidelines for in-hospital evaluation of a family's readiness for a child on home PN:

1. Is the family able to comfortably initiate the technical procedures in the hospital?
2. Are the parents ready to perform these procedures at home?
3. Are the parents able to interact with the child in the hospital by providing nurturance, comfort, and other care that they will need to provide at home?
4. Can the parents respond to cues from the child and deal with them comfortably?
5. Has the family the support of a nuclear and extended family in conducting home PN therapy?
6. Does the family have community support systems available, such as church and friends?

AGE APPROPRIATE CONSIDERATIONS IN PN THERAPY

Individual as well as age-appropriate considerations should be applied to the care of the child receiving PN. The following developmental approach is based on Colley and co-workers' (13) original recommendations for children receiving PN. It is applicable for either the hospitalized or home PN patient. While in the hospital, nurses are responsible for monitoring the child's developmental level, the individual child's needs, and the parents' need to be included in caretaking. If PN therapy is provided in the home, the family should be reminded and encouraged to use these age-appropriate guidelines.

Neonate and Infant. The infant on PN has a tremendous need for sucking and stimulation. Feeding time is a special time for nurturing the parent–child relationship; usually an infant is held in the "en-face" position, talked to and cuddled for 15–20 minutes every 3–4 hours. When the PN infant is not being fed orally, definite intervals during the day should be specified for providing stimulation, holding, talking to, rocking, and touching the infant (preferably by the parents to promote parent–infant bonding). A pacifier is ideal for satisfying an infant's sucking needs. Auditory, visual, kinesthetic, and tactile stimulation (e.g., water-beds and mobiles) have been shown to have a positive impact on weight gain and development.

Toddler.   To the toddler who is gaining some autonomy, PN restricts mobility and prohibits oral intake. Although restraints may be needed to prevent the child from interfering with the PN apparatus, special efforts should be made to allow the child as much freedom as possible. Safe, age-appropriate play activities should be provided as opportunities to expend energy and work out frustrations (e.g., splashing in water, catching a ball, putting objects into containers). Ideally, food should not be prepared or eaten in front of the child. During mealtime, the child should be given special attention (e.g., a ride in a cart, holding or rocking). Lollipops are usually not contraindicated and may be quite pacifying. If limited oral intake is permitted, the child's *favorite* food should be offered at intervals. In the hospital, parents should be encouraged to feed or entertain their child if they are present at mealtime; mealtime interaction nurtures the parent–child relationship.

Preschooler.   Problems particular to the preschooler on PN are immobility, fears, fantasies, and a rudimentary understanding of bodily functions. The PN apparatus limits the active play of this age-group. Appropriate play activities that provide an outlet for energy and aggression might include racing toy cars across the blankets or demolishing block towers on the overbed table. Under supervision, and within the limits imposed by the child's illness, activities such as riding a tricycle or joining in playroom activities should be encouraged. Simple, concrete explanations of the PN treatment regimen are adequate for the preschooler's cognitive level of understanding. Supervision of play with hospital IV equipment and dolls is beneficial for this age-group. The complexity of body physiology is a mystery to a preschooler and a source of fears and fantasies. Gentle discussion and repeated reassurances can calm anticipated or expressed fears. Mealtimes can be frustrating for the preschooler. Although he is not allowed to eat, he may desire to talk about favorite foods and will need reassurance concerning *how difficult* it is to be deprived of favorite foods. A preschooler's moral developmental level of understanding may lead him to believe he was "bad" and is being punished with PN and being NPO. Although the child may not be able to express these fears, he should be reassured that PN and being NPO are not punitive measures. To provide the preschooler with some control over his care, he should be encouraged to perform a little self-care (e.g., bathing, dressing, brushing teeth).

Older School-Aged Children and Adolescents.   Older children and adolescents have different needs as their sense of identity, values, self-esteem, control over their lives, and maturing cognitive abilities emerge. School-aged children should be given rational explanations for their problems. Opportunities should be made for older children to express their thoughts, feelings, and questions. Although the older child may appear happy and calm, separation from friends, loss of activity, and food deprivation are stressful. Self-esteem and body image are of heightened concern in this age group. A child requiring PN may have suffered nutritional deficiencies that contribute to poor growth with short stature, delayed puberty and an unattractive appearance (dry skin, pallor, acne, lack-lustre hair, and thinness). Assisting the child to improve his or her appearance can promote the child's self esteem. This may involve overseeing careful body hygiene, suggesting applications of moisture lotion or makeup, and maintaining clean, styled hair. Allowing the older child to wear his or her own clothes provides freedom of choice and may disguise or enhance the child's figure. Because adolescents need independence and control over their environment, their wishes should be included in the daily plan of care (i.e., choosing particular times for treatment, study, and free time). Room arrangements can enhance peer socialization. Friends should be encouraged to visit. The older child is capable of understanding basic body physiology. Detailed PN information should be offered and discussed as frequently as needed. Concrete explanations may be facilitated with the use of dummies, pictures, or actual equipment.

PEER SUPPORT

An additional way of promoting a child's adaptation to PN is to introduce the child to others who have experienced PN or to a peer support group. A self-help group for PN patients and their families is the Lifeline Foundation (see Appendix III for address). The address should be offered to children who receive long-term or home PN. Contact the child's school to discuss the child's needs and plans for reentry. Follow-up contact with the school is also a means of understanding the child's adaptation to home PN. The school is one of the most influential social systems outside the family; it provides the setting within which the child is measured and in which the child measures himself or herself academically, socially, emotionally, and physically.

Conclusion

Since PN for children is in its infancy, future research is needed to more fully understand children's reactions to therapy. Not only does a larger sample of children need to be studied, but their parents and siblings should be interviewed to define their impact on the PN child's adaptation. Health professionals should be aware that children receiving PN therapy have unique psychosocial needs. Anticipatory guidance is needed as are age-appropriate interventions to ameliorate detrimental reactions and to promote a healthy adaptation to PN.

References

1. Dudrick SJ, Englert DM: Total care of the patient receiving total parenteral nutrition. *Psychosomatics* 21(2):109, 1980.
2. Prugh Dg, Taguiri CK: Emotional aspects of respirator care of patients with poliomyelitis. *Psychosom Med* 16:104, 1954.
3. Holland JC, Coles MR: Neuropsychiatric aspects of acute poliomyelitis. *Am J Psychiatry* 114:54, 1957.
4. Abram HS: Survival by machine: The psychological stress of chronic hemodialysis. *Am J Psychiatry* 124:37, 1968.

5. Gulledge AD: Social and psychiatric implications of HPN, in Steiger E (ed): *Home Parenteral Nutrition.* New York, Pro Clinica, 1981, p 39.

6. Jordan HA, Moses H, MacFayden BV, et al: Hunger and satiety in humans during parenteral hyperalimentation. *Psychosom Med* 36(2):144, 1974.

7. MacRitchie KH: Life without eating or drinking. Total parenteral nutrition outside hospital. *Can Psychiatr Assoc J* 23:373, 1978.

8. Malcolm R, Robson RK, Vanderveen TW, et al: Psychosocial aspects of total parenteral nutrition. *Psychosomatics* 21:115, 1980.

9. Peteet JR, Medeiros C, Slavin L, et al: Psychological aspects of artificial feeding in cancer patients. *JPEN* 5:138, 1981.

10. Perl M, Hall RC, Dudrick SJ, et al: Psychological aspects of long-term home hyperalimentation. *JPEN* 4:554, 1980.

11. Price BS, Levine EL: Permanent total parenteral nutrition: Psychological and social responses of the early stages. *JPEN* 3:48, 1979.

12. Parfitt DM, Thompson VD: Pediatric home hyperalimentation: Educating the family. *MCN* 5:196, 1980.

13. Colley R, Wilson JM, Wilhem MP: Intravenous nutrition—Nursing considerations. *Issues in Comprehensive Pediatric Nursing* 1(5):50, 1977.

19

The Nutrition Support Team

Robert L. Poole
John A. Kerner, Jr.

Although parenteral nutrition (PN) can be a life-saving therapy, it is potentially hazardous when used by personnel unfamiliar with its associated complications. This awareness has led to the development of multidisciplinary nutrition support teams. The potential benefits of such teams have been described in a prospective study by Nehme (1) and a retrospective review by Skoutakis et al. (2). Both studies reported very low complication rates when total parenteral nutrition (TPN) was administered with strict adherence to established protocols. The fundamental details of establishing a nutritional support team (NST) have been well described previously (2–10).

The structure of an NST depends on a hospital's individual needs. A very small hospital dealing with acutely ill medical and surgical patients may require only a full-time nurse and a therapeutic dietitian working under the supervision of a properly trained and interested physician. The other extreme is a large university hospital, such as Boston Children's Hospital, where the nutrition support service has a physician coordinator, at least one clinical nutrition fellow on service at any time, a full-time hyperalimentation nurse, a research dietitian, a pharmacist, and a secretary/coordinator (4). Additional departments that may be incorporated into an NST are physical therapy and social services.

Program Development

At Stanford University Hospital our attention was focused first on the intensive care nursery (ICN), where the number of infants receiving PN ranges from eight to 15 per day—approximately one half of patients receiving PN in the entire hospital. Our program began with informal discussions between an attending physician and a clinical pharmacist. Subsequently, a nutritionist (clinical dietitian), funded by a Maternal and Child Health Training Grant (MCT-000984-04-0), and a nutrition support nurse, funded by the hospital's pharmacy, were added to the core group.

Table 1. Roles of Nutrition Support Team Members

Physician-Director

To conduct nutrition rounds and supervise administration of the program

To provide consultations and patient assessments

To participate in and coordinate the nutrition education of health care professionals

To develop and update guidelines for the use of parenteral nutrition[a]

To develop relevant research projects in clinical nutrition[b]

To participate in national and international nutrition conferences to update knowledge. (All members of the team attend such conferences.)

Clinical pharmacist

To assist house officers in initiating, maintaining, and monitoring patients on parenteral nutrition. Such monitoring includes maintaining flow sheets of pertinent laboratory values and calculating the specific intake per kilogram of all relevant intravenous nutrients.

To provide formal education to health care professionals on selected parenteral nutrition topics

To assist with the continuous update of parenteral nutrition guidelines

To perform and assist with research projects dealing with specific aspects of parenteral nutrition

Clinical dietitian

To complete full nutritional assessments of individual patients, including thorough anthropometric measurements: length, weight, head circumference, weight for length, triceps skinfold thickness, mid upper arm circumference, arm muscle circumference, and arm muscle area

To recommend patient-specific enteral feeding regimens, especially during the transition from parenteral to enteral nutrition

To provide inservice education to health care professionals on topics regarding clinical nutrition

To assist with nutrition research projects

To work with the nurse, social worker, and family on a nutritional care plan for discharge

To develop guidelines for feeding progression and for evaluation of feeding skills

Nutrition support nurse

To conduct daily rounds on all patients receiving parenteral nutrition

To coordinate the uniform application of parenteral nutrition throughout all areas of the hospital

To coordinate and assist in inservice education of nursing staff in the insertion and maintenance of central venous catheters, operation of infusion devices, and prevention and management of parenteral nutrition complications

To coordinate and assist in the training of patients and families to be discharged on home parenteral nutrition

To review microbiology data in cooperation with infection control nurses, and laboratory data in cooperation with the satellite pharmacists

To write and update standards of nursing care for those patients receiving parenteral and enteral nutrition

To conduct patient care audits

To coordinate and participate in nutritional research

---

[a]Kerner JA, Sunshine P: Parenteral alimentation. *Semin Perinatol* 3:417, 1979.

[b]Kerner JA, Cassani C, Hurwitz R, et al: Monitoring intravenous fat in neonates with the fatty acid/serum albumin molar ratio. *JPEN* 5:517, 1981; Poole R, Rupp C, Kerner J: Calcium and phosphorus in neonatal TPN solutions. *JPEN* 5:580, 1981; D'Harlingue A, Stevenson DK, Shahin SM, et al: Monitoring the use of intravenous fat in neonates. *Pediatr Res* 16:487, 1982.

The specifics of our nutrition support service for the ICN were recently reported (11).

Briefly, the initial goals of our NST were to: (1) assess and improve the nutritional care of the hospitalized neonate; (2) educate fellows, housestaff, medical students, nurses, and other health care professionals concerning the intricacies of PN, including the potential advantages and disadvantages of this technique; (3) provide formal written consults upon request; (4) conduct weekly teaching rounds on patients with nutritional problems; (5) develop research projects involving clinical nutrition questions or problems; and (6) promote cost containment by providing a better understanding of PN, resulting in more efficient use of PN and fewer complications.

Member Functions and Responsibilities

Our NST now serves the pediatric ward as well as the ICN. The roles of our individual team members are listed in Table 1.

The responsibilities of the physician-director (2–5,12) and clinical dietitian (3–5) are relatively constant in various hospital settings, but those of the pharmacist (13–18) and nurse (19) may vary considerably. With increasing frequency larger institutions are establishing NSTs with full-time directors. The director's specialty interest is of little importance; the major requirements are an interest in the general problems of PN and a knowledge of metabolism and nutrition.

Conclusion

Providing adequate nutrition to neonates, infants, and older pediatric patients is a challenge that requires the skillful input of several disciplines. A nutrition support team can provide the guidelines, monitoring, consultations, and education that are necessary for the safe and effective administration of both parenteral and enteral nutrition. The team concept of nutritional support is becoming the standard of care for the hospitalized patient to promote health and healing.

References

1. Nehme AE: Nutritional support of the hospitalized patient: The team concept. *JAMA* 243:1906, 1980.
2. Skoutakis VA, Martinez DR, Miller WA, et al: Team approach to total parenteral nutrition. *Am J Hosp Pharm* 32:693, 1975.
3. Blackburn GL, Bothe A, Lahey MA: Organization and administration of a nutrition support service. *Surg Clin North Am* 61:709, 1981.
4. Suskind RM: The nutrition support service: An organized approach to the nutritional care of the hospitalized and ambulatory pediatric patient, in Suskind RM (ed): *Textbook of Pediatric Nutrition*. New York, Raven Press, 1981, p 375.
5. *Establishing a Nutritional Support Service*. Chicago, Abbott Laboratories, 1980.

6. Naccarto DV: Developing a nutrition support service. *Nutritional Support Services* 1:13, 1981.

7. Fletcher AB: Implementation of the neonatal TPN system, in *The Compromised Neonate.* Berkeley, Cutter Labortories, 1980, p 16.

8. *Fundamentals of Nutritional Support.* Deerfield, Illinois, Travenol Laboratories, 1981.

9. Sutphen JL: Nutritional support of the pediatric patient. *Clinical Consultations in Nutritional Support* 1(4):1, 1981.

10. Merritt RJ: Neonatal nutritional support. *Clinical Consultations in Nutritional Support* 1(4):5, 1981.

11. Poole R, Kerner JA: Establishing a nutritional support team for an intensive care nursery. *Nutritional Support Services* 3(2), February 1983.

12. Levy JS, Winters RW, Heird WC: Total parenteral nutrition in pediatric patients. *Pediatrics in Review* 2:99, 1980.

13. Greenlaw CW: Pharmacist as team leader for total parenteral nutrition therapy. *Am J Hosp Pharm* 36:648, 1979.

14. Mutchie KD, Smith KA, MacKay MW, et al: Pharmacist monitoring of parenteral nutrition: Clinical and cost effectiveness. *Am J Hosp Pharm* 36:785, 1979.

15. Vanderveen TW: Drug-nutrition interrelationships—An expanded role for the nutritional support team pharmacist. *ASPEN Update* 3:1, 1981.

16. Powell JR, Cupit GC: Developing the pharmacist's role in monitoring total parenteral nutrition. *Drug Intelligence and Clinical Pharmacology* 8:576, 1974.

17. Maslakowski CJ: Drug-nutrient interactions/interrelationships. *Nutritional Support Services* 1:14, 1981.

18. Griggs B: The monitoring and administration of total parenteral nutrition. *NITA* 4:220, 1981.

19. Heird WC: Total parenteral nutrition, in Lebenthal E (ed): *Textbook of Gastroenterology and Nutrition in Infancy.* New York, Raven Press, 1981, p 659.

20
The Transition from Parenteral to Enteral Feedings

John A. Kerner, Jr.

Health care personnel who work with parenteral feedings must be versed thoroughly in the proper delivery of enteral feedings. An extensive discussion of routes of administration (e.g., oral; tube—nasogastric, transpyloric; needle catheter jejunostomy), methods of administration, and complications of enteral feedings is beyond the scope of this chapter but is present in a number of excellent review articles (1–7).

Great care must be taken during the transition from parenteral to enteral feedings. One must avoid giving either excessive or insufficient fluids during the transition period by carefully calculating the portions to be administered via the enteral and parenteral routes combined. Selection of an appropriate enteral feeding regimen designed specifically for the patient's special needs is crucial for a successful transition. Table 1 lists a number of medical conditions and recommendations for possible enteral dietary regimens. Table 1 is a general guide, since the list is not complete, and patients with these illnesses do not always respond favorably to the listed recommendations. Ideally, the choice of enteral regimen should be discussed with a nutritionist to enhance the chance of success.

Enteral Formulations Available

Available infant formulas are depicted in Table 2. Terms used to describe various enteral products for children, such as *elemental, chemically defined, low residue,* or *supplemental,* are often confusing. The following classification of enteral products is based on guidelines issued by the American Society for Parenteral and Enteral Nutrition at its third Clinical Congress in 1979.

Table 1. Conditions for Which Defined-Formula Diets May be Considered

Condition	Method of Management
INFANTS AND TODDLERS	
Chronic diarrhea and malnutrition	Hospitalized patient: Continuous infusion of dilute Vivonex HN; Pregestimil; Nutramigen, Flexical.
Short bowel syndrome	Hospitalized patient: Continuous infusion of dilute Vivonex HN; Pregestimil; Nutramigen, Flexical.
Postinfectious chronic diarrhea, with inappropriate weight gain	Low lactose, no-milk protein formula as small, frequent feedings—soy bean formulas, Nutramigen if soy bean sensitivity is suspected.
Celiac disease	Dietary supplement of low lactose formula between regular meals—Ensure, with flavor packs (cherry, strawberry, orange, lemon, and so forth).
Cystic fibrosis	Hydrolyzed protein formula, possibly with medium-chain triglycerides.
Chronic congestive heart failure	Increase in caloric density may be achieved with Polycose (2 teaspoons of liquid to 4 oz of milk increases from 80 to 110 calories) and additional calories may be added as medium-chain triglycerides (8.2 calories/ml).
OLDER CHILDREN	
Regional enteritis	Dietary supplement to maintain good calorie–protein intake with low fat, low lactose, and low residue. Precision L-R; rarely, patients may improve nutrition with continuous nocturnal feedings of Vivonex for short periods.
Ulcerative colitis	Same management as for regional enteritis.
Chronic liver disease Renal disease without azotemia Chronic neurologic syndromes Cardiopulmonary disease	Patients with chronic disease frequently are prone to undernutrition. Because of a higher incidence of lactose intolerance with malnutrition, dietary supplements with low lactose formula (e.g., Ensure or Sustacal) may be advantageous.

SOURCE: Greene H, Schubert W: Diarrhea and malabsorption. *Pediatric Nutrition Handbook*, Evanston, Ill. American Academy of Pediatrics, 1979, pp 198–199. Copyright © 1979 by American Academy of Pediatrics. Reprinted with permission.

DEFINED FORMULA DIETS

Defined formula diets are also known as *elemental, chemically defined,* or *predigested* diets. Components of the diet are absorbed rapidly in the proximal portion of the small intestine and require little or no digestion due to the amino acid and carbohydrate sources.

These preparations have low viscosity and residue, are lactose-free, have high osmolality (450–800 mOsm/kg), have approximately 1 cal/ml, are high in carbohydrate (50–90% of calories) and low in fat, and are low to normal in protein (8–16% of calories). Since the concentration of carbohydrate is high, patients must be monitored carefully for glucose intolerance. When these formulas are given in volumes needed to meet caloric requirements, the Recommended Dietary Allowances for *adult* patients for vitamins and minerals are met or exceeded. Vitamin supplementation may be required in the pediatric patient.

Because these products are hyperosmolar they should be initiated at one-quarter to one-half strength and very gradually increased to prevent diarrhea and cramping. The formulas containing hydrolyzed protein or amino acids are not very palatable; if given orally these products should be taken in sips throughout the day. Ideally the product is given chilled, in a covered container (to minimize the smell), and is taken by straw. Otherwise, the product may be given by tube. Table 3 gives a breakdown of available defined formula diets.

MEAL REPLACEMENT DIETS

Meal replacement diets are made with blenderized natural foods or with intact isolated nutrients. These diets require intact digestive and absorptive capacity because the nutrient sources are more complex than those in the defined formula diets. They are suitable as the sole source of nutrition for patients whose gastrointestinal tracts are functioning fairly well. The diets can be provided both orally and by tube. They may or may not be lactose-free. Most have approximately 1 cal/ml (exceptions are Magnacal—2 cal/ml, Isocal HCN—2 cal/ml, Ensure Plus—1.5 cal/ml, Sustacal HC—1.5 cal/ml). They have a wide range of osmolalities and variable amount of residue. Added flavorings increase palatability and variety. These products are often better tolerated if started at half strength.

Tables 4 and 5 give a breakdown of available meal replacement diets. Table 4 shows intact protein, milk or meat based, lactose containing products; Table 5 shows lactose-free products.

SUPPLEMENTS

Supplements are designed to be used in addition to other food intake to increase the intake of one or more nutrients. They are not nutritionally complete formulations and should not be used as the sole source of nutrition. Vitamins and minerals are provided in varying amounts, but the amounts are generally inadequate. Supplements may vary in residue and nutrient content. They may contain concentrated sources of one nutrient, such as protein, fat, or carbohydrate. These "feeding module" products can be used to meet specific patient requirements or to adapt one of the commercial formulas. Changes in caloric density and changes in osmolality caused by these products should be taken into account. See Table 6 for a breakdown of available supplemental products.

Table 2. Approximate Composition of Infant Formulae

Formula/Milk	kcal/oz	Protein g/dl	Protein Source	Fat g/dl	Fat Source	Carbohydrate g/dl	Carbohydrate Source	Na mEq/dl	K mEq/dl	P mg/dl	Ca mg/dl	Osmolality mOsm/kg water
Human milk	20	1.0–1.2	Human milk	4.5	Human milk	7.0	Lactose	0.7	1.3	16	34	300
Enfamil	20	1.5	Nonfat milk	3.7	Soy oil, coconut oil	7.0	Lactose	1.0	1.7	44	53	278
Enfamil Premature	24	2.4	Nonfat milk, whey	4.1	Corn oil, MCT, coconut oil	8.9	Corn syrup solids, lactose	1.4	2.3	48	95	300
Isomil	20	2.0	Soy protein isolate with L-methionine	3.6	Coconut oil, soy oil	6.8	Corn syrup, sucrose	1.3	1.8	50	70	250
Isomil SF	20	2.0	Soy protein isolate with L-methionine	3.6	Coconut oil, soy oil	6.8	Corn syrup solids	1.3	1.8	50	70	150
Meat Base	20	2.6	Beef hearts	3.4	Sesame oil	6.2	Cane sugar, tapioca starch	1.2	1.4	65	98	280
Nursoy	20	2.1	Soy protein isolate with L-methionine	3.6	Oleo, coconut oil, oleic, soy oil	6.9	Sucrose	0.9	1.9	44	63	296
Nutramigen	20	2.2	Casein hydrolysate	2.6	Corn oil	8.8	Sucrose, modified tapioca starch	1.4	1.8	48	63	479
Portagen	20	2.4	Sodium caseinate	3.2	MCT, corn oil	7.8	Corn syrup solids, sucrose	1.4	2.2	48	63	220
Pregestimil	20	1.9	Casein hydrolysate with added amino acids	2.7	Corn oil, MCT	9.1	Corn syrup solids, modified tapioca starch	1.4	1.9	42	63	348
Prosobee	20	2.0	Soy protein isolate with L-methionine	3.6	Soy oil, Coconut oil	6.9	Corn syrup solids	1.3	2.1	50	63	200
Similac	20	1.6	Nonfat milk	3.6	Coconut oil, soy oil	7.2	Lactose	1.1	2.0	39	51	290
Similac-LBW	24	2.2	Nonfat milk	4.5	MCT, coconut oil, soy oil	8.5	Corn syrup solids, lactose	1.6	3.1	56	73	300

Product											
Similac PM/60/40	20	Whey, sodium caseinate	1.6	Coconut oil, corn oil	3.7	Lactose	6.9	0.7	1.5	20	40	260
Similac Special Care	24	Whey, casein	2.2	MCT, corn oil, coconut oil	4.4	Lactose, polycose	8.6	1.5	2.6	72	144	300
SMA	20	Whey, casein	1.5	Oleo, coconut oil, safflower oil, soy oil	3.6	Lactose	7.2	0.7	1.4	33	44	300
SMA-Preemie	24	Whey, casein	2.0	Oleo, coconut oil, oleic, soy oil, MCT	4.4	Lactose, maltodextrins	8.6	1.4	1.9	40	75	268
Soyalac	20	Soybean solids	2.1	Soy oil	3.7	Sucrose, corn syrup solids	6.6	1.3	1.9	50	60	210
I-Soyalac	20	Soy protein isolate with L-methionine	2.1	Soy oil	3.7	Sucrose, tapioca starch	6.6	1.6	1.8	50	60	230

FOR ADVANCED FEEDING BEYOND INFANCY

Product											
Similac Advance	16	Nonfat milk, soy protein isolate	2.0	Soy oil, corn oil	2.7	Corn syrup, lactose	5.5	1.3	2.2	39	51	210
Cow's Milk	20	Cow's milk	3.3	Cow's milk	3.7	Lactose	4.8	2.5	3.5	95	124	288

FOR SPECIAL FEEDING PROBLEMS[a]

Product											
RCF CHO-Free Formula Base (Without CHO source)	12	Soy protein isolate with L-methionine	2.0	Coconut oil, soy oil	3.6	May add: polycose, dextrose, fructose	—	1.3	1.8	50	70	Dependent upon CHO source
Product 3232A (Using 83.5 g powder & water to make 1 quart)	13	Casein Hydrolysate	2.2	MCT, Corn Oil	2.8	Modified tapioca starch; May Add CHO: corn syrup solids, dextrose, fructose	2.3	1.4	1.7	48	63	Dependent upon additional CHO source

[a]Informational sources: Mead Johnson Nutritional Division, Evansville, Indiana, 5/82; Ross Laboratories, Columbus, Ohio, 5/82.

Table 3. Defined Formula Diets

| Product | Cal/ml | Protein | | Fat | | Carbohydrate | | Na mEq/liter | K mEq/liter | P mg% | Ca mg% | Osmolality mOsm/kg water |
		g%	Source	g%	Source	g%	Source					
Flexical (Mead Johnson)	1.0	2.3	Enzymatically hydrolyzed casein, amino acids (70% free amino acids, 30% peptides)	3.4	MCT (20%), soy oil, soy lecithin	15.2	Corn syrup solids, modified tapioca starch	15	32	50	60	550 mOsm/kg
Vital High Nitrogen (Ross)	1.0	4.2	Peptides from enzymatically hydrolyzed soy, whey, and meat protein, free amino acids	1.1	MCT (45%), safflower oil	18.8	Hydrolyzed corn syrup solids, sucrose	17	30	66.7	66.7	460 (flavored) mOsm/kg
Vipep (Cutter)	1.0	2.5	Enzymatic digest of fish protein (peptides); supplemented with amino acids	2.5	MCT (80%), corn oil	17.6	Corn syrup solids, sucrose, corn starch, tapioca flour	32.6	21.8	60	60	520 mOsm/kg
Vivonex-standard (Eaton)	1.0	2.0	Free crystalline L-amino acids	0.1	Safflower oil	23.0	Glucose, oligosaccharides	37.4	29.9	55.6	55.6	550 mOsm/kg (unflavored)
Vivonex-HN (Eaton)	1.0	4.2	Free crystalline L-amino acids	0.1	Safflower oil	21.0	Glucose, oligosaccharides	34	18	33	33	810 mOsm/kg (unflavored)
Precision-LR (Doyle)	1.1	2.6	Egg albumin (egg white solids)	0.1	MCT, partially hydrogenated soybean oil, mono and di-glycerides	22.3	Maltodextrin, sucrose	30	22	52.6	52.6	525 mOsm/kg

Product	cal/ml	Protein source		Fat source		Carbohydrate source						Osmolality
Precision Isotonic (Doyle)	1.0	Egg albumin (egg white solids), Na caseinate	3.0	Partially hydrolyzed soy bean oil with BHA, mono, di-glycerides	3.1	Glucose oligosaccharides, sucrose	15.0	35	26	66.6	66.6	300 mOsm/kg
Precision HN (Doyle)	1.05	Egg albumin (egg white solids)	4.4	MCT, partially hydrogenated soybean oil, mono, diglyc-erides	0.19	Maltodextrin, sucrose	21.8	42.8	23.2	33	33	557 mOsm/kg
Travasorb MCT (Travenol)	1.0–2.0	Whey, lactalbumin, K caseinate	4.9	MCT (80%), sunflower oil	3.3	Corn syrup solids	12.2	15.2	44.5	50 (at 250 mOsm/liter) 100 (at 475 mOsm/liter)	50 (at 250 mOsm/liter) 100 (at 475 mOsm/liter)	250 mOsm/liter (at 1 cal/ml) 475 mOsm/liter (at 2 cal/ml)
Travasorb Standard (Travenol)	1.0	Hydrolyzed lactalbumin, L-methionine (di- and tripeptides and free amino acids)	3.0	MCT, sunflower oil	1.3	Glucose, oligosaccharides	19.0	40	30	50	50	450 mOsm/liter
Travasorb HN (Travenol)	1.0	Hydrolyzed lactalbumin, L-methionine (di- and tripeptides and free amino acids)	4.5	MCT, sunflower oil	1.3	Glucose, oligosaccharides	17.5	40	30	50	50	450 mOsm/liter
Criticare-HN (Mead Johnson) comes in liquid form	1.06	Enzymatically hydro-lyzed casein, amino acids (70% free amino acids 30% small peptides)	3.8	Safflower oil	0.3	Maltodextrin, modified corn starch	22.2	27.7	33.9	53	53	650 mOsm/kg

Table 4. Intact Protein—Milk or Meat Base (*Containing Lactose*)

Product	Cal/ml	Protein Source	g%	Fat Source	g%	Carbohydrate Source	g%	Na mEq/liter	K mEq/liter	P mg%	Ca mg%	Osmolality mOsm/ kg water
Formula 2 (Cutter)	1.0	Beef, skim milk, egg yolk	3.8	Corn oil, egg yolks, beef fat	4.0	Sucrose, orange juice, vegetables, wheat, farina, lactose	12.4	26.1	45.1	95	110	510
Liquid Meritene (Doyle)	1.0	Skim milk	6.0	Corn oil, mono- and diglycerides	3.3	Corn syrup solids, sucrose, lactose	11.5	39.9	42.7	125	125	560
Carnation Instant Breakfast	1.2	Milk, soy isolate, NF milk solids, Na caseinate	5.8	Milk fat	3.1	Corn syrup solids, sucrose, lactose	13.5	40	70	148.5	156.5	2000
Compleat-B (Doyle)	1.0	Beef puree skim milk	4.0	Corn oil, mono- and diglycerides	4.0	Hydrolyzed cereal solids, green bean puree, pea puree, nonfat dry milk, lactose, maltodextrin, peach puree, orange juice	12.0	51.6	33.7	125	62.5	390

Table 5. Intact Protein—Lactose Free

Product	Cal/ml	Protein Source	g%	Fat Source	g%	Carbohydrate Source	g%	Na mEq/liter	K mEq/liter	P mg%	Ca mg%	Osmolality mOsm/kg water
Isocal (Mead Johnson)	1.06	Na + Ca caseinate, soy protein isolate	3.4	Soy oil, MCT (20%)	4.4	Maltodextrins	13.2	23	34	52.1	62.5	300
Isocal HCN (Mead Johnson)	2.0	Na + Ca caseinate	7.5	MCT (30%) Soy oil	9.1	Corn syrup	22.5	34.8	35.9	66.6	66.6	740
Sustacal (Mead Johnson)	1.0	Na + Ca caseinate, soy protein isolate	6.1	Partially hydrogenated soy oil	2.3	Corn syrup, sucrose	14.0	40	53	92	100	625
Sustacal HC (Mead Johnson)	1.5	Na + Ca caseinate	6.1	Partially hydrogenated soybean oil	5.8	Corn syrup solids, sucrose	19.0	36.2	37.5	83.3	83.3	650
Ensure (Ross)	1.06	Na + Ca caseinates, soy protein isolate	3.7	Corn oil	3.7	Corn syrup solids, sucrose	14.5	32.2	32.5	50	50	450
Ensure Plus (Ross)	1.5	Na + Ca caseinates, soy protein isolate	5.5	Corn oil	5.3	Corn syrup solids, sucrose	19.7	46.1	48.6	63	63	600
Osmolite (Ross)	1.06	Na + Ca caseinates, soy protein isolate	3.7	MCT (50%), corn oil, soy oil	3.85	Glucose polymers	14.5	23.5	27.1	50	50	300
Magnacal (Organon)	2.0	Na + Ca caseinate	7.0	Partially hydrogenated soy oil, mono- and diglycerides	8.0	Maltodextrin, sucrose	25.0	43.5	32.0	100	100	590
Renu (Organon)	1.0	Na + Ca caseinate	3.5	Partially hydrogenated soy oil, mono and di-glycerides	4.0	Maltodextrin, sucrose	12.5	22	32	50	50	300
Vitaneed (Organon)	1.0	Puree beef, Na + Ca caseinate	3.5	Partially hydrogenated soy oil, beef fat, mono- and diglycerides	4.0	Maltodextrin	12.5	22	32	50	50	375
Travasorb (Travenol)	1.06	Na + Ca caseinate, soy protein isolate	3.5	Corn oil, soy oil, mono- and diglycerides	3.5	Sucrose, corn syrup solids	13.6	30	31	50	50	450 mOsm/liter

Table 6. Modular Products—Single Nutrient Additives and Supplements

Product	Cal/ml (or g)	Protein Source	g%	Fat Source	g%	Carbohydrate Source	g%	Na mEq/liter	K mEq/liter	P mg%	Ca mg%	Osmolality mOsm/kg water
FAT												
MCT oil (Mead Johnson)	7.75	—	0	MCT oil (fractionated coconut oil)	93.3	—	0	0	0	0	0	N/A
Microlipid (Organon)	4.5	—	0	Safflower oil	50	—	0	0	0	0	0	80
CHO												
Moducal (Mead Johnson)	2.0	—	0	—	0	Maltodextrin	50	1.3	0.1	0	0	N/A
Polycose (Ross)	2.0	—	0	—	0	Modified corn starch	50	2.5	0.5	6	30	850
Sumacal (Organon)	2.0	—	0	—	0	Maltodextrin	50	28.3	2.0	—	—	860
PROTEIN[a]												
Casec (Mead Johnson)	3.7/g	Ca caseinate	24 g/100 cal	Butterfat	0.54	—	0	6.6	2.1	0	0	N/A
Pro-Mix (Navaco)	1.0	Whey	22.7	—	0	Lactose	2.27	18.5	16.5	—	—	N/A
PROTEIN–CALORIE												
Citrotein (Doyle)	0.66	Egg albumin (egg white solids)	4.0	Partially hydrogenated soy oil	0.17	Sucrose, maltodextrins	12.1	29.7	17.2	104	104	496 (orange) 514 (grape)
CALORIE												
Controlyte (Doyle)	2.0	Trace	—	Soybean oil	9.6	Maltodextrins	28.6	2.6	0.4	3.2	3.2	590
Sustacal pudding (Mead Johnson)	1.6	Nonfat milk	4.8/100 g	Partially hydrogenated soy oil	6.7/100 g	Modified food starch, sucrose	22.6/100g	37	55	146.6	146.6	N/A
CHO-FREE												
RCF—Ross Carbohydrate Free (Ross)	Varies on amount of CHO added (0.4, if no CHO added)	Soy protein isolate	2.0	Coconut oil, soy oil	3.6	(Polycose, dextrose, or fructose can be added as per product information)	0	0.30 g/L	0.71 g/L	50	70	Varies based on amount of CHO added

[a]An additional modular protein supplement is now available—Propac (Organon).

Specific Guidelines

It is crucial that the transition from total parenteral nutrition (TPN) to enteral nutrition be *gradual*. Advancing enteral feedings too quickly may overtax the previously inactive gastrointestinal tract and may result in significant setbacks.

In general, infants and children with preexisting intestinal disease (e.g., intractable diarrhea) will not tolerate lactose-containing formulas; if there has been sufficient damage to the intestinal brush border, they may not tolerate sucrose containing formulas either. On the other hand, a large number of infants who have required TPN following surgical correction of a congenital intestinal anomaly can tolerate standard cow's milk-based formulas, which contain lactose.

Levy and associates have described helpful guidelines for the initiation of enteral feedings in patients who have been maintained solely on TPN (8). Once an appropriate enteral feeding regimen is selected, they begin feedings in small amounts (90–120 ml/day for a 3 kg infant = 30–40 ml/kg/day) *without* changing the composition or infusion rate of the parenteral nutrients. At Stanford University Hospital enteral feedings are also begun in small amounts. Initially diluted feedings are offered; the concentration increases each day while maintaining a constant volume (i.e., one quarter-strength feedings are given and increased by one-quarter strength each day until achieving full strength).

If the initial small volumes of full strength enteral feedings are tolerated, the volume of enteral feedings is slowly increased and the volume of the parenteral nutrients is proportionately decreased. Ideally, an attempt is made to maintain intravenous plus oral intake that will provide an amino acid plus protein intake of approximately 3 g/kg/day, a total fluid intake of 150–160 ml/kg/day, and a total caloric intake of 120–130 cal/kg/day (8).

When Levy and co-workers reach an enteral intake of 2–2.5 g/kg/day of protein and more than 100 cal/kg/day, the dextrose–amino acid solution is discontinued and replaced with 10% dextrose. The dextrose is decreased to 5% and subsequently discontinued when the infant is clearly tolerating the oral feeding regimen and is beginning to gain weight (8).

If there are no complications, the transition period lasts approximately 1 week. Enteral nutrient intolerance, requiring change in the feeding regimen or change in the route of delivery, may prolong the transition period. In some patients with short bowel syndrome or intractable diarrhea it may take a month or more to wean a child off TPN.

During the transition period feeding difficulties are common; they are not well understood. Many infants refuse the chosen enteral regimen, even when a standard formula is offered. Older children and adolescents complain of nausea, anorexia, and occasionally, vomiting. These symptoms, which apparently are not related to any documented intestinal dysfunction, require variable time periods for resolution (8).

To begin oral feedings in older infants and children, one follows the same principles previously discussed for a young infant. Small volume feedings are begun, starting with dilute feedings and advancing gradually to full strength. As the small volume feedings are advanced in strength, parenteral fluids remain constant. Once full strength feedings have been reached, oral feeds are gradually increased, and parenteral solutions are proportionately decreased (see Clinical Examples that follow for further details).

Table 7. Patients on Parenteral Nutrition

I. May have
  A. Bowel intact
  B. Bowel not intact

II. May be on
  A. Complete bowel rest
  B. Incomplete bowel rest

III. May be classified as patients who

A. Can't eat	B. Won't eat	C. Can't eat enough
Examples: intractable diarrhea; post-op complications; secretory diarrhea; coma; swallowing dysfunction; nausea/vomiting; GI fistulas; ulcerative colitis; Crohn's disease; obstruction	Examples: anorexia nervosa; depression; cancer	Examples: Crohn's disease; ulcerative colitis; cystic fibrosis; short bowel syndrome; immature gut (premature infants)

Harry Greene and co-workers studied seven adult volunteers fed a 3000 calorie diet that was either free of oral carbohydrate or contained 50% of calories as glucose (9). During the period when no oral carbohydrate was given, the activities of the intestinal disaccharidases (sucrase and maltase) decreased significantly. The sucrase and maltase responded only to high intraluminal concentrations of glucose and not to moderate changes in blood glucose concentration produced by intravenous glucose infusions (9).

Enzyme activities would thus be expected to be lower during TPN than after oral feeds are begun. Infants with intractable diarrhea fed enterally with dilute elemental diets achieved higher activities of sucrase, maltase, and trypsin than infants receiving solely TPN (10).

The above studies provide experimental evidence to recommend the gradual introduction of diet to patients being weaned from parenteral to enteral feedings. The gradual introduction of feedings should provide time for adaptive increases in carbohydrate digestive and metabolizing enzymes (9) and possibly for other adaptive enzymes involved in the assimilation of protein and fat (11–15).

Table 7 lists a few examples of the variety of types of patients who are receiving parenteral nutrition. For each type, the transition to complete enteral feedings will require individualized consideration. In some conditions transition from clear liquids to full liquids to soft diet to regular diet may be accomplished relatively quickly. In others it is necessary to progress very cautiously (Fig. 1). In short bowel syndrome, for example, patients initially receive TPN. Transitional enteral feedings are necessary to enhance cellular regeneration and adaptation of the remaining bowel. As bowel function returns postoperatively, tube feedings of elemental or defined formula diets are begun, using a very slow rate of infusion and carefully monitoring fluid and electrolyte balance and intake and output. As the patient's condition permits, the parenteral nutrition is decreased and tube feeding increased, since the bowel is beginning to adapt. Finally, appropriate oral intake is started and tube feeding reduced and discontinued as adequate absorption of the oral diet

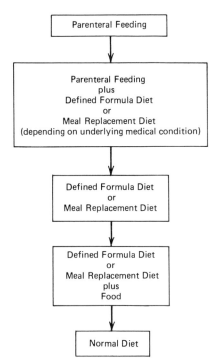

Figure 1 Transition from parenteral to enteral feedings. The time to progress from one step to the next depends on the patient's underlying condition.

occurs. The duration of each sequence is determined by the individual patient's need and progress.

Nutritionists can be extremely helpful when trying to determine a suitable diet plan for a patient. They have the expertise to choose from "standard diets" (clear liquids, full liquids, soft diet, low residue diet, regular diet, etc.), modifications of the standard diet (such as "small frequent feedings" in the anorectic child or adolescent), standard diet plus nutritional supplements (shown in Table 6), or "defined formula" or "meal replacement" diets (Tables 3–5) in complicated patients. They can help teach the health care team about the benefits and side effects of various regimens. For example, a more predigested and elemental formula (i.e., it contains more low molecular weight nutrients) has increased osmolality. Thus, large bolus feedings of such a formula are more prone to produce "dumping." To avoid such side effects either small frequent feedings or continuous tube feedings (by intragastric, intraduodenal, or jejunal route) can be used. Each diet, when tailored to the individual, should meet the patient's nutritional and emotional needs and should not adversely affect the patient's particular medical condition.

Clinical Examples

CASE 1

P. R. weighed 6 lb 10 oz at birth. He was begun on Isomil feedings (since three previous siblings had cow's milk intolerance). At 2 weeks of age he was well and his weight was 6 lb 12 oz. But at 4 weeks of age he had a history of vomiting and loose stools, and his weight had fallen to 6 lb 11½ oz. Initially, he improved with smaller feedings (the mother had been giving 4–6 oz per feeding). Five days later loose stools returned with no further emesis. The stools became explosive and his weight dropped to 6 lb 5 oz.

The child was admitted to the hospital and responded to being placed NPO and on IV fluids. The next day oral D₅W feedings caused increased stooling; CHO-free formula was then started. When fructose was added to the CHO-free, explosive stools occurred. Enteropathogenic *Escherichia coli* was isolated on stool culture and treated with neomycin. A second challenge with CHO-free with minimal additional fructose again caused profuse diarrhea. Twelve days after his initial admission, he was transferred to Stanford University Hospital for further treatment. His length was 49.5 cm (<5%), weight 6 lb 2 oz (<5%), head circumference 34.5 cm (<5%), triceps skinfold thickness was 5%, mid-upper arm circumference was also 5%. CBC and electrolytes were normal. The child tolerated Pedialyte but could not tolerate half-strength breast milk. Our initial impression was possible soy protein intolerance, possible viral gastroenteritis with secondary mucosal damage and intolerance to rapid early advancement of feedings, and a history of pathogenic *E. coli* isolated from the stool and appropriately treated.

A central line was placed and parenteral nutrition (PN) including Intralipid was begun. The child was eventually advanced to a maximum of 127 cal/kg/day from the parenteral nutrients.

After 1 week of PN while receiving nothing by mouth, the patient was started on half-strength Pedialyte at 15 ml every 2 hr (the patient's weight then was 3 kg, so the oral fluids were supplying *60 ml/kg/day*). The PN fluids were held at *100 ml/kg/day*. Therefore, total fluids were held at *160 ml/kg/day*. The PN fluids remained at 100 ml/kg/day and the oral feedings were kept at *constant volume* (15 ml q2h) progressing from one half-strength Pedialyte to one quarter-strength Pregestimil; we then increased by one quarter-strength per day (i.e., one-quarter-strength to one half strength to three quarter strength to full strength Pregestimil).

When the patient was on 15 ml every 2 hr of full strength Pregestimil, the oral feedings were gradually increased and the parenteral nutrition fluids proportionately decreased. Thirteen days after admission (6 days after oral feedings were begun) he was taking all his feedings orally. His weight was up to 3.185 kg (7 lb). His triceps skinfold thickness and mid-upper arm circumference were both up to fifteenth percentile. He was tolerating full-strength Pregestimil well in volumes of 60 ml every 3 hr, so his central line was discontinued. He was then advanced by 5 ml/feed to a maximum of 75 ml every 3 hr. He tolerated this regimen (600 ml/day; 189 ml/kg/day = 126 cal/kg/day) well without abnormal stools. The child was discharged on this regimen with a discharge weight of 3.2 kg (7 lb 2 oz) up 0.4 kg from admission. Two weeks after discharge the child's weight was up to 4.2 kg (9 lb 4 oz).

CASE 2

C.M. was a 17-year-old boy with cystic fibrosis. One year before admission he developed anal pain, which increased over the 3 mo before his admission. The pain was associated with an 8 lb weight loss as well as with blood-streaked stools. Barium enema had been normal. There was no family history of inflammatory bowel disease. Physical exam was normal except for four mucosal tags protruding from the patient's anus; there was also a surrounding area of of marked erythema.

On admission to the hospital, sigmoidoscopy to 15 cm under spinal anesthesia revealed an edematous and friable mucosa, and a biopsy of this area revealed mild chronic, nonspecific inflammation. In addition, there were multiple deep chronic linear ulcerations around the entire circumference of the anus. A biopsy taken through one of the chronic ulcers revealed granulomatous reaction. There were foreign body giant cells with polarizable crystalline material within the giant cells. An ulcerated fissure was also seen as well as acute and chronic inflammation. The pathologists felt a foreign body reaction was a possibility since the patient had been treating the anal area with local products such as Wyanoid HC suppositories, but they could not rule out Crohn's disease. A subsequent upper GI series with small bowel follow-through more than 1 year later was normal. Sedimentation rates were elevated during his hospitalization to a maximum of 47 mm/hr.

After the biopsy, because of the extreme anal pain he was placed NPO and started on parenteral nutrition (PN). *After 3 wk of PN,* the perianal area had improved considerably but was still erythematous and angry in appearance. Steroids were given IV and later switched to orally, and a *transition to oral feedings was initiated.* After a taste test of three available elemental diets, he was started on one elemental diet (ED) at a fixed volume per day–300 ml/day initially at one-quarter strength. The PN fluids were kept constant. Each day the concentration of the ED was increased (i.e., one-quarter strength to one-half strength to three-quarter strength to full strength). Four days after initiation of this regimen, he was at full strength of the ED. Six days after the initiation of the program his PN fluids had been discontinued, and he was taking three Flexical packets (flavored with Hawaiian punch), three packets of Vital, and 15 ml tid of MCT oil per day—providing 1920 cal from the EDs and 405 cal from the MCT oil, which totalled 2325 cal/day.

After 2 wk of receiving the EDs he was advanced to Isocal because of its low osmolality (300 mOsm/kg) and low residue content. He remained on Isocal until discharge (approximately 7 wk after admission). His perianal area was dramatically improved at discharge.

As an outpatient he was very gradually progressed from Isocal to minimal residue diet to a low residue diet and finally to a low roughage, moderate residue diet.

CASE 3

C.S. was a 16-year-old female who presented at the Children's Hospital at Stanford in September of 1981 with recently diagnosed ulcerative colitis, unresponsive to previous therapy. In April of 1981 she developed fatigue and weakness. In May she developed diarrhea. By June she was having seven to eight bloody stools per day. On 7/10/81 she presented to her private physician with symptoms of weakness and fatigue. CBC at that visit revealed a Hgb of 6.8. At home she was experiencing seven to eight bloody stools per day and abdominal cramps upon each bowel movement.

On 7/25/81 she was admitted to a local hospital. Sigmoidoscopy revealed an acute colitis. Upper GI with small bowel follow-through was normal and her sedimentation rate was 70 mm/hr. She was treated with ampicillin and prednisone and transfused with a total of 10 units of packed red blood cells over 2 wk. Multiple stool cultures and stools for ova and parasites were negative. Over the 2 wk there was a slight decrease in the bloody stools and she was discharged on prednisone and Azulfidine.

After discharge she continued to have bloody diarrhea, weakness, and a low-grade fever. A Hgb of 7.9 on 8/17/81 prompted readmission. Barium enema at this time was consistent with severe ulcerative colitis. She received 6 units of packed red blood cells over the next 2 wk, and remained on steroids and Azulfidine. A subclavian line was placed for PN but she was still allowed to eat.

On 8/28/81 Azulfidine was stopped because of no apparent benefit, cortisone enemas were begun, and oral metronidazole was empirically initiated. This regimen resulted in decreased frequency of bloody stools and decreased stool volume.

On her admission to The Children's Hospital on 9/1/81 we continued her metronidazole and prednisone but placed her NPO and switched her to TPN. Stool volume continued to decrease and no blood transfusions were necessary. By 9/29/81 her sedimentation rate was down to 27 mm/hr. At that time we changed her from continuous to cyclic TPN (gradually tapering her to 16 hr of PN infusion per day, with 8 hr "off" to be free of the TPN equipment).

On 10/1/81 after being NPO for 30 days a "clear liquid diet" without caffeine or citrus was begun. This feeding was well tolerated so PN fluid volume was decreased to three fourths of maintenance with $D_{17.5}W$ (reduced from $D_{20}W$) on 10/4. On 10/5 PN was decreased to one half of maintenance fluids, and the dextrose was decreased to $D_{15}W$; the patient was advanced to a low residue diet. On 10/6 PN was further decreased to one quarter of maintenance with $D_{12.5}W$. On 10/7 PN was decreased to $D_{10}W$. By 10/8 she was on a low residue diet and off PN.

For the last week of September (while NPO) her TPN calories averaged 3591 per day. By 10/5 her PN calories had been weaned to 1330; her oral calories had been increased to 2230 (total 3560 cal). By 10/6 she was up to 2680 oral cal. Her weight at that time was 81.9 kg (admission weight was 83.7 kg). She was discharged home 10/13 on a low residue diet and on steroids orally and by enema. Sedimentation rate was 28 mm/hr and Hct 31%.

References

1. Leleiko NS, Murray C, Munro HN: Enteral support of the hospitalized child, in Suskind RM (ed): *Textbook of Pediatric Nutrition.* New York, Raven Press, 1981, p 357.

2. Hoover HC, Ryan JA, Anderson EJ, et al: Nutritional benefits of immediate postoperative jejunal feeding of an elemental diet. *Am J Surg* 139:153, 1980.

3. Moss G: Early enteral feeding after abdominal surgery, in Deitel (ed): *Nutrition in Clinical Surgery.* Williams & Wilkins, 1980, p 161.

4. Heymsfield SB, Bethel RA: Enteral hyperalimentation—An alternative to central venous hyperalimentation. *Curr Concepts in Gastro* 4:13, 1979.

5. Heymsfield SB, Bethel RA, Ansley JD, et al: Enteral hyperalimentation: An alternative to central venous hyperalimentation. *Ann Intern Med* 90:63, 1979.

6. Andrassy RJ, Page CP, Feldtman RW, et al: Continual catheter administration of an elemental diet in infants and children. *Surgery* 82:205, 1977.

7. Koretz RL, Meyer JH: Elemental diets—Facts and fantasies. *Gastroenterology* 78:393, 1980.

8. Levy JS, Winters RW, Heird WC: Total parenteral nutrition in pediatric patients. *Pediatrics in Review* 2:99, 1980.

9. Greene HL, Stifel FB, Hagler L, et al: Comparison of the adaptive changes in disaccharidase, glycolytic enzyme and fructose diphosphatase activities after intravenous and oral glucose in normal men. *Am J Clin Nutr* 28:1122, 1975.

10. Greene HL, McCabe DR, Merenstein GB: Protracted diarrhea and malnutrition in infancy: Changes in intestinal morphology and disaccharidase activities during treatment with total intravenous nutrition or oral elemental diets. *J Pediatr* 87:695, 1975.

11. Alpers DH: Protein synthesis in intestinal mucosa: The effect of route of administration of precursor amino acids. *J Clin Invest* 51:167, 1972.

12. Kumar VO, Ghai P, Chase HP: Intestinal dipeptide hydrolase activities in undernourished children. *Arch Dis Child* 46:801, 1971.

13. Mansbach CM: Effect of fat feeding on complex lipid synthesis in hamster intestine. *Gastroenterology* 64:866, 1973.

14. Nicholson JA, McCarthy D, Kim YS: Differential response of intestinal brush border and cytosol peptide hydrolase activities to variation of dietary protein content. *Gastroenterology* 64:778, 1973.

15. Dowling RH: Compensatory changes in intestinal absorption. *Brit Med Bull* 23:275, 1967.

Part V
Special Considerations

21
The Use of Umbilical Catheters for Parenteral Nutrition

John A. Kerner, Jr.

The umbilical artery catheter is commonly used for infusing parenteral nutrition (PN) solutions in the neonate (1). Few studies exist regarding the safety of this practice.

Higgs and co-workers (2) described a controlled trial of total parenteral nutrition (TPN) versus formula feeding (Nan, Nestlé) by continuous nasogastric drip. The study included 86 infants weighing from 500–1500 g. The TPN, including glucose, amino acids, and fat emulsion, was administered by umbilical artery (UA) catheter for the first 2 weeks of life. There was no difference in neonatal morbidity or mortality between the two groups. Specifically, there was no difference in septicemia, although four of the 43 TPN babies had "catheter problems," described in the text only as "blockage" of the catheter.

Hall and Rhodes (3) wished to test the feasibility of perfusing parenteral nutrients (hypertonic dextrose, amino acids, vitamins, and minerals) into already existing lines inserted primarily for monitoring arterial blood gases (using UA lines). TPN delivered by umbilical catheter was initiated at an average of 4.5 days of age and continued for a mean of 7 days. The UA lines were removed when assisted ventilation was no longer required, oxygen requirements fell to ambient air, and enteral feedings were started. The authors delivered TPN to 80 infants by UA lines and to nine infants by indwelling umbilical venous catheters—these 89 infants were all "high risk" infants unable to tolerate enteral feedings. Results were compared to those for 23 infants with tunneled jugular catheters for chronic medical or surgical problems preventing use of the gastrointestinal tract. All infants studied ranged in weight from under 1000 g to over 2500 g.

As in the study of Higgs, Hall and Rhodes found that morbidity, mortality, and the common complications, such as infection and thrombosis, were similar in both groups.

In the umbilical catheter group 14 of 89 (16%) had positive blood cultures; eight of 89 (9%) had interruption of blood flow secondary to catheter thrombosis. Cyanotic legs were noted in three infants; this symptom disappeared within hours

303

after catheter removal. One infant died with a thrombus extending from the thoracic aorta down to and including the right renal artery. Death occurred only 8 hours after starting the TPN infusion (3).

Hall and Rhodes conclude that TPN by indwelling umbilical catheters presents no greater risk than infusion through tunneled jugular catheters. However, careful analysis of the authors' data raises questions about their conclusions. According to the authors, "Six deaths may have been catheter-related" (3). Five of those deaths occurred in the *umbilical artery catheter* group; death resulted from the thrombosis of the aorta described above, candidal septicemia in two, streptococcal septicemia in one, enterococcal septicemia in one. One death occurred in the jugular venous catheter group, with right atrial thrombosis superior vena cava syndrome, and *Staphylococcus epidermidis* on blood culture.

Finally, Yu et al. (4) studied 34 preterm infants with birth weights under 1200 g and randomly assigned them to TPN—including dextrose, amino acids, fat emulsion, electrolytes, vitamins, and trace elements all delivered by UA line—or milk feedings for the first 2 weeks after birth. Bacterial or fungal septicemia was not a complication in infants in either group during the study period. One infant in the TPN group who continued to require TPN for 10 weeks subsequently developed candidal septicemia but recovered on systemic amphotericin B. The TPN group had a greater nitrogen intake, improved weight gain, no necrotizing enterocolitis, and an unchanged mortality rate compared to the conventional milk-fed group. The group fed enterally was given freshly expressed breast milk from the infant's own mother or Similac 20 if the mother's milk was not available. Four infants developed necrotizing enterocolitis. No data on catheter-related complications were presented. Three infants in the TPN group developed cholestatic jaundice associated with elevated transaminase levels (the association of TPN and cholestasis is discussed in Chapter 13).

Hall and Rhodes (3) found that the rate of complication associated with *using TPN* in umbilical catheters was similar to that for long-term umbilical vessel catheterization *without* TPN infusion (5–9). Hall and Rhodes' study as well as the other two studies mentioned above address only the *short-term* side effects of the use of TPN through umbilical catheters. The short-term risk of serious complication from umbilical catheterization is probably between 2% and 5% and may be slightly greater with venous than with arterial placement (10).

The *long-term* risks of catheterization of the umbilical artery or umbilical vein are as yet unknown. It is known that umbilical vein catheterization employed for infusing intravenous fluids or for exchange transfusions in the newborn infant has been implicated as a cause of portal vein thrombosis (11). Umbilical venous catheterization has also resulted in candidal septicemia and the development of a right atrial mass (12).

In current review of PN in the neonate, Denson et al. state that although their greatest experience has been with venous catheters placed into the superior vena cava, they have successfully used the *UA catheter* for the first few weeks of PN in the most critically ill neonates (13). Merritt suggests caution with such use (14). He does not recommend using the UA line for infants requiring long-term PN for three major reasons (14):

1. UA catheters are associated with a very high incidence of arterial thrombosis. Fortunately, most of these thromboses do not precipitate life-threatening sequelae (15).

2. Because of the laminar flow characteristics of large arteries, arterial blood may not dilute the PN solution as effectively as venous blood. Thus, the patient may develop localized areas of hypertonic infusion.

3. Malpositioning the UA catheter can result in severe consequences. Placement too near the renal arteries, for example, has been associated with the onset of severe glucosuria and dehydration.

Dr. Arnold Coran, a pediatric surgeon, strongly recommends that PN *not* be given through either umbilical arteries or umbilical veins. PN through umbilical veins causes phlebitis, which may lead to venous thrombosis and portal hypertension. He is especially concerned about infusing PN solutions into a UA line, since this practice can lead to thrombosis of the aorta or iliac vessels. Furthermore, *severe damage* can occur to an artery *without being recognized.* There may even be thrombosis of the aorta without recognition. Only over an extensive period of time will the side effects of UA catheter use—such as inappropriate growth of one limb (16)—be known. Even the use of 12.5% dextrose infused through a UA line has increased osmolality that is clearly shown to cause thrombophlebitis (16). Although the first three studies described earlier all claimed there were no short-term complications, they did not address the problem of long-term complications.

Coran states that if PN is required and peripheral veins are not usable or if peripheral vein delivery is inadequate to provide necessary calories, he would consider percutaneous subclavian vein catheterization, which he can perform successfully even in a 900 g infant (16).

Like Coran and Merritt, we are reluctant to use umbilical catheters for the infusion of parenteral nutrients. We attempt to provide needed calories by peripheral vein. If more calories are needed or if PN must be provided for longer than 2 weeks, a central venous line is placed using the techniques described in Chapter 17.

References

1. Merritt RJ: Neonatal nutritional support. *Clinical Consultations in Nutritional Support* 1(4):10, 1981.

2. Higgs SC, Malan AF, Heese H DeV, et al: A comparison of oral feeding and total parenteral nutrition in infants of very low birthweight. *S Afr Med J* 48:2169, 1974.

3. Hall RT, Rhodes PG: Total parenteral alimentation via indwelling umbilical catheters in the newborn period. *Arch Dis Child* 51:929, 1976.

4. Yu VYH, James B, Hendry P, et al: Total parenteral nutrition in very low birthweight infants: A controlled trial. *Arch Dis Child* 54:653, 1979.

5. Balagtas RC, Bell CE, Edwards LD, et al: Risk of local and systemic infections associated with umbilical vein catheterization: A prospective study in 86 newborn patients. *Pediatrics* 48:359, 1971.

6. Peter G, Lloyd-Still JD, Lovejoy FH Jr: Local infection and bacteremia from scalp vein needles and polyethylene catheters in children. *J Pediatr* 80:78, 1972.

7. Van Vliet PKJ, Gupta JM: Prophylactic antibiotics in umbilical artery catheterization in the newborn. *Arch Dis Child* 48:296, 1973.

8. Bard H, Albert G, Teasdale F, et al: Prophylactic antibiotics in chronic umbilical artery catheterization in respiratory distress syndrome. *Arch Dis Child* 48:630, 1973.

9. Goetzman BW, Stadalnik RC, Bogren HG, et al: Thrombotic complications of umbilical artery catheters: A clinical and radiographic study. *Pediatrics* 56: 374, 1975.

10. Behrman RE: The fetus and the neonatal infant, in Vaughan VC, McKay RJ, Behrman RE (eds): *Nelson Textbook of Pediatrics.* Philadelphia, WB Saunders Co, 1979, p 434.

11. Roy CC, Silverman A, Cozzetto FJ: Portal hypertension, in *Pediatric Clinical Gastroenterology,* 2nd ed. St Louis, CV Mosby, 1975, p 583.

12. Johnson DE, Base JL, Thompson TR, et al: Candida septicemia and right atrial mass secondary to umbilical vein catheterization. *Am J Dis Child* 135:275, 1981.

13. Denson SE, Palma PA, Adcock EW III: TPN for the neonate. Part 1. Macronutrients. *Nutritional Support Services* 1(8):24, 1981.

14. Merritt RJ: Neonatal nutritional support. *Clinical Consultations in Nutritional Support.* 1(4):10, 1981.

15. Neal WA, Reynolds JW, Jarvis CW, et al: Umbilical artery catheterization: Demonstration of arterial thrombosis by aortography. *Pediatrics* 50:6, 1972.

16. Coran AG: Parenteral nutritional support of the neonate. *Tele Session* (a group telephone workshop), Tele Session Corporation, New York, August 17, 1981.

22
Cyclic TPN for Hospitalized Pediatric Patients

John A. Kerner, Jr.

Cyclic total parenteral nutrition (TPN), also referred to as *intermittent* or *discontinuous TPN*, refers to TPN in which for a period of time, usually 8–12 hours, administration of hypertonic dextrose is discontinued. There are several different ways to administer cyclic TPN: (1) administration of dextrose and amino acids for a certain number of hours followed by the infusion of fat emulsion; (2) simultaneous infusion of dextrose, amino acids, and fat followed by the administration of a dextrose-free solution (e.g., saline); (3) administration of dextrose, amino acids, and fat followed by infusion of amino acids without dextrose; (4) infusion of dextrose, amino acids, and fat concurrently followed by a *fasting period* of up to 10 hours (1).

The standard way to administer TPN is to deliver a continuous infusion through a large-caliber vein. The constant infusion of hypertonic dextrose results in high circulating levels of insulin (2). The hyperinsulinism leads to lipogenesis (conversion of dextrose to fat especially in the liver, the major site for *de novo* lipogenesis in humans [2,3]). The release of free fatty acids from adipose tissue is largely prevented due to the high insulin levels, even to the point where signs of essential fatty acid deficiency become apparent in the serum (4). In addition, constant lipogenesis and excessive glycogen deposition cause the hepatocytes to become engorged with fat and glycogen, leading to hepatomegaly and fatty infiltration of the liver, with possible evidence of liver dysfunction as well (see the section on hepatic dysfunction in Chapter 13).

Advantages of Cyclic TPN

The pioneer article regarding the use of cyclic TPN was by Maini and co-workers (5). They felt it would be desirable "to use a therapy that would allow a period each day during which lipogenic signals could be diminished and lipolysis could occur. In addition, fat mobilization from the liver and from peripheral adipose tissue stores, which contain a significant reserve of essential fatty acids, could be expected to diminish the potential for essential fatty acid deficiency" (5). During 8–10 hours of the day the infusion of hypertonic dextrose and amino acids was discontinued in their adult patients after reducing the infusion rate to 75–80 ml/hr for the last hour. During the "time off" of hypertonic dextrose and amino acids, patients received 3% amino acid solutions alone, saline, or oral protein alone. They documented improvement in liver function tests in patients on cyclic TPN (the liver function tests had become abnormal on continuous TPN), which in many patients was associated with resolution of hepatomegaly (5). A striking decrease in serum insulin occurred while on dextrose-free solutions. Serum albumin and transferrin levels returned to normal while on cyclic TPN, implying improved visceral protein status on this regimen.

Theoretical advantages for the use of cyclic TPN therefore include:

Prevention or treatment of TPN-induced fatty infiltration of the liver

Prevention or treatment of essential fatty acid deficiency

Raising or maintaining serum albumin since fat calories are the preferred source for visceral protein synthesis

Prevention of hyperinsulinism of continuous TPN

Prevention of lipogenesis

Prevention of the energy expense of triglyceride synthesis which increases the respiratory quotient (see Chapter 5)

In addition to the theoretical benefits of cyclic TPN, there is a very practical psychological benefit. As performed at the University of Michigan Medical Center (1), we also provide cyclic TPN using the fourth regimen described previously— infusing dextrose, amino acids, and fat emulsion all simultaneously, followed by a fasting period of up to 10 hours. The fasting period allows the patient to be free from the intravenous infusion pumps, tubing, and poles. Freedom from the TPN equipment provides a sense of normalcy, allowing the patient the opportunity for greater activity and more social interaction. The free time can be utilized to attend the hospital school, go to physical or occupational therapy, or even leave the hospital on an outing.

Hospital Use of Cyclic TPN

Although cyclic TPN is well established for home TPN patients (6–9), its use in the hospital is limited. Home TPN patients at the initiation of cyclic TPN are usually in satisfactory nutritional status, as opposed to malnourished hospitalized patients. Fleming et al. (10) recently described the use of cyclic TPN at home in severely malnourished patients.

Matuchansky and co-workers (11) designed a prospective study of nocturnal cyclic TPN over 12-hour infusion periods as a primary method of nutritional support in 27 consecutive acute patients hospitalized for severe malnutrition due to various gastrointestinal disorders. The nonprotein energy source was provided by fat (40%) and hypertonic dextrose (60%). The patients were totally starved during the day and were able to perform various physical activities including washing, dressing, and walking on the wards. Cyclic TPN was associated with a significant improvement in nutritional status. There was a low incidence of catheter-related infection (one case of septicemia due to *Staphylococcus epidermidis*) and metabolic complications (four cases of consistent, reversible hypertriglyceridemia) (11).

Matuchansky's study showed that his method of cyclic TPN was safe and efficient. Mechanical complications were very few. The main positive effect of their method was the improved comfort of their hospitalized patients with improvement of patient morale (11).

Faubion et al. (1) described eight patients ranging in age from 6 months to 17 years. Conditions necessary for instituting cyclic TPN included: stable metabolic status, stable electrolytes, steady weight gain for at least 2–4 days on continuous TPN, no requirements for subcutaneous or intravenous insulin, and well-positioned central catheters. They described no major complications. At the Children's Hospital at Stanford we have used cyclic TPN in five adolescents (two with Crohn's disease, two with ulcerative colitis, and one with hypogammaglobulinemia with a secretory diarrhea caused by the protozoan parasite, *Cryptosporidium*) without complications. Like Faubion and co-workers, we feel that cyclic TPN provides a more normal and less stressful environment for the patient. The patients enjoy their freedom away from a constant TPN infusion, as well as being given the autonomy to decide when their "time off" time will be.

Practical Guidelines

Prior to initiation of cyclic TPN the patient must

1. Have stable electrolytes and stable metabolic status
2. Demonstrate at least 2–4 days of weight gain on continuous TPN
3. Have a well-positioned central venous catheter.

ADMINISTRATION SCHEDULE (using the recommendations of Faubion et al. [1])

1. Day One (20-hr infusion; 4 hr "off"): Two hours before the central line is heparin-locked, the infusion rate is decreased by one-half. One hour before heparin-locking the line the rate is further reduced by half. For details of how to heparin-lock the line, see Chapter 17.
2. Day Two (18-hr infusion; 6 hr "off"): The infusion rate is calculated by dividing 90% of the desired volume of PN solution by 14. This will give you the hourly infusion rate for 14 of the 18 hours. The infusion schedule is depicted in Table 1.
3. Day Three (16-hr infusion; 8 hr "off"): In this case 90% of the desired volume is divided by 12 (instead of 14) to find the steady infusion rate.
4. To decrease "time off" of TPN
   a. Divide 90% of the desired volume by 10 for a 14-hr infusion period (10 hr "off") to generate steady infusion rate.
   b. Divide 90% of the desired volume by eight for a 12-hr infusion period (12 hr "off") to calculate the steady infusion rate.

Table 1. Example of Cyclic TPN Schedule (18 hr on, 6 hr off)

INFUSION PERIOD	18 HOURS
Starting	2 hours
Steady infusion rate	14 hours[a]
Tapering	2 hours
VOLUME NEEDED	1000 ml[a]
SCHEDULE	
1st hr	16 ml
2nd hr	32 ml
3rd–16th hr	64 ml
17th hr	32 ml
18th hr	16 ml
Heparin-lock TPN line for 6 hr	

SOURCE: Modified from Faubion WC, Baker WL, Iotl BA, et al: Cyclic TPN for hospitalized pediatric patients. *Nutritional Support Services* 1:24, 1981.

[a]To calculate the steady infusion rate, divide 90% of the volume needed (1000 ml) by 14 (90% of 1000 ml = 900; 900 ÷ 14 = 64 ml/hr)

5.   The amount of fat emulsion is not tapered up or down. The daily amount needed is given at a constant rate for the entire time that the TPN infuses.

MONITORING

The family and patient are taught the signs of hypoglycemia. Initially, for the first few days of cyclic TPN, blood glucose (or Dextrostix) determinations are performed 30–60 minutes after the infusion has ceased to check for rebound hypoglycemia. If no problems occur, additional glucose monitoring is not necessary.

COMPLICATIONS

Complications of cyclic TPN are similar to those of continuous TPN, although there may be decreased incidence of hepatomegaly and liver dysfunction as well as decreased incidence of essential fatty acid deficiency. The more frequent manipulation of the catheter theoretically increases the risk of sepsis and line clotting. Thus, strict protocols are necessary for catheter care in cyclic TPN (see Chapter 17).

References

1.   Faubion WC, Baker WL, Iotl BA, et al: Cyclic TPN for hospitalized pediatric patients. *Nutritional Support Services* 1:24, 1981.
2.   DenBesten L, Reyna RH, Connor WE, et al: The different effects on the serum lipids and fecal steroids of high carbohydrate diets given orally or intravenously. *J Clin Invest* 52:1384, 1973.

3. Chang S, Silvis SE: Fatty liver produced by hyperalimentation of rats. *Gastroenterology* 64:178, 1973.

4. Wene JD, Connor WE, DenBesten L: The development of essential fatty acid deficiency in healthy men fed fat free diets intravenously and orally. *J Clin Invest* 56:127, 1975.

5. Maini B, Blackburn GL, Bistrian BR, et al: Cyclic hyperalimentation: An optimal technique for preservation of visceral protein. *J Surg Res* 20:515, 1976.

6. Scribner BH, Cole JJ, Christopher TG: Long-term total parenteral nutrition: The concept of an artificial gut. *JAMA* 212, 457, 1970.

7. Broviac JW, Scribner BH: Prolonged parenteral nutrition at home. *Surg Gynecol Obstet* 139:24, 1974.

8. Jeejeebhoy KN, Zohrad WJ, Langer B, et al: Total parenteral nutrition at home for 23 months without complication and with good rehabilitation. *Gastroenterology* 65:811, 1973.

9. Jeejeebhoy KN, Langer B, Tsallas G, et al: Total parenteral nutrition at home: Studies in patients surviving 4 months to 5 years. *Gastroenterology* 71:943, 1976.

10. Fleming CR, Beart RW, Sharon JB, et al: Home parenteral nutrition for management of the severely malnourished adult patient. *Gastroenterology* 79:11, 1980.

11. Matuchansky C, Morichau-Beauchant M, Druart F, et al: Cyclic (nocturnal) total parenteral nutrition in hospitalized adult patients with severe digestive diseases: Report of a prospective study. *Gastroenterology* 81:433, 1981.

23
Home Parenteral Nutrition

John A. Kerner, Jr.

In the early 1970's Joyeaux and Solassol in France, Scribner in the United States, and Jeejeebhoy in Canada pioneered the use of intravenous feeding at home for the patient with gastrointestinal tract failure. Since that time, home parenteral nutrition (HPN) programs have been developed in many major medical centers (1). There are approximately 400 patients in the United States on HPN at any one time (2).

Many HPN candidates have reached a point at which their medical condition and nutritional requirements are reasonably stable. For these patients, who require less frequent monitoring, the benefits of HPN are enormous. Prolonged hospitalization causes not only a financial stress but also an emotional one for all involved. Returning the patient to family, friends, and some normal activities of daily living, with resultant increased independence, has a profoundly positive psychological effect. It is the purpose of this chapter to provide an overview of the use of HPN in pediatric patients. More detailed descriptions of HPN, including a booklet from the proceedings of a comprehensive symposium on total parenteral nutrition in the home (3), are available to the interested reader (3–10).

Indications

HPN for a pediatric patient is considered if the child is unable to maintain adequate nutritional and fluid balance on enteral feedings and is expected to require prolonged in-hospital PN. Ament has managed over 200 patients on HPN, 25% of whom have been infants and children. He describes five major categories of disorders in pediatric patients that may qualify them for HPN (11);

1. Short bowel syndrome, with and without the potential for bowel adaptation
2. Primary motility disorders (e.g., pseudoobstruction syndrome)

3. Severe mucosal injury
4. Congenital failure of villus formation
5. Crohn's disease
   a. Growth failure refractory to medical management
   b. Short bowel syndrome secondary to multiple surgical resections
   c. Intractable diffuse disease
   d. Enterocutaneous fistulas (12)

We have found that a sixth category for possible HPN is complex secretory diarrhea. In such cases, either the cause is unknown or unusual, such as congenital villus atrophy or *Cryptosporidium*-induced diarrhea.

Venous Access

In infants and children who are to receive HPN, the silastic tunneled Hickman and Broviac catheters allow for safe venous access for continuous or intermittent PN delivery. In the operating room under local or general anesthesia, the Broviac or Hickman catheter is usually inserted by a cutdown over the cephalic vein or, occasionally, the external jugular vein terminating at the junction of the superior vena cava and the right atrium (1). At UCLA approximately 80% of the catheters are placed in the saphenous or femoral vein, since their pediatric surgeon believes these veins are the most accessible and because they are concerned about their patients' future appearance, wishing to avoid scars on the upper chest (11).

HPN Methods of Delivery

There are two types of pediatric HPN delivery—cyclic (intermittent) and continuous. All of the patients managed by the team at UCLA are on cyclic HPN (11). Cyclic PN can be accomplished as described in Chapter 22. Alternatively, once the patient is stabilized on an optimal PN solution, the number of hours the patient receives the PN solution is gradually decreased by one hour each day until the same volume of solution is being administered over a 10–16 hour period encompassing the sleeping hours, allowing the patient to pursue reasonably normal daytime activities. During the time the PN is not infusing, the catheter is filled with a heparin-saline solution and capped (see Chapter 17). Considerations that might favor continuous infusion include situations in which large volumes of fluid (> 4 liters/day) are required, or where rapid fluid shifts would not be tolerated, for example, in patients with congestive heart failure (1). Such patients can be freed from multiple intravenous poles, bottles, and tubing with the use of a lightweight ambulatory hyperalimentation vest developed by Dudrick and associates (6) (Fig. 1). The vest has storage space for the PN solutions and is complete with a miniature volumetric pump powered by rechargeable batteries.

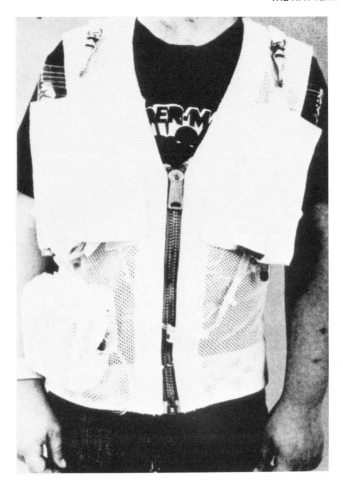

Figure 1 Ambulatory hyperalimentation vest.

The HPN Team

At the heart of a successful home parenteral nutrition program is a well organized teaching program that incorporates a highly committed nutritional support team. Effective teaching will lead to a successful transition from hospital to home care.

Maintaining a child on HPN is a 24-hour responsibility that requires two physicians, knowledgeable in the management of patients on PN, to share the responsibility year-round. A pharmacist well trained in the preparation of intravenous admixtures and nutritional solutions is essential. A social worker, experienced in dealing with chronically ill children, is needed not only to help with the financial aspects of the case, but also to be sure the family is able to cope with the responsibilities of the HPN program, not to mention the emotional stress regarding the ultimate prognosis for their child. A nutritionist is needed for counseling, since a number of HPN patients may be able to receive at least some of their nutrients enterally. The nutritionist is best able to determine the foods or enteral products most appropriate for the individual patient's underlying disease state. In addition, the nutritionist can provide follow-up nutritional assessment (11).

A nurse is needed for teaching the patient or designated family member about all aspects of HPN care and for discharge planning. Various procedures and techniques must be taught[a] so that the patient or designated family member can assume home care responsibility. In addition, one reliable family member should learn the practice so as to provide backup.

The patient should be hospitalized at the initiation of the HPN program. The inpatient approach allows the entire HPN team to work with the patient and designated family member. Instruction should ideally take place outside of the patient's room in a place where distractions will be minimal. Each teaching session should be no longer than 1 hour so that all the information can be understood and remembered. The matter covered should also be provided in print for reinforcement, and for quick reference. The sessions should include return demonstrations.

The patient or designated family member will have to become skilled at handling all the equipment involved, as well as proficient in

Catheter dressing change

Flushing technique and the heparin-locking procedure

Use of an infusion apparatus

Attachment of fresh PN solutions, and home admixing, if applicable*

Metabolic monitoring, which includes recording intake and output, testing urine for glucose and acetone, daily weights, and checking body temperature

Techniques for emergency repair of the catheter

Finally, a visiting nurse service that understands the HPN process would be ideal in order to evaluate the home situation, maintain communication and support, and aid the HPN team in assessing the effectiveness of the home program (11).

Frequently in adult HPN programs, a psychiatrist joins the HPN team to perform an initial evaluation including patient's orientation, memory functions, basic knowledge, and presence or absence of anxiety or depression, and to be available for support.

Follow-up Visits

At UCLA follow-up visits are usually scheduled weekly during the first month and monthly thereafter for growing infants. For the older child, visits may be scheduled monthly or bi-monthly. At each visit blood specimens for monitoring are obtained

---

[a]At Stanford University Medical Center we have a training manual for HPN patients— Cheung T: *Home parenteral nutrition training manual*. Chicago, Abbott Laboratories, 1982.

*Not all people have the ability to mix PN solutions or perform certain procedures; therefore, community resources such as the Visiting Nurses Association or the local pharmacies may be used.

to be sure the patient is in metabolic balance. These include complete blood count, tests for electrolytes, calcium, phosphorus, and magnesium, and for liver function. Height and weight are also measured to determine if nutritional support is adequate (13). The management of infants and children on HPN differs from that for adult HPN in that nutritional requirements must be constantly readjusted to meet the pediatric patient's changing growth requirements.

General Results of HPN

The Mayo Clinic's experience with adult HPN patients has shown that the nutritional repletion of chronically malnourished patients has been dramatic; the average weight gain in patients treated has been 13 kg, properly proportioned between fat and lean body mass. Serial studies have shown impressive increases in visceral proteins, albumin and transferrin, and skeletal muscle mass reflected by the creatinine height index. There has been a 60% reduction in hospitalization for this group since HPN was started as compared to comparable periods before HPN was practiced. Seventy percent of patients have clearly been rehabilitated. Although the other patients improved nutritionally, rehabilitation failed secondary to combinations of effects of their primary disease, depression, and narcotic addiction (2).

In the first extensive experience of HPN reported in pediatrics, Strobel et al. described 34 patients (ages 1.5 months to 20.5 years) on an HPN program for periods ranging from 23–786 days (10). All patients improved their nutritional status. Twenty-three out of 29 on the program for more than 2 months showed an increase in height. All had significant decreases in symptomatology. All were able to resume their education or work. At the time the paper was submitted, 24 patients, including 15 with Crohn's disease, no longer required HPN (10).

Goldberger and associates (9) described three children (aged 4 months, 5 months, and 14 years) on HPN for 10, 23, and 44 months respectively. Normal skeletal development and weight gain were achieved while allowing normal social and psychological development outside the hospital. The duration of catheter patency ranged from 3–22 months. Catheter-related sepsis or mechanical failure occasionally required catheter removal and replacement (9).

Cannon and co-workers (14) looked at the effects of prolonged HPN on growth and psychomotor development in eight infants, each begun on HPN in the first 60 days of life. Normalization of somatic growth was observed in all patients during the study period. Six of eight patients had normal psychomotor development following discharge from the hospital to home. Catheter-related complications were infrequent, although there was one episode of sepsis during 121 patient-months. The major complication was rickets despite provision of recommended doses of vitamin D.

In Ament's experience, HPN infants have had normal neurologic development. Motor and language skills show some compromise for unknown reasons (11). Motor skills may be diminished owing to the time that a patient's movement is restricted while receiving the HPN infusion; language skills may be delayed because of lack of normal oral stimulation, since many receive no foods by mouth.

Strobel et al. (15) described the use of HPN in Crohn's disease in 17 pediatric patients (aged 9.25–20.5 years) for severe symptomatic disease unresponsive to sulfasalazine in 14, steroids in 12, inpatient TPN in seven, and surgical resections in six. Remission was achieved in 12 of the 17 patients after one course of HPN alone. All 17 had a marked improvement in disease symptoms while on HPN. Ten patients demonstrated "catch-up" growth. There was only one episode of sepsis per 5.8 catheter-experience years (15).

Complications

All the same complications inherent to in-hospital parenteral nutrition can occur on HPN, but the metabolic and catheter-related complications appear to be much less frequent. The greatest risk during inpatient or outpatient PN is the *risk of sepsis.* Parents of HPN patients must be aware of temperature elevation in their children and must notify their physician at once. Physicians must make a judgment on the seriousness of the fever and must always examine the children when they develop fever to determine if there is a potential for sepsis (13). Catheter-related infection is the main indication for catheter removal and one of the main reasons for readmission to the hospital. This complication is easily treated by catheter removal but must be diagnosed correctly. Because venous access may be limited in some patients, it is important to be certain one is dealing with catheter-related infection before removing the catheter.

Steiger and associates obtain blood cultures through peripheral veins as well as through the central catheter when catheter-related sepsis is suspected; then the catheter is "capped off" and not used. A positive blood culture requires catheter removal. Repeated catheter cultures may be necessary to document infection. If the patient remains febrile or septic despite not using the catheter and no other source of fever can be found they recommend that the catheter be removed. If an infected catheter is removed, the temperature usually returns to normal and subsequent blood cultures are negative. Systemic antibiotics are only necessary if the fever does not resolve within 24 hours (1).

Catheter occlusion by thrombosis is not uncommon, especially with the smaller lumen of the Broviac catheter (Lees and co-workers using the larger bore Hickman catheter have not noted any instances of catheter blockage [4]). The use of urokinase to dissolve the thrombus has been reported to be of value, and a number of centers have found that the instillation of urokinase saved several occluded catheters from being removed and replaced (1,13,16).

Frequent catheter complications include cracking and breaking either from long-term use or by inadvertent misuse of catheter clamping devices. Such damage is managed with a catheter repair kit, either at the hospital that trained the HPN patient or by the patient's local physician. Eighty per cent of Ament's patients have had successful repair of damaged catheters (2,13).

Metabolic complications are surprisingly few on HPN if careful attention is paid to the child's nutritional assessment and biochemical parameters. Ament did find that three of eight infants started on HPN at less than 60 days of age developed frank clinical rickets, thought to be secondary to the infants' inability to metabolize enough of the 400 IU of vitamin D provided daily (11). He found that administering 1000 IU of vitamin D per day to those infants resulted in positive balance for both calcium and phosphorus. In Ament's early experience, only one HPN patient developed chronic jaundice or cirrhosis (11). His group's more recent data are more discouraging (17). All their patients on long-term TPN developed hepatic fibrosis and 11% had cirrhosis. The etiology of this wide spectrum of damage is unknown but did not correlate directly with time on TPN.

Psychosocial Issues

Little is known about the psychosocial aspects of pediatric HPN. The literature on adults has more information in this area. Steiger feels that psychological issues in adults should be recognized and discussed during the intensive in-hospital training program, focusing on fear of the underlying disease, fear of death, costs of the program, and return to a reasonably functional lifestyle (1). Those patients most likely to accept the adult HPN program are those who have had prolonged malnutrition and who for the first time in a long while feel well on parenteral feedings. Those who find it most difficult to accept, at least initially, are those who were previously healthy and then developed a sudden catastrophic event, such as a mesenteric infarction, requiring a PN program (1).

Psychiatric problems in adult HPN patients at the start of their training program include both acute (38% of patients) and chronic (4%) organic brain syndrome secondary to therapeutic drugs, metabolic abnormalities, sepsis, or a combination of these factors (18). Other problems requiring psychiatric treatment were anxiety regarding the catheter and the infusion apparatus, depression (22% of patients), drug dependency, and interpersonal conflicts (18). Additional psychosocial problems are described in detail by Gulledge (19).

In the pediatric HPN patients for whom Ament has cared, he has seen limited emotional stress in the families. In fact, in all of his cases, Ament has not seen divorce or separation because of the child. Data regarding the effect of HPN on siblings has not been reported (13). I can add only one anecdotal report: In one of our HPN patients from Stanford who was 1½ years old, one of his older siblings *deliberately* cut the patient's PN catheter. There is no question that more studies are needed on the impact of HPN on the child, the parents, and the siblings.

Cost

A full term infant on PN at UCLA as of February, 1980 incurred a daily hospital bill of $400 resulting in a yearly cost of $146,000. For an infant on HPN the cost was $36,500 per year—a substantial savings (11). The average cost per year for the HPN program in adults is approximately $20,000 versus approximately $73,000 if they were to remain in the hospital (4).

The recent establishment of private companies to deliver equipment and supplies to the home, maintain inventory, directly bill the patient, help with insurance problems, and provide other services to the patient and physician, has significantly reduced the financial and logistic burdens that in the past were borne by the training center (4). The experience at the Cleveland Clinic is that payment for HPN depends on the insurance coverage of the patient and his or her financial status. If the patient has a major medical clause in a health insurance policy from a private insurance company, it will usually cover 80–100% of expenses.

HPN Versus Home Enteral Nutrition

Prior to instituting HPN the entire nutrition support team must be convinced that a home enteral nutrition (HEN) program is not a viable alternative. HPN and HEN were recently compared in 18 patients (20). Both groups studied demonstrated marked increases in weight, triceps skinfold thickness, arm muscle circumference, and serum albumin. Three of the nine HPN patients developed one episode of catheter-related sepsis. No significant side effects were seen in the HEN patients receiving their nutrition by micro-feeding jejunostomy tubes. The cost of HEN per day averaged $20–$40 versus $150–$250 for HPN. Chrysomilides and Kaminski concluded that HEN should be selected over HPN in all *possible* cases and that the micro-feeding jejunostomy route is safe, useful, and cost-effective (20). Obviously, an inflamed or nonfunctioning gastrointestinal tract cannot be used for HEN. On the other hand, for a patient with Crohn's disease who has growth failure and quiescent disease (i.e., no evidence of significant active intestinal inflammation), HEN may be a viable alternative to HPN.

Conclusion

HPN is a feasible alternative for selected pediatric patients who have a motivated and devoted family and support of a medical institution committed to meeting patient needs. HPN is a therapeutic technique that permits normal growth and development to take place in children who might not thrive or survive without it, and allows others to regain normal or near normal intestinal function over weeks or months while in a loving home environment.

References

1. Steiger E: Home parenteral nutrition. *ASPEN Update* 3(4):1, 1981.
2. Fleming CR: Home parenteral nutrition. *Mayo Clin Proc* 56:132, 1981.
3. Steiger E (ed): *Home parenteral nutrition.* New York, Pro Clinica, 1981.
4. Lees CD, Steiger E, Hooley RA, et al: Home parenteral nutrition. *Surg Clin North Am* 61:621, 1981.
5. Fleeman CM, Wright RA: Concepts of home parenteral nutrition. *Nutritional Support Services* 1(6):16, 1981.
6. Dudrick SJ, Englert DM, Barroso AO, et al: Update on ambulatory home hyperalimentation. *Nutritional Support Services* 1(1):18, 1981.
7. Srp F, Steiger E, Montague N, et al: Patient preparation for cyclic home parenteral nutrition: A team approach. *Nutritional Support Services* 1(1):30, 1981.
8. Byrne WJ, Ament ME, Burke M, et al: Home parenteral nutrition. *Surg Gynecol Obstet* 149:593, 1979.
9. Goldberger JH, DeLuca FG, Wesselhoeft CW, et al: A home program of long-term total parenteral nutrition in children. *J Pediatr* 94:325, 1979.
10. Strobel CT, Byrne WJ, Fonkalsrud EW, et al: Home parenteral nutrition: Results in 34 pediatric patients. *Ann Surg* 188:394, 1978.

11. Ament ME: Pediatric HPN, in Steiger E (ed): *Home Parenteral Nutrition.* New York, Pro Clinica, 1981, p 10.

12. Byrne WJ, Burke M, Fonkalsrud EW, et al: Home parenteral nutrition: An alternative approach to the management of complicated gastrointestinal fistulas, not responding to conventional medical or surgical therapy. *JPEN* 3:355, 1979.

13. Ament ME: Home parenteral nutrition in infants and children. Course in Intravenous Nutrition in the Pediatric Patient. Letterman Army Medical Center, San Francisco, February 13, 1981, p 326.

14. Cannon RA, Byrne WJ, Ament ME, et al: Home parenteral nutrition in infants. *J Pediatr* 96:1098, 1980.

15. Strobel CT, Byrne WJ, Ament ME: Home parenteral nutrition in children with Crohn's disease: An effective management alternative. *Gastroenterology* 77:272, 1979.

16. Glynn MFX, Langer B, Jeejeebhoy KN: Therapy for thrombotic occlusion of long-term intravenous alimentation catheters. *JPEN* 4:387, 1980.

17. Kibort PM, Ulich TR, Berquist WE, et al: Hepatic fibrosis and cirrhosis in children on long-term parenteral nutrition. *Clin Res* 30:115A, 1982.

18. Gulledge AD, Gipson WT, Steiger E, et al: Short bowel syndrome and psychological issues for home parenteral nutrition. *Gen Hosp Psychiatry* 2:271, 1980.

19. Gulledge AD: Social and psychiatric implications of HPN, in Steiger E (ed): *Home Parenteral Nutrition.* New York, Pro Clinica, 1981, p 39.

20. Chrysomilides SA, Kaminski MV Jr: Home enteral and parenteral nutritional support: A comparison. *Am J Clin Nutr* 34:2271, 1981.

24

The Role of Parenteral Nutrition in Pediatric Oncology

Michael D. Amylon

Inadequate caloric intake, weight loss, decreased lean body mass, and severe protein–calorie malnutrition are relatively common in the pediatric patient with cancer (1–3). Factors that exacerbate such nutritional depletion include the local and systemic effects of the tumor cells, as well as the many toxic side effects of therapy. The syndrome of cancer cachexia is well recognized, and many patients present to the oncologist with anorexia, tissue wasting, and organ dysfunction. In other cases, the complications and side effects of therapy lead directly to a significant decrease in food intake and the development of severe malnutrition. In either situation, the malnutrition increases morbidity and mortality or alters the tolerance of the host, preventing the delivery of optimal therapy. Even the patient who presents to the oncologist in a state of good nutrition is placed at great risk for the development of malnutrition as a consequence of the toxicities of current aggressive multimodality treatment. Therefore, it is worthwhile to examine the potential of parenteral nutrition (PN) to ameliorate morbidity, permit the delivery of effective therapy, and, hopefully, contribute to improving the prognosis of the child with a malignancy.

Interference With Adequate Nutritional Intake

Many patients with cancer are anorectic. Although it has not been proven directly, it has been suggested that a humoral substance is elaborated that acts directly on the hunger center in the hypothalamus (4,5). Many patients also seem to experience perturbations of taste and smell, which may contribute to appetite reduction (6,7). Solid tumors (e.g., tumors of the head, neck, or gastrointestinal tract) can cause a direct mechanical obstruction and limit food intake. Additionally, hypermetabolic states, energy trapping, and altered (inefficient) metabolic pathways within a large tumor cell population may lead to a catabolic state despite the patient's intake of adequate nutriments (8,11). Surgical intervention for tumors of the head and neck

323

or tumors within the abdomen or pelvis can prevent the ingestion of adequate nutrition for a considerable period of time postoperatively.

Most chemotherapeutic agents have side effects, including nausea and vomiting, that decrease the patient's ability to maintain adequate oral nutrition. Mucositis is likely to occur in patients treated with high doses of a variety of agents and contributes to poor intake as well as to malabsorption and diarrhea. Infection in patients with chemotherapy-induced neutropenia also contributes to the total number of days of unsatisfactory nutritional intake.

Radiation of a large area of tissue anywhere in the body can lead to symptoms of radiation sickness, which include nausea and vomiting with anorexia. Radiation therapy to the abdomen is particulary toxic. There is a direct toxic effect on the gastrointestinal tract with alteration in mucosal architecture that becomes manifest very soon after the initiation of therapy and can lead to malabsorption (12,13). Radiation to the mouth or esophagus may result in severe mucositis that prevents adequate oral intake.

The cancer patient has impaired ability to heal wounds or to repair damage to normal tissues induced by radiation or chemotherapy (14). The immune system is compromised, host defense mechanisms function poorly, and infection is common (15–17). Reduction in lean body mass results in muscle wasting that can limit physical activity substantially. Changes in the mucosal lining of the intestines, noted in severely malnourished patients, result in further malabsorption; consequently, a vicious cycle evolves.

There is often a very narrow margin of safety protecting the patient who is being treated aggressively for a malignant disease from unacceptable toxicity. In the face of malnutrition and its consequent physiological derangements, this margin may be reduced or eliminated, thereby either preventing the delivery of optimal therapy or precipitating unacceptable morbidity, or both.

The Use of Parenteral Nutrition

Several studies have demonstrated that PN can reverse many of the observed physical effects of malnutrition in the patient with cancer. Weight loss can be reversed, the concentrations of serum proteins can be increased, and positive nitrogen balance can be achieved (3,11,12,18). Subjective responses such as an improved sense of well-being and increased energy and activity have been reported (19–21). Even altered immune function can be restored with improvement in nutritional status (15,22).

Many have questioned the ability of the cancer patient to tolerate intravenous nutritional support without developing significant side effects, and certainly the risks must be evaluated before recommending its use. In the already severely compromised oncology patient whose course will be further complicated by immunosuppressive and myelosuppressive chemotherapy and/or radiation therapy, the risk of infectious complications may be quite high. Similarly, there may be additive or even synergistic hepatic or renal toxicities. In addition, mechanical complications such as thrombosis or hemorrhage are potential hazards in these patients with long-term use of indwelling central venous catheters. Interestingly, with improved techniques of catheter care and with careful monitoring and avoidance of metabolic derangements, the complication rates for PN use in these individuals do not exceed those reported for other patient populations (19,20,23–27).

Another potential barrier to the delivery of PN in the patient with a malignant disease is the possibility that tumor growth might be stimulated by the provision of adequate nutrients. The tumor often seems to have a selective advantage over the host in the competition for nutrients, as evidenced by the continued growth of large tumors even when the patient is losing weight rapidly. Additionally, some animal models have suggested that nutritional deprivation slows tumor growth, and conversely that nutritional repletion stimulates growth (28,29). To date, no studies in humans have shown any appreciable acceleration of tumor growth in patients receiving PN (21,30). Thus, it appears possible to reverse many of the metabolic derangements and to restore and maintain nutritional balance in the pediatric oncology patient without unacceptable risk or adverse effect on tumor growth.

Support with PN in the oncology patient has not been shown *conclusively* to improve the patient's ability to tolerate anticancer treatment (29–33). However, studies have suggested that postsurgical morbidity is reduced, chemotherapy-induced myelosuppression may be modified slightly, and the ability of the radiation therapist to deliver a planned dose of therapy may be improved (12,20,21,34–36).

It has also been difficult to document improvement in the long-term survival rate of patients treated with nutritional support programs. Several authors have suggested that a nutritionally replete host is more likely to have a favorable response to therapy (12,31,37), although others have been unable to demonstrate such a benefit (33,38–40). In the final analysis, the ultimate prognostic indicator is the efficacy of the antineoplastic therapy. If the cancer is eradicated, then the patient will be expected to recover eventually to a normal state of well-being, including nutritional repletion; if the therapy is unsuccessful, then the patient will ultimately succumb regardless of nutritional status. As yet, there are no data to suggest whether providing or withholding PN will effect long-term survival.

References

1. van Eys J: Malnutrition in children with cancer: Incidence and consequence. *Cancer* 43:2030, 1979.

2. Filler RM, Jaffe N, Cassady JR, et al: Parenteral nutritional support in children with cancer. *Cancer* 39:2665, 1977.

3. Rickard KA, Grosfeld JL, Kirksey A, et al: Reversal of protein-energy malnutrition in children during treatment of advanced neoplastic disease. *Ann Surg* 190:771, 1979.

4. Theologides A: The anorexia-cachexia syndrome: A new hypothesis. *Ann NY Acad Sci* 230:14, 1974.

5. Morrison SD: Control of food intake in cancer cachexia: A challenge and a tool. *Physiol Behav* 17:705, 1976.

6. De Wys WD: Abnormalities of taste as a remote effect of a neoplasm. *Ann NY Acad Sci* 230:427, 1974.

7. De Wys WD, Walters K: Abnormalities of taste sensation in cancer patients. *Cancer* 36:1888, 1975.

8. Gold J: Proposed treatment of cancer by inhibition of gluconeogenesis. *Oncology* 22:185, 1968.

9. Brennan MF: Uncomplicated starvation versus cancer cachexia. *Cancer Res* 37:2359, 1977.

10. Bozzetti F, Pagnoni AM, Del Vecchio M: Excessive caloric expenditure as a cause of malnutrition in patients with cancer. *Surg Gynecol Obstet* 150:229, 1980.

11. Brennan MF: Total parenteral nutrition in the cancer patient. *N Engl J Med* 305:375, 1981.

12. Copeland EM, Souchon EA, MacFadyen BV, et al: Intravenous hyperalimentation as an adjunct to radiation therapy. *Cancer* 39:609, 1977.

13. Newman A, Katsaris J, Blendis LM, et al: Small intestinal injury in women who have had pelvic radiotherapy. *Lancet* II:1471, 1973.

14. Devereux DF, Triche TJ, Webber LB, et al: A study of adriamycin-reduced wound breaking strength in rats: An evaluation by light and electron microscopy, induction of collagen maturation, and hydroxyproline content. *Cancer* 45:2811, 1980.

15. Daly JM, Dudrick SJ, Copeland EM: Intravenous hyperalimentation: Effects on delayed cutaneous hypersensitivity in cancer patients. *Ann Surg* 192:587, 1980.

16. Donaldson SS, Lennon RA: Alterations of nutritional status: Impact of chemotherapy and radiation therapy. *Cancer* 43(Suppl):2036, 1979.

17. Pizzo PA: Infectious complications in the child with cancer. I. Pathophysiology of the compromised host and the initial evaluation and management of the febrile cancer patient. *J Pediatr* 98:341, 1981.

18. Richard KA, Kirksey A, Baehner RL, et al: Effectiveness of enteral and parenteral nutrition in the nutritional management of children with Wilm's tumors. *Am J Clin Nutr* 33:2622, 1980.

19. Copeland EM, Daly JM, Dudrick SJ: Nutrition as an adjunct to cancer treatment in the adult. *Cancer Res* 37:2451, 1977.

20. Filler RM, Dietz W, Suskind RM, et al: Parenteral feeding in the management of children with cancer. *Cancer* 43(Suppl):2117, 1979.

21. Copeland EM, Daly JM, Ota DM, et al: Nutrition, cancer, and intravenous hyperalimentation. *Cancer* 43:2108, 1979.

22. Copeland EM, MacFadyen BV, Dudrick SJ: Effect of intravenous hyperalimentation on established delayed hypersensitivity in the cancer patient. *Ann Surg* 184:60, 1976.

23. Merritt RJ, Ennis CE, Andrassy RJ, et al: Use of Hickman right atrial catheters in pediatric oncology patients. *JPEN* 5:83, 1981.

24. Pollack PF, Kadden M, Byrne WJ, et al: 100 patients years' experience with the Broviac silastic catheter for central venous nutrition. *JPEN* 5:32, 1981.

25. Hickman RO, Buckner CD, Clift RA, et al: A modified right atrial catheter for access to the venous system in marrow transplant recipients. *Surg Gynecol Obstet* 148:871, 1979.

26. Dindogru A, Pasick S, Rutkowski Z, et al: Total parenteral nutrition in cancer patients. *JPEN* 5:243, 1981.

27. Dindogru A, Pasick S, Rutkowski Z, et al: Total parenteral nutrition in leukopenic cancer patients. *JAMA* 244:680, 1980.

28. Buzby GP, Mullen JL, Stein TP, et al: Host-tumor interaction and nutrient supply. *Cancer* 45:2940, 1980.

29. Steiger E, Oram-Smith J, Miller E, et al: Effects of nutrition on tumor growth and tolerance to chemotherapy. *J Surg Res* 18:455, 1975.

30. Brennan MF, Copeland EM: Panel report on nutritional support of the cancer patient: Proceedings of an NIH sponsored conference. *Am J Clin Nutr* 34(Suppl):1199, 1981.

31. Lanzotti VJ, Copeland EM, George SL, et al: Cancer chemotherapeutic response and intravenous hyperalimentation. *Cancer Chemother Rep* 59:437, 1975.

32. Deitel M, Vasic V, Alexander MA: Specialized nutritional support in the cancer patient: Is it worthwhile? *Cancer* 41:2359, 1978.

33. Popp MB, Fisher RI, Wesley R, et al: A prospective randomized study of adjuvant parenteral nutrition in the treatment of advanced diffuse lymphoma: Influence on survival. *Surgery* 90:195, 1981.

34. Issell BF, Valdivieso M, Zaren HA, et al: Protection against chemotherapy toxicity by IV hyperalimentation. *Cancer Treat Rep* 62:1139, 1978.

35. Johnston ID: Parenteral nutrition in the cancer patient. *J Hum Nutr* 33:189, 1979.

36. Sobol SM, Conoyer JM, Sessions DG: Enteral and parenteral nutrition in patients with head and neck cancer. *Ann Otol Rhinol Laryngol* 88:495, 1979.

37. Copeland EM, Daly JM, Dudrick SJ: Nutrition and cancer. *Int Adv Surg Oncol* 4:1, 1981.

38. Sako K, Lore JM, Kaufman S, et al: Parenteral hyperalimentation in surgical patients with head and neck cancer: A randomized study. *J Surg Oncol* 16:391, 1981.

39. Valerio D, Overett L, Malcolm A, et al: Nutritional support for cancer patients receiving abdominal and pelvic radiotherapy: A randomized prospective clinical experiment of intravenous versus oral feeding. *Surg Forum* 29:145, 1978.

40. Lanzotti V, Copeland E, Bhuchar V, et al: A randomized trial of total parenteral nutrition (TPN) with chemotherapy for non-oat cell lung cancer (NOCLC). *Proc Am Assoc Cancer Res Am Soc Clin Oncol* 21:377, 1980.

25

The Use of Computers in Parenteral Nutrition

Nick Mackenzie
Robert L. Poole

Advantages of Computer-Assisted Parenteral Nutrition

Computers are being used with increasing frequency in the delivery of parenteral nutrition (PN). Their use is saving physician and pharmacist time in solution ordering and preparation and is also beneficial in clinical and nutritional assessment and diet analysis.

SOLUTION PREPARATION

Baker et al. (1) described the use of a computer to assist the pharmacy in formulating pediatric PN solutions. A computer program for the preparation of tailored PN solutions for neonates employing a standardized order sheet for the physician was reported by May and Robbins (2). Once ordered, the data was fed into the computer by pharmacy staff to generate (1) a formula for pharmacy use in solution preparation, (2) a label with the bottle contents per fluid volume ordered, and (3) a summary sheet reviewing the patient's nutritional input of the past 24 hours.

Giacoia et al. (3) addressed the issue of saving pharmacy time. Given an average of 350 formulations per month, they reported an annual savings of approximately 900 hours of pharmacist time by using computer-assisted PN.

CLINICAL MONITORING

Although a reduction in manpower is an obvious advantage of using computers, programs have also been developed to store and analyze important clinical data.

329

Sharp and German (4) developed a program for continuous data processing of the important numerical data used in the monitoring of infants on intravenous nutrition. Following analysis of the data, the computer generated graphs of caloric intake over time and plotted daily weight gain on a growth grid. Fisher and Munro (5) described a computer program developed to assess and monitor the nutritional status of hospitalized patients. Their program permitted the nutritional assessment of large numbers of patients and also provided detailed evaluations of the efficacy of PN. Storage of accumulated data and its subsequent analysis will make it possible to determine the effects of nutritional correction on morbidity and mortality. Some institutions employ computer-assisted diet analysis programs to identify nutrient deficiencies based on input of their patients' daily nutritional intake (6).

ORDERING SOLUTIONS

Computer technology has much to offer in the provision of PN not only in solution preparation and clinical monitoring, but also in solution ordering based on analysis of important patient variables. Giacoia and Chopra (7) are using a program to arrive at final PN solution orders that take into account the following factors: insensible water loss; normal water loss (e.g., stool, urine); abnormal water loss (e.g., gastric, excessive urine output); surplus of water (e.g., blood transfusions); and carbohydrate, protein, fat, vitamin, and trace element requirements. This type of detailed program has been used only for a short period of time but appears to be quite promising.

The use of computers to assist allied health professionals in the provision of PN is still in its infancy. As computer programs to assist clinicians in the provision of PN become more sophisticated, the patient's nutritional status will undoubtedly improve.

The PN Computer Program

The following is a description of how we are using computers to assist us in the provision of PN to pediatric patients. TPNPGM is a computer program that generates PN solution mixing instructions, bottle labels, and a record for the patient chart describing the contents of the PN solution. This program was designed to meet several goals: (1) to automate the repetitive and tedious calculations required to provide PN tailored to the needs of the individual infant in the Stanford intensive care nursery; (2) to reduce the time required for pharmacy personnel to formulate each PN solution order by automatically generating a set of PN mixing instructions and bottle labels; (3) to produce a record for the patient's chart describing the amounts of each PN constituent per kilogram bodyweight as well as the total amounts of fat emulsion, protein, and calories received; and (4) to save a record of the PN formulation on a floppy disk for later reference.

The program first establishes the standard concentrations of each of the ingredients that may constitute PN. It then requests the patient's identifying information, weight, and total fluid requirements. Next, the amount of oral formula is determined as well as the amounts of any other intravenous lines, such as central venous pressure lines, which may contribute to the fluid load. This fluid assessment is done to prevent accidental fluid volume overload.

```
FAT EMULSION BOTTLE LABEL
Patient: DOE, JOHN  MED REC #123456  Unit: ICN
Date Ordered 10/20/82    Date/Time Due 10/20 @ 12:00 Hours
DISCARD 24 HOURS AFTER HANGING !!!
10 % FAT EMULSION CONCENTRATION
Patient to receive    5 mls. FAT EMULSION
TO RUN AT  0.2 mls/hr.
```

Figure 1 Fat emulsion bottle label.

After the fluid status is determined, the program requests the amounts of all the PN components per kilogram bodyweight. These amounts are categorized by fat emulsion, amino acid, electrolytes, vitamins, trace elements, and "other." This last category is provided in the event that some constituent not normally a component of the PN solution needs to be added. Heparin and insulin amounts may also be specified as well as the amount of solution needed to flush the line and the container size in which the PN solution will be prepared. The actual computations occur next with no noticeable delay, followed by printing of the mixing instructions, bottle labels, and PN solution content record for the patient chart. At this point the user is offered the opportunity to correct any entry that may have been incorrect and to print the instructions, labels, and content records again. If no corrections need to be made, another set of PN solution calculations for another patient may be made.

The program has four other features to facilitate the correction of data entry errors. Typing "HELP" will cause the computer to list the options available for editing data entry errors. The user may return to a previous entry by simply typing "BACKUP" to the current program prompt. This will cause the previously entered parameter to be requested again. Once entered, the program resumes normal execution. Typing "JUMP" will invoke a menu of sections of the program to return to for data entry correction. For example, while entering electrolyte data, the user

```
TPN BOTTLE LABEL
Patient: DOE, JOHN  MED REC #123456
Unit: ICN  Bottle    1 which is    1 of    1
Date Ordered 10/20/82    Date/Time Due 10/20 @ 12:00 Hours
DISCARD 24 HOURS AFTER HANGING !!!
KEEP REFRIGERATED UNTIL ONE HOUR BEFORE USE
Total bottle volume    305 mls
Patient to receive    205 mls to flow at    8.5 mls/hr
Dextrose   7.5% final concentration
              CONTENTS OF THIS BOTTLE
Sodium        3.1 mEq    Pediatric Trace Elements    1.6 mls
Potassium     3.1 mEq    Multiple Vitamin  1.5 mls
Chloride      3.4 mEq    Vitamin B12    7.4 mcgm
Acetate       0.8 mEq    Vitamin K    0.7 mg
Phosphate     1.6 mM     Folic Acid  74.4 mcgm
Magnesium     0.4 mEq    Heparin 152.4 units
Calcium gluc    313 mg   Zinc  312.6 mcgm
Regular Insulin    0 units
Amino Acid    1.6 gms
Screened by:_____    Made/Checked by:_____
```

Figure 2 TPN bottle label.

```
PEDIATRIC TPN MIXING INSTRUCTIONS
Patient: DOE, JOHN  MED REC #123456
Unit: ICN  Bottle  1 which is  1 of  1 bottles
Date ordered 10/20/82    Date/Time Due 10/20 @ 12:00 Hours
Total bottle Volume   304.8 mls
Place  45.7 mls of D 50.0 in bottle
             PLACE THE FOLLOWING IN THE BOTTLE
NaCl     0.1 mls        Pediatric Trace Elements    1.6 mls
NaPO4    0.5 mls        Multiple Vitamin   1.5 mls
Na Acetate   0.4 mls    Vitamin B12    7.4 mls
KCl      1.6 mls        Vitamin K      0.7 mls
KPO4     0.0 mls        Folic Acid     0.7 mls
K Acetate   0.0 mls     Magnesium      0.4 mls
Zinc     0.3 mls        Heparin        1.5 mls
Calcium gluc     3.1 mls Regular Insulin    0 mls
Amino Acid  15.6 mls
Q.S. with 223.5 mls sterile water to total volume  304.8 mls
```

Figure 3 Pediatric TPN mixing instructions.

may realize that the wrong weight was entered for the patient. This feature allows the correct weight to be entered. When the error has been corrected, typing "RE-TURN" will cause the prompting of the question that was being asked when the user decided to "jump." In this manner, normal program execution may resume (Figs. 1–4). The complete computer program appears in Appendix of this manual.

The PN solution order forms are filled out by physicians (see Figure 1, Chapter 16). Later, pharmacy personnel enter the information into the computer from the order forms. The output is all printed on adhesive-backed labels for easy application to the pharmacy work books, the PN solution bottles, and the patient chart.

```
CONTENT OF PEDIATRIC TPN
Patient: DOE, JOHN  MED REC #123456
Unit: ICN  Bottle  1 to  1
Date Ordered 10/20/82    Date/Time Due 10/20 @ 12:00 Hours
Total IV Volume   205 mls to flow at   8.5 mls/hr
Patient weighs   1.05 kgs and will receive 200 mls/kg/day
Dextrose  7.5% final concentration
              ADDITIVES Per (Units)/Day
Sodium     2.0 mEq/kg  Pediatric Trace Elements   1.0 mls/kg
Potassium  2.0 mEq/kg  Multiple Vitamin   1.0 mls
Chloride   2.2 mEq/kg  Vitamin B12    5.0 mcgm
Acetate    0.5 mEq/kg  Vitamin K    0.5 mg
Phosphate  1.0 mM/kg   Folic Acid   50.0 mcgm
Magnesium  0.25 mEq/kg Heparin 102.4 units
Calcium gluc   200 mg/kg    Zinc  200.0 mcgm/kg
Regular Insulin   0 units
Amino Acid   1.0 gms/kg     Fat Emulsion 0.5 gms/kg
TPN and FAT EMULSION provide  59 calories/kg/day
Screened by: _____
```

Figure 4 Contents of pediatric TPN solution.

The primary responsibility for input errors rests with the physician ordering the PN solution and the nursing staff, which administers the fluid after verifying the order against the PN solution content label. Pharmacy personnel review the PN solution orders looking for obviously anomalous requests. In addition, pharmacists review the printed reports to verify that what was ordered was provided in the PN solution. However, it must be remembered that what may seem like an abnormally large amount of particular ingredient may be appropriate in certain circumstances.

This program is written in Microsoft's version 5.2 of the BASIC language and will run in unmodified form on any microcomputer supporting the CP/M operating system. A version of BASIC has been written for virtually all computers manufactured at the present time; therefore, this program will run in modified form on any computer. The output may be produced on any printer. The typical retail hardware cost of implementing this program is approximately $2500 and may be as low as $200 for a version implemented on a hand-held computer.

At Stanford University Medical Center we currently use the Osborne 1 microcomputer and the Okidata Microline 82 A printer.

References

1. Baker JS, Kirkman H, Woodley C, et al: Computer-assisted pediatric hyperalimentation. *Am J Hosp Pharm* 31:752, 1974.

2. May F, Robbins G: A computer program for parenteral nutrition solution preparation. *JPEN* 2:646, 1978.

3. Giacoia GP, Warden LK, Canfield BG: Computerized total parenteral nutrition formulas for newborn infants (letter). *Am J Hosp Pharm* 37:22, 1980.

4. Sharp DS, German JC: Computer utilization for intravenous nutrition in surgical neonates: Preliminary report. *J Pediatr Surg* 12:189, 1977.

5. Fisher M, Munro I: A computer programme for nutritional surveillance. *Aust NZ J Surg* 50:512, 1980.

6. Danford DE: Computer applications to medical nutrition problems. *JPEN* 5:441, 1981.

7. Giacoia GP, Chopra R: The use of a computer in parenteral alimentation of low birth weight infants. *JPEN* 5:328, 1981.

Appendix I

The Revised Recommended Dietary Allowances (1980)

Estimated Safe and Adequate Daily Dietary Intakes of Additional Selected Vitamins and Minerals[a]

		Vitamins			Trace Elements[b]						Electrolytes		
	Age (years)	Vitamin K (µg)	Biotin (µg)	Panto-thenic Acid (mg)	Copper (mg)	Manga-nese (mg)	Fluoride (mg)	Chromium (mg)	Selenium (mg)	Molyb-denum (mg)	Sodium (mg)	Potassium (mg)	Chloride (mg)
Infants	0–0.5	12	35	2	0.5–0.7	0.5–0.7	0.1–0.5	0.01–0.04	0.01–0.04	0.03–0.06	115–350	350–925	275–700
	0.5–1	10–20	50	3	0.7–1.0	.7–1.0	0.2–1.0	0.02–0.06	0.02–0.06	0.04–0.08	250–750	425–1275	400–1200
Children	1–3	15–30	65	3	1.0–1.5	1.0–1.5	0.5–1.5	0.02–0.08	0.02–0.08	0.05–0.1	325–975	550–1650	500–1500
and	4–6	20–40	85	3–4	1.5–2.0	1.5–2.0	1.0–2.5	0.03–0.12	0.03–0.12	0.06–0.15	450–1350	775–2325	700–2100
Adolescents	7–10	30–60	120	4–5	2.0–2.5	2.0–3.0	1.5–2.5	0.05–0.2	0.05–0.2	0.1–0.3	600–1800	1000–3000	925–2775
	11 +	50–100	100–200	4–7	2.0–3.0	2.5–5.0	1.5–2.5	0.05–0.2	0.05–0.2	0.15–0.5	900–2700	1525–4575	1400–4200
Adults		70–140	100–200	4–7	2.0–3.0	2.5–5.0	1.5–4.0	0.05–0.2	0.05–0.2	0.15–0.5	1100–3300	1875–5625	1700–5100

Reproduced from Recommended Dietary Allowances, 9th ed (1980), with the permission of the National Academy of Sciences, Washington, DC.

[a]Because there is less information on which to base allowances, these figures are not given in the main table of the RDA and are provided here in the form of ranges of recommended intakes.

[b]Since the toxic levels for many trace elements may be only several times usual intakes, the upper levels for the trace elements given in this table should not be habitually exceeded.

Mean Heights and Weights and Recommended Energy Intake[a]

Category	Age (years)	Weight (kg)	Weight (lb)	Height (cm)	Height (in)	Energy Needs (with range) (kcal)	(MJ)
Infants	0.0–0.5	6	13	60	24	kg × 115 (95–145)	kg × .48
	0.5–1.0	9	20	71	28	kg × 105 (80–135)	kg × .44
Children	1–3	13	29	90	35	1300 (900–1800)	5.5
	4–6	20	44	112	44	1700 (1300–2300)	7.1
	7–10	28	62	132	52	2400 (1650–3300)	10.1
Males	11–14	45	99	157	62	2700 (2000–3700)	11.3
	15–18	66	145	176	69	2800 (2100–3900)	11.8
	19–22	70	154	177	70	2900 (2500–3300)	12.2
	23–50	70	154	178	70	2700 (2300–3100)	11.3
	51–75	70	154	178	70	2400 (2000–2800)	10.1
	76 +	70	154	178	70	2050 (1650–2450)	8.6
Females	11–14	46	101	157	62	2200 (1500–3000)	9.2
	15–18	55	120	163	64	2100 (1200–3000)	8.8
	19–22	55	120	163	64	2100 (1700–2500)	8.8
	23–50	55	120	163	64	2000 (1600–2400)	8.4
	51–75	55	120	163	64	1800 (1400–2200)	7.6
	76 +	55	120	163	64	1600 (1200–2000)	6.7
Pregnancy						+300	
Lactation						+500	

Reproduced from Recommended Dietary Allowances, 9th ed (1980), with the permission of the National Academy of Sciences, Washington, DC.

[a]The data in this table have been assembled from the observed median heights and weights of children together with desirable weights for adults for the mean heights of men (70 inches) and women (64 inches) between the ages of 18 and 34 years as surveyed in the U.S. population (HEW/NCHS data).

The energy allowances for the young adults are for men and women doing light work. The allowances for the two older age groups represent mean energy needs over these age spans, allowing for a 2% decrease in basal (resting) metabolic rate per decade and a reduction in activity of 200 kcal/day for men and women between 51 and 75 years, 500 kcal for men over 75 years and 400 kcal for women over 75 (see text). The customary range of daily energy output is shown for adults in parentheses, and is based on a variation in energy needs of ±400 kcal at any one age, emphasizing the wide range of energy intakes appropriate for any group of people.

Energy allowances for children through age 18 are based on median energy intakes of children these ages followed in longitudinal growth studies. The values in parentheses are 10th and 90th percentiles of energy intake, to indicate the range of energy consumption among children of these ages.

Food and Nutrition Board, National Academy of Sciences–National Research Council Recommended Daily Dietary Allowances,[a] Revised 1980
(Designed for the maintenance of good nutrition of practically all healthy people in the U.S.A.)

	Age (years)	Weight (kg)	Weight (lb)	Height (cm)	Height (in)	Protein (g)	Fat-Soluble Vitamins: Vitamin A (μg RE)[b]	Vitamin D (μg)[c]	Vitamin E (mg α-TE)[d]	Water-Soluble Vitamins: Vitamin C (mg)	Thiamin (mg)	Riboflavin (mg)	Niacin (mg NE)[e]	Vitamin B-6 (mg)	Folacin (μg)[f]	Vitamin B-12 (μg)	Minerals: Calcium (mg)	Phosphorus (mg)	Magnesium (mg)	Iron (mg)	Zinc (mg)	Iodine (μg)
Infants	0.0–0.5	6	13	60	24	kg × 2.2	420	10	3	35	0.3	0.4	6	0.3	30	0.5[g]	360	240	50	10	3	40
	0.5–1.0	9	20	71	28	kg × 2.0	400	10	4	35	0.5	0.6	8	0.6	45	1.5	540	360	70	15	5	50
Children	1–3	13	29	90	35	23	400	10	5	45	0.7	0.8	9	0.9	100	2.0	800	800	150	15	10	70
	4–6	20	44	112	44	30	500	10	6	45	0.9	1.0	11	1.3	200	2.5	800	800	200	10	10	90
	7–10	28	62	132	52	34	700	10	7	45	1.2	1.4	16	1.6	300	3.0	800	800	250	10	10	120
Males	11–14	45	99	157	62	45	1000	10	8	50	1.4	1.6	18	1.8	400	3.0	1200	1200	350	18	15	150
	15–18	66	145	176	69	56	1000	10	10	60	1.4	1.7	18	2.0	400	3.0	1200	1200	400	18	15	150
	19–22	70	154	177	70	56	1000	7.5	10	60	1.5	1.7	19	2.2	400	3.0	800	800	350	10	15	150
	23–50	70	154	178	70	56	1000	5	10	60	1.4	1.6	18	2.2	400	3.0	800	800	350	10	15	150
	51+	70	154	178	70	56	1000	5	10	60	1.2	1.4	16	2.2	400	3.0	800	800	350	10	15	150
Females	11–14	46	101	157	62	46	800	10	8	50	1.1	1.3	15	1.8	400	3.0	1200	1200	300	18	15	150
	15–18	55	120	163	64	46	800	10	8	60	1.1	1.3	14	2.0	400	3.0	1200	1200	300	18	15	150
	19–22	55	120	163	64	44	800	7.5	8	60	1.1	1.3	14	2.0	400	3.0	800	800	300	18	15	150
	23–50	55	120	163	64	44	800	5	8	60	1.0	1.2	13	2.0	400	3.0	800	800	300	18	15	150
	51+	55	120	163	64	44	800	5	8	60	1.0	1.2	13	2.0	400	3.0	800	800	300	10	15	150
Pregnant						+30	+200	+5	+2	+20	+0.4	+0.3	+2	+0.6	+400	+1.0	+400	+400	+150	[h]	+5	+25
Lactating						+20	+400	+5	+3	+40	+0.5	+0.5	+5	+0.5	+100	+1.0	+400	+400	+150	[h]	+10	+50

Reproduced from Recommended Dietary Allowances, 9th ed (1980), with the permission of the National Academy of Sciences, Washington, DC.

[a] The allowances are intended to provide for individual variations among most normal persons as they live in the United States under usual environmental stresses. Diets should be based on a variety of common foods in order to provide other nutrients for which human requirements have been less well defined.

[b] Retinol equivalents. 1 retinol equivalent = 1 μg retinol or 6 μg β carotene. See text for calculation of vitamin A activity of diets as retinol equivalents.

[c] As cholecalciferol. 10 μg cholecalciferol = 400 IU of vitamin D.

[d] α-tocopherol equivalents. 1 mg d-α-tocopherol = 1 α-TE. See text for variation in allowances and calculation of vitamin E activity of the diet as α-tocopherol equivalents.

[e] 1 NE (niacin equivalent) is equal to 1 mg of niacin or 60 mg of dietary tryptophan.

[f] The folacin allowances refer to dietary sources as determined by Lactobacillus casei assay after treatment with enzymes (conjugases) to make polyglutamyl forms of the vitamin available to the test organism.

[g] The recommended dietary allowance for vitamin B-12 in infants is based on average concentration of the vitamin in human milk. The allowances after weaning are based on energy intake (as recommended by the American Academy of Pediatrics) and consideration of other factors, such as intestinal absorption; see text.

[h] The increased requirement during pregnancy cannot be met by the iron content of habitual American diets nor by the existing iron stores of many women; therefore the use of 30–60 mg of supplemental iron is recommended. Iron needs during lactation are not substantially different from those of nonpregnant women, but continued supplementation of the mother for 2–3 months after parturition is advisable in order to replenish stores depleted by pregnancy.

337

Appendix II

Terminology

"Calories"

In this manual the word *calorie* (abbreviation *cal*) is used as nutrition shorthand. Nutrient requirements are described in terms of calories/kilogram/day (cal/kg/day).

In research, or whenever scientific precision is needed, the correct term is *kilocalorie* or *Calorie* (abbreviated as *kcal* or *Cal;* note the use of capital C). For convenience in this text, the word kilocalorie is abbreviated to calorie.

The word calorie originated in chemistry and physics as a measure of heat and represents the amount of heat necessary to raise the temperature of 1 g water by 1°C. This unit can measure very small amounts of heat.

Food has a relatively high heat potential. The "scientific" calorie is too small a unit of measure to use in nutrition. Therefore, nutritionists use the kilocalorie, which equals 1000 of the small calories of physics. The kilocalorie is the amount of heat required to raise the temperature of 1 kg of water 1°C (from 15°C to 16°C).

"Total parenteral nutrition"

The terms *hyperalimentation, total parenteral nutrition, central vein parenteral nutrition,* and *total parenteral alimentation* have all been used to describe modifications of the technique originally described by Dudrick and co-workers (1). The word *total* was chosen over *complete* since current parenteral nutrition infusates are not necessarily complete for *all* nutrients. We agree with Levy and co-workers (2) that *total parenteral nutrition* appears to be the best term to describe the situation in which parenteral nutrients supply the sole (total) nutritional support, and that it should be further modified to designate the route of delivery (i.e., central vein or peripheral vein). When enteral nutrients are supplemented with intravenously administered nutrients, the best description is *parenteral supplementation of tolerated enteral nutrients.*

References

1. Dudrick SJ, Wilmore DW, Vars HM, et al: Long-term total parenteral nutrition with growth, development, and positive nitrogen balance. *Surgery* 64:134, 1968.
2. Levy JS, Winters RW, Heird WC: Total parenteral nutrition. *Pediatrics in Review* 2:99, 1980.

Information on Parenteral Nutrition and Drug Compatibility and Stability

The texts and journals listed below are sources for information on stability and compatibility of parenteral nutrition solution components and other parenteral medications.

Texts

Trissel LA: *Handbook on Injectable Drugs,* 2nd ed. Washington, DC, American Society of Hospital Pharmacists, 1980.

King JC: *Guide to Parenteral Admixtures.* St Louis, Cutter Laboratories Inc, 1980. (Three volumes supplemented as new information is available.)

Journals

American Journal of Hospital Pharmacy
Hospital Formulary
Hospital Pharmacy
Drug Intelligence and Clinical Pharmacy
Journal of Parenteral and Enteral Nutrition
Nutritional Support Services
American Journal of Intravenous Therapy and Clinical Nutrition
Journal of the Parenteral Drug Association

The following are commonly used references for parenteral nutrition and drug compatibilities:

Bergman HD: Incompatibilities in large volume parenterals. *Drug Intell Clin Pharm* 11:345, 1977.

Chiou WL, Moorhatch P: Interaction between vitamin A and plastic intravenous fluid bags. *JAMA* 223:328, 1973.

Cluxton RJ: Some complexities of making compatibility studies in hyperalimentation solutions. *Drug Intell Clin Pharm* 5:177, 1971.

Feigin RD, Moss KS, Shackelford PG: Antibiotic stability in solutions used for intravenous nutrition and fluid therapy. *Pediatrics* 51:1016, 1973.

Giovanoni R: The manufacturing of pharmacy solutions and incompatibilities, in Fisher JE (ed): *Total Parenteral Nutrition.* Boston, Little, Brown and Co, 1976.

Hartline JV, Zachman RD: Vitamin A delivery in total parenteral nutrition solution. *Pediatrics* 58:448, 1976.

Henry RS, Jurgens RW, Sturgeon R, et al: Compatibility of calcium gluconate with sodium phosphate in a mixed TPN solution. *Am J Hosp Pharm* 37:673, 1980.

Hull RL: Physicochemical considerations in intravenous hyperalimentation. *Am J Hosp Pharm* 31:236, 1974.

Jurgens RW, Henry RS, Welco A: Amino acid stability in a mixed parenteral nutrition solution. *Am J Hosp Pharm* 38:1358, 1981.

Kleinman LM, Tangrea JA, Gallelli JF, et al: Stability of solutions of essential amino acids. *Am J Hosp Pharm* 30:1054, 1973.

Laegeler WL, Tio JM, Blake MI: Stability of certain amino acids in a parenteral nutrition solution. *Am J Hosp Pharm* 31:776, 1974.

Mirtallo JM, Rogers KR, Johnson JA, et al: Stability of amino acids and the availability of acid in total parenteral nutrition solutions containing hydrochloric acid. *Am J Hosp Pharm* 38:1729, 1981.

Moorhatch P, Chiou WL: Interactions between drugs and plastic intravenous fluid bags. Part 1. Sorption studies on 17 drugs. *Am J Hosp Pharm* 31:72, 1974.

Nedich RL: Vitamin A absorption from plastic I.V. bags. *JAMA* 224:1531, 1973.

Newton DW: Physiocochemical determinants of incompatibility and instability in injectable drug solutions and admixtures, in Trissel LA (cd): *Handbook on Injectable Drugs*, ed 2. Washington, DC, American Society of Hospital Pharmacists, 1980.

Rowlands DA, Wilkinson WR, Yoshimura N: Storage stability of mixed hyperalimentation solutions. *Am J Hosp Pharm* 30:436, 1973.

Rupp CA, Kotabe SE: Common sense guidelines for compatibility. *Drug Intell Clin Pharm* 9:155, 1975.

Appendix IV

Home Parenteral Nutrition

The Lifeline Foundation

This foundation was established for support of patients on home parenteral or enteral nutrition. To accomplish this, the foundation publishes a newsletter to keep members in touch with one another and to allow them to share experiences and problems (as well as their possible solutions). The newsletter is free to patients on home nutrition programs.

Education is an essential function of the foundation since many hospitals do not yet have nutrition support teams for in-hospital therapy and even fewer hospitals are currently prepared to provide home parenteral or enteral nutrition. Research in the area of developing practical products for home patients and research on the psychosocial attitudes of patients requiring enteral and parenteral nutrition are both fundamental goals of the Foundation.

For health personnel interested in the foundation or for your patients on home nutrition programs who wish more information, they may contact:

> The Lifeline Foundation
> Two Osprey Road
> Sharon, Massachusetts 02067
> (617) 784-3250

Registry of Patients on Home Total Parenteral Nutrition

This international registry provides summary information about the patients being maintained at home on parenteral nutrition. The headquarters for the Registry is located at

> New York Academy of Medicine
> 2 East 103rd Street
> New York, NY 10029

Since its development in 1976, the registry has distributed questionnaires to obtain summary information from each cooperating hospital rather than specific data on individual patients. The information from a specific hospital is kept confidential. The only data distributed are the total summaries from all responders.

The Registry and its data are useful to anyone interested in the indications for and results of home parenteral nutrition, to those who wish to know the names of hospitals where home TPN programs exist, and to legislative committees and insurance companies requesting background data in this field. The responding institutions are in the United States and Canada, and information from the United Kingdom will soon be available as well.

Those wishing further information about the Registry or those who have a home parenteral nutrition program and wish to participate may write to the Registry or call Ms. Judith Skolnik, (212) 876-8200, ext. 253.

TPNPGM: A Computer Program to Help Provide PN in Pediatric Patients

```
100 REM *********************************************
110 REM *                TPN:
120 REM * This program generates TPN mixing
130 REM * instrucions for the Stanford Pediatric
140 REM * Pharmacy.
150 REM *
160 REM *    Written by: Nick Mackenzie, MD
170 REM * Stanford Department of Anesthesia, S280
180 REM *       Stanford, California  94305
190 REM *          Copyright 25/October/82
200 REM *********************************************
210 REM * This program and user manual are available on
220 REM * floppy disk in a number of computer formats.
230 REM * Please address requests for information on
240 REM * TPN to the author at the above address.
250 REM *********************************************
260 REM * This program is composed of two programs : TPN and TPN2.
270 REM * TPN initializes variables and "conditions" the
280 REM * printer.  TPN2 requests user input, generates the bottle
290 REM * labels, mixing instructions, and nutritional summary.
300 REM *
310 REM * If your computer system has sufficient memory, TPN and
320 REM * TPN2 may be combined into a single program.  In that
330 REM * case you may wish to implement MBASIC with the "no files
340 REM * option" : i.e.
350 REM * A> MBASIC /F:0
360 REM * as this will "free up" some more RAM
370 REM *
380 REM * If you encounter problems while running this program,
390 REM * type "HELP" and you will be instructed in the ways
400 REM * that errors may be corrected.  Esentially, the BACKUP
410 REM * command issued as a response to any prompt except that
420 REM * requesting ( y/n ) will cause the previous prompt to
430 REM * be displayed.  The command JUMP will allow for reentry
440 REM * of a previously completed section and RETURN will
450 REM * bring the user back to the place where JUMP was requested.
460 REM * The COMPUTE command will dirrect the program to begin
470 REM * generating Labels.  However, the results will be nonsense
480 REM * unless all the data entries have been made.  Therefore,
490 REM * use the COMPUTE command with caution.
500 REM *********************************************
510 REM * Define constants specific to the terminal
520 REM * on which program is running
530 REM *********************************************
540 BLANK$="
550 CS$=CHR$(26): REM    clear screen
560 UP$=CHR$(11): REM    move cursor up one line
570 CR$=CHR$(13): REM    carriage return
580 LF$=CHR$(10): REM    linefeed without carriage return
590 DLF$=LF$: REM    double linefeed
600 ESC$=CHR$(27): REM   escape character
610 SUL$=ESC$+CHR$(108): REM   start underline or reverse video
620 EUL$=ESC$+CHR$(109): REM   end underline or reverse video
630 SLO$=ESC$+CHR$(41): REM   start low intensity
640 ELO$=ESC$+CHR$(40): REM   end low intensity
650 REM *********************************************
660 REM * define constants for standard concentratons
670 REM * of TPN ingredients
680 REM *********************************************
690 FOLCONC=100:    REM   mcgm/ml    of  FOLATE
700 ZINCONC=1000:   REM   mcgm/ml        ZINC
710 VITB12CONC=1:   REM   mcgm/ml        VIT B12
720 VITKCONC=1:     REM   mg/ml          VIT K
730 NAACTCONC=2:    REM   mEq/ml         Na ACETATE
740 NACLCONC=4:     REM   mEq/ml         Na Cl
750 NAPO4CNC=4:     REM   mEq Na/3 mM/ml Na PO4
760 KACTCONC=2:     REM   mEq/ml         K ACETATE
```

```
770 KCLCONC=2:       REM  mEq/ml      K Cl
780 KP04CNC=4.4:     REM  mEq K/3 mM/ml K P04
790 MGCONC=1:        REM  mEq/ml      Mg
800 CACONC=100:      REM  mg/ml       CALCIUM GLUCONATE
810 HPRNCONC=100:    REM  units/ml    HEPARIN
820 INSULINCNC=100:  REM  units/ml    INSULIN
830 AACONC=.1:       REM  gm/1 ml     AMINO ACID
840 DEXCNC=50:       REM  gm/100 ml   DEXTROSE
850 FATCONC=10:      REM  gm/100 ml   FAT EMULSION
860 REM **********************************************
870 REM * DEFINE YEAR & "LENGTH" OF MEDICAL RECORD NUMBER
880 REM **********************************************
890 YEAR = 82:       REM * This line needs to be changed at years end.
900 MEDREC.LEN%=6: REM * That is, 6 characters in length
910 REM **********************************************
920 REM * CONDITION OKIDATA PRINTER:
930 REM *   THIS COMMAND WILL "HANG UP" THE COMPUTER IF THE PRINTER
940 REM *   HAS NOT BEEN "SELECTED".  YOU MAY WISH TO MOVE THIS
950 REM *   COMMAND TO LINE 535 AND THEN IT WOULD ONLY BE EXECUTED
960 REM *   ONCE DURING A PROGRAM RUN INSTEAD OF BEFORE EACH NEW PATIENT.
970 REM **********************************************
980 LPRINT CHR$(29);
990 REM * CALL IN THE I/O PART OF TPN, TPN2.
1000 CHAIN "TPN2",100,ALL


100 REM TPN2: CALLED BY TPN AFTER VARIABLE INITIALIZATION
110 DIM IV(10): REM array to contain rates for other IV & IA lines
120 I=3:  REM i is the number of 'other' constituents needed
130 DIM OTHER$(I),OTHER.UNITS$(I),OTHER.CNC(I),OTHER.AMT(I),OTHER.VOL(I)
140 REM **********************************************
150 REM * start of main program:    Version 10/25/82
160 REM **********************************************
170 SECTION%=1:PRINT CS$;TAB(20);SUL$;"TPN";EUL$;LF$;LF$
180 PRINT "A program to generate mixing instructions for"
190 PRINT "Pediatric TPN formula.";LF$;LF$
200 PRINT "Do you wish to change any of the"
210 PRINT "Standard Concentrations (y/n)?";
220 REM **********************************************
230 REM * ask for changes in standard concentrations
240 REM **********************************************
250 GOSUB 6550:IF C$="n" OR C$="N" GOTO 970
260 PRINT "Enter the Standard Concentratons of the following"
270 PRINT "solutions.  Concentrations are expressed as"
280 PRINT "(unit)/ml.";LF$;LF$
290 SECTION%=1:REM entry point 1 for JUMP routine
300 REM ***********
310 PRINT "Folate (mcgm) ";:GOSUB 6390:PRINT FOLCONC
320 GOSUB 6400:ON EFLAG% GOTO 310,3430,6750,170
330 IF FLAG%=0 THEN FOLCONC=VAL(A$)
340 REM ***********
350 PRINT "Zinc (mcgm) ";:GOSUB 6390:PRINT ZINCONC
360 GOSUB 6400:ON EFLAG% GOTO 350,3430,6750,310
370 IF FLAG%=0 THEN ZINCONC=VAL(A$)
380 REM ***********
390 PRINT "Vitamin B12 (mcgm) ";:GOSUB 6390:PRINT VITB12CONC
400 GOSUB 6400:ON EFLAG% GOTO 390,3430,6750,350
410 IF FLAG%=0 THEN VITB12CONC=VAL(A$)
420 REM ***********
430 PRINT "Vitamin K (mg) ";:GOSUB 6390:PRINT VITKCONC
440 GOSUB 6400:ON EFLAG% GOTO 430,3430,6750,390
450 IF FLAG%=0 THEN VITKCONC=VAL(A$)
460 REM ***********
470 PRINT "Na Acetate (mEq) ";:GOSUB 6390:PRINT NAACTCONC
480 GOSUB 6400:ON EFLAG% GOTO 470,3430,6750,430
490 IF FLAG%=0 THEN NAACTCONC=VAL(A$)
500 REM ***********
```

```
510 PRINT "NaCl (mEq) ";:GOSUB 6390:PRINT NACLCONC
520 GOSUB 6400:ON EFLAGZ GOTO 510,3430,6750,470
530 IF FLAGZ=0 THEN NACLCONC=VAL(A$)
540 REM ***********
550 PRINT "NaPO4 (mEq Na/3 mM PO4) ";:GOSUB 6390:PRINT NAPO4CNC
560 GOSUB 6400:ON EFLAGZ GOTO 550,3430,6750,510
570 IF FLAGZ=0 THEN NAPO4CNC=VAL(A$)
580 REM ***********
590 PRINT "K Acetate (mEq) ";:GOSUB 6390:PRINT KACTCONC
600 GOSUB 6400:ON EFLAGZ GOTO 590,3430,6750,550
610 IF FLAGZ=0 THEN KACTCONC=VAL(A$)
620 REM ***********
630 PRINT "KCl (mEq) ";:GOSUB 6390:PRINT KCLCONC
640 GOSUB 6400:ON EFLAGZ GOTO 630,3430,6750,590
650 IF FLAGZ=0 THEN KCLCONC=VAL(A$)
660 REM ***********
670 PRINT "KPO4 (mEq K/3 mM PO4) ";:GOSUB 6390:PRINT KPO4CNC
680 GOSUB 6400:ON EFLAGZ GOTO 670,3430,6750,630
690 IF FLAGZ=0 THEN KPO4CNC=VAL(A$)
700 REM ***********
710 PRINT "Magnesium (mEq) ";:GOSUB 6390:PRINT MGCONC
720 GOSUB 6400:ON EFLAGZ GOTO 710,3430,6750,670
730 IF FLAGZ=0 THEN MGCONC=VAL(A$)
740 REM ***********
750 PRINT "Calcium gluconate (mg) ";:GOSUB 6390:PRINT CACONC
760 GOSUB 6400:ON EFLAGZ GOTO 750,3430,6750,710
770 IF FLAGZ=0 THEN CACONC=VAL(A$)
780 REM ***********
790 PRINT "Heparin (Units) ";:GOSUB 6390:PRINT HPRNCONC
800 GOSUB 6400:ON EFLAGZ GOTO 790,3430,6750,750
810 IF FLAGZ=0 THEN HPRNCONC=VAL(A$)
820 REM ***********
830 PRINT "Insulin (Units) ";:GOSUB 6390:PRINT INSULINCNC
840 GOSUB 6400:ON EFLAGZ GOTO 830,3430,6750,790
850 IF FLAGZ=0 THEN INSULINCNC=VAL(A$)
860 REM ***********
870 PRINT "Amino Acid (gm/100 ml) ";:GOSUB 6390:PRINT AACONC
880 GOSUB 6400:ON EFLAGZ GOTO 870,3430,6750,830
890 IF FLAGZ=0 THEN AACONC=VAL(A$)
900 REM ***********
910 PRINT "Dextrose (gm/100 ml)";:GOSUB 6390:PRINT DEXCNC
920 GOSUB 6400:ON EFLAGZ GOTO 910,3430,6750,870
930 IF FLAGZ=0 THEN DEXCNC=VAL(A$)
940 REM *******************************************
950 REM * find name, med rec num, unit & bottle
960 REM *******************************************
970 SECTIONZ=2:PRINT CS$;TAB(15)"TPN COMPUTATIONS:";DLF$;DLF$
980 INPUT "Enter patient's LAST NAME";A$:PRINT
990 GOSUB 6770:ON EFLAGZ GOTO 980,3430,6750,910:LASTN$=A$
1000 INPUT "Enter patient's FIRST NAME";A$:PRINT
1010 GOSUB 6770:ON EFLAGZ GOTO 1000,3430,6750,980:FIRSTN$=A$
1020 INPUT "Enter MEDICAL RECORD NUMBER";A$:PRINT
1030 GOSUB 6770:ON EFLAGZ GOTO 1020,3430,6750,1000:MEDREC$=A$
1040 IF LEN(MEDREC$)<>MEDREC.LENZ THEN GOSUB 6530:GOTO 1020
1050 INPUT "Enter the WEIGHT (kg)";A$:PRINT
1060 GOSUB 6770:ON EFLAGZ GOTO 1050,3430,6750,1020:WEIGHT=VAL(A$)
1070 INPUT "Enter the UNIT NUMBER";A$:PRINT
1080 GOSUB 6770:ON EFLAGZ GOTO 1070,3430,6750,1050:UNITNUM$=A$
1090 INPUT "Enter the BOTTLE NUMBER";A$:PRINT
1100 GOSUB 6770:ON EFLAGZ GOTO 1090,3430,6750,1070:BOTNUM=VAL(A$)
1110 PRINT TAB(5);SUL$;"Numbers of each month:";EUL$
1120 PRINT "1 - January        7 - July"
1130 PRINT "2 - February       8 - August"
1140 PRINT "3 - March          9 - September"
1150 PRINT "4 - April         10 - October"
1160 PRINT "5 - May           11 - November"
1170 PRINT "6 - June          12 - December"
```

```
1180 PRINT DLF$
1190 INPUT "Enter MONTH ORDERED";A$:PRINT
1200 GOSUB 6770:ON EFLAG% GOTO 1190,3430,6750,1090:MONTH=VAL(A$)
1210 IF MONTH<1 OR MONTH>12 THEN GOSUB 6530:GOTO 1190
1220 INPUT "Enter DAY ORDERED";A$:PRINT
1230 GOSUB 6770:ON EFLAG% GOTO 1220,3430,6750,1190:DAY=VAL(A$)
1240 IF DAY<1 OR DAY>31 THEN GOSUB 6530:GOTO 1220
1250 PRINT "YEAR ";:GOSUB 6390:PRINT YEAR
1260 GOSUB 6400:ON EFLAG% GOTO 1250,3430,6750,1220
1270 IF FLAG%=0 THEN YEAR=VAL(A$)
1280 PRINT "Enter MONTH DUE ";:GOSUB 6390:PRINT MONTH
1290 GOSUB 6400:ON EFLAG% GOTO 1280,3430,6750,1250
1300 IF FLAG%=0 THEN MONTHDUE=VAL(A$) ELSE MONTHDUE=MONTH
1310 IF MONTHDUE<1 OR MONTHDUE>31 THEN GOSUB 6530:GOTO 1280
1320 INPUT "Enter DAY DUE";A$:PRINT
1330 GOSUB 6770:ON EFLAG% GOTO 1320,3430,6750,1280:DAYDUE=VAL(A$)
1340 IF DAYDUE<1 OR DAYDUE>31 THEN GOSUB 6530:GOTO 1320
1350 INPUT "Enter HOUR DUE";A$:PRINT
1360 GOSUB 6770:ON EFLAG% GOTO 1350,3430,6750,1320:HOURDUE=VAL(A$)
1370 IF HOURDUE<1 OR HOURDUE>24 THEN GOSUB 6530:GOTO 1350
1380 REM ****************************************
1390 REM * fluid input: IV & PO
1400 REM ****************************************
1410 SECTION%=3:PRINT CS$
1420 PRINT "We need to determine the total fluid load to be"
1430 PRINT "given to the patient and how much of this will be"
1440 PRINT "TPN, FAT EMULSION, PO and other IV or IA lines."
1450 PRINT:INPUT "Enter TOTAL FLUID intake (ml/kg/day)";A$:PRINT
1460 GOSUB 6770:ON EFLAG% GOTO 1450,3430,6750,1350:TOTFLD=VAL(A$)
1470 MLS.KG.DAY=TOTFLD
1480 TOTFLD=TOTFLD*WEIGHT
1490 INPUT "Enter AMOUNT of FAT EMULSION (gm/kg/day)";A$:PRINT
1500 GOSUB 6770:ON EFLAG% GOTO 1490,3430,6750,1450:FAT.EMULSION=VAL(A$)
1510 IF FAT.EMULSION = 0 THEN GOTO 1560
1520 PRINT "Enter CONCENTRATION OF FAT EMULSION ";:GOSUB 6390:PRINT FATCONC
1530 GOSUB 6400:ON EFLAG% GOTO 1520,3430,6750,1490
1540 IF FLAG%=0 THEN FATCONC=VAL(A$)
1550 FAT.EMULSION=(FAT.EMULSION/(FATCONC/100))*WEIGHT
1560 LINES=0:TOTIV=0
1570 PRINT "How many IV and IA lines exist which will NOT be"
1580 INPUT "used for TPN or FAT EMULSION";A$:PRINT
1590 GOSUB 6770:ON EFLAG% GOTO 1560,3430,6750,1520:LINES=VAL(A$)
1600 TOTIV.NACL = 0
1610 IF LINES>0 THEN FOR I=1 TO LINES ELSE TOTIV=0:GOTO 1730
1620  PRINT USING "Enter FLOW RATE (mls/hr) of line ##";I;
1630  INPUT A$:PRINT
1640  GOSUB 6770:ON EFLAG% GOTO 1560,3430,6750,1560:IV(I)=VAL(A$)
1650  TOTIV=TOTIV+IV(I)*24
1660  PRINT "  Enter its % SALINE ( ie. 0.9, 0.45, 0.225 )";
1670  INPUT A$:PRINT
1680  GOSUB 6770:ON EFLAG% GOTO 1560,3430,6750,1560:SALINE=VAL(A$)
1690  IF SALINE > .9 THEN PRINT "**** ERROR IN NaCl concentration.":GOTO 1660
1700  TOTIV.NACL = TOTIV.NACL + ( SALINE * ( .154/.9) * IV(I) * 24 )
1710  PRINT
1720 NEXT I
1730 TOTFLD=TOTFLD-FAT.EMULSION-TOTIV
1740 IF TOTFLD>50 THEN GOTO 1760
1750   GOSUB 6530:PRINT USING "### mls is FAT EMULSION and OTHER IV's":GOTO 1420
1760 PRINT CS$
1770 POFLD=0
1780 PRINT "Will PO feeds be given (y/n)";:GOSUB 6550
1790 IF C$="n" THEN IVFLD=TOTFLD:PO$="n":GOTO 2160 ELSE PO$="y"
1800 PRINT CS$;"When PO feeds are given in addition to TPN,"
1810 PRINT "TPN calculatons can be based on:"
1820 PRINT LF$;"1 - IV + PO ORDERS, where electrolytes are"
1830 PRINT"calculated assuming all fluids are IV, although a"
1840 PRINT "portion may actually be PO."
```

```
1850 PRINT LF$;"2 - IV REGARDLESS OF PO, in this case IV rate is"
1860 PRINT "constant and does not depend upon the amount of PO"
1870 PRINT "intake.  IV electrolytes are calculated"
1880 PRINT "for the 24 hour volume of IV solution."
1890 PRINT LF$;"Are these orders IV REGARDLES OF PO (y/n)";
1900 GOSUB 6550:ORDER$=C$
1910 PRINT CS$;TAB(15);"PO FLUID INTAKE"
1920 IF ORDER$="n" GOTO 1950
1930 PRINT DLF$;"For purposes of calorie calculaton we need to know"
1940 PRINT "PO fluid intake.":GOTO 1960
1950 PRINT DLF$;"Now we need to know PO fluid intake."
1960 PRINT LF$;"First you will be asked for the AMOUNT, i.e. 6 ml."
1970 PRINT LF$;"Then, the FREQUENCY of administraton, ie. q 2 hours";LF$
1980 INPUT "Enter the AMOUNT (ml)";A$:PRINT LF$
1990 AMOUNT=0
2000 GOSUB 6770:ON EFLAG% GOTO 1980,3430,6750,1560:AMOUNT=VAL(A$)
2010 IF AMOUNT=0 GOTO 1980
2020 Q=0
2030 INPUT "Enter the FREQUENCY (q Hrs)";A$:PRINT LF$
2040 GOSUB 6770:ON EFLAG% GOTO 2030,3430,6750,1980:Q=VAL(A$)
2050 IF Q=0 GOTO 2030
2060 POFLD=AMOUNT*(24/Q)
2070 IF ORDER$="y" THEN IVFLD=TOTFLD ELSE IVFLD=TOTFLD-POFLD
2080 CALOZ=20
2090 PRINT "Enter the NUMBER OF CALORIES/OZ ";:GOSUB 6390:PRINT CALOZ
2100 GOSUB 6400:ON EFLAG% GOTO 2090,3430,6750,2030
2110 IF FLAG%=0 THEN CALOZ=VAL(A$) ELSE CALOZ=20
2120 PRINT LF$
2130 REM **********************************************
2140 REM * amino acids and dextrose
2150 REM **********************************************
2160 SECTION%=4:PRINT CS$
2170 PRINT SUL$;"Amino acid dose (.5 - 2.5) gm/kg/day.";EUL$:PRINT
2180 INPUT "Enter AMINO ACID (gm/kg/day)";A$
2190 IF PO$="y" THEN GOSUB 6770:ON EFLAG% GOTO 2170,3430,6750,2090:AMNACD=VAL(A$)
2200 IF PO$="n" THEN GOSUB 6770:ON EFLAG% GOTO 2170,3430,6750,1560:AMNACD=VAL(A$)
2210 AMNACD=AMNACD*WEIGHT
2220 PRINT:PRINT:INPUT "Enter DEXTROSE CONCENTRATION (mg%)";A$
2230 GOSUB 6770:ON EFLAG% GOTO 2220,3430,6750,2160:DEXTROSE=VAL(A$)
2240 DEXTROSE=DEXTROSE/100
2250 REM **********************************************
2260 REM * trace elements and vitamins
2270 REM **********************************************
2280 SECTION%=5:PRINT CS$
2290 PRINT "Do you wish to add ROUTINE TRACE ELEMENTS or"
2300 PRINT "VITAMIN SUPLEMENTS (y/n)";
2310 GOSUB 6550:IF C$="n" GOTO 2730
2320 PRINT:PRINT "Do you wish:"
2330 PRINT "1 - Pediatric trace elements"
2340 PRINT "2 - Adult trace elements"
2350 PRINT "3 - No trace elements"
2360 TE.TYPE=1
2370 PRINT:PRINT "Which do you wish ";:GOSUB 6390:PRINT TE.TYPE
2380 GOSUB 6400:ON EFLAG% GOTO 2320,3430,6750,2220
2390 IF FLAG%=0 THEN TE.TYPE=VAL(A$)
2400 IF TE.TYPE<1 OR TE.TYPE>3 GOTO 2370 ELSE ON TE.TYPE GOTO 2410,2420
2410 TRCELM=1:TE.TYPE$="Pediatric":TE.UNITS$="mls/kg":GOTO 2430
2420 TRCELM=5:TE.TYPE$="Adult":TE.UNITS$="mls"
2430 PRINT:PRINT TE.TYPE$;" trace elements (";TE.UNITS$;") ";:GOSUB 6390:PRINT TRCELM
2440 GOSUB 6400:ON EFLAG% GOTO 2430,3430,6750,2290
2450 IF FLAG%=0 THEN TRCELM=VAL(A$)
2460 IF TE.TYPE=1 THEN TRCELM=TRCELM*WEIGHT
2470 MVTS=1
2480 PRINT "Multiple vitamins (mls) ";:GOSUB 6390: PRINT MVTS
2490 GOSUB 6400:ON EFLAG% GOTO 2480,3430,6750,2430
2500 IF FLAG%=0 THEN MVTS=VAL(A$)
2510 FOLATE=50
```

```
2520 PRINT "Folate (mcgm) ";:GOSUB 6390: PRINT FOLATE
2530 GOSUB 6400:ON EFLAG% GOTO 2520,3430,6750,2480
2540 IF FLAG%=0 THEN FOLTE=VAL(A$)
2550 ZINC=200
2560 PRINT SUL$;"1 ml of Trace Elements supplies 100 mcgm/kg Zinc.";EUL$:PRINT
2570 PRINT "Enter amount of ADDITIONAL ZINC (mcgm/kg)";:GOSUB 6390:PRINT ZINC
2580 GOSUB 6400:ON EFLAG% GOTO 2560,3430,6750,2520
2590 IF FLAG%=0 THEN ZINC=VAL(A$)
2600 ZINC=ZINC*WEIGHT
2610 VITK=.5
2620 PRINT SUL$;"Vitamin K dose: [ 0.5 - 1 ] mg";EUL$:PRINT
2630 PRINT "Vitamin K (mg) ";:GOSUB 6390:PRINT VITK
2640 GOSUB 6400:ON EFLAG% GOTO 2620,3430,6750,2560
2650 IF FLAG%=0 THEN VITK=VAL(A$)
2660 VITB12=5
2670 PRINT "Vitamin B12 (mcgm) ";:GOSUB 6390:PRINT VITB12
2680 GOSUB 6400:ON EFLAG% GOTO 2670,3430,6750,2620
2690 IF FLAG%=0 THEN VITB12=VAL(A$)
2700 REM ******************************************
2710 REM * electrolytes
2720 REM ******************************************
2730 SECTION%=6:PRINT CS$
2740 PRINT TAB(10)"ELECTROLYTES AND ADDITIVES"
2750 PRINT LF$
2760 PO4FLG%=0
2770 PRINT "Enter the AMOUNT of the following:";PRINT
2780 INPUT "PO4 [2 - 3] (mM/kg/day)";A$:PRINT
2790 GOSUB 6770:ON EFLAG% GOTO 2780,3430,6750,2670:PO4=VAL(A$)
2800    PO4=PO4*WEIGHT:NAPO4=PO4*(NAPO4CNC/3)
2810 INPUT "Na [2 - 3] mEq/kg/day";A$:PRINT
2820 GOSUB 6770:ON EFLAG% GOTO 2810,3430,6750,2780:NA=VAL(A$)
2830    NA=NA-(TOTIV.NACL/WEIGHT): IF NA>=0 THEN GOTO 2860
2840    PRINT "**** OTHER IV & IA LINES ALREADY SUPPLY MORE Na THAN"
2850    PRINT "REQUESTED.  PLEASE EVALUATE. ***":GOTO 2810
2860    NA=NA*WEIGHT:IF NAPO4>NA THEN NAPO4=NA:PO4FLG%=1 ELSE NA=NA-NAPO4
2870 INPUT "K  [2 - 3] mEq/kg/day";A$:PRINT
2880 GOSUB 6770:ON EFLAG% GOTO 2870,3430,6750,2810:K=VAL(A$)
2890    K=K*WEIGHT
2900    IF PO4FLG%=1 THEN KPO4=(PO4-(NA*(3/NAPO4CNC)))*(KPO4CNC/3):NA=0:K=K-KPO4
2910    IF K<0 THEN GOSUB 6530:PRINT"More PO4 was requested than Na & K":GOTO 2740
2920 INPUT "Acetate [2 - 3] mEq/kg/day";A$:PRINT
2930 GOSUB 6770:ON EFLAG% GOTO 2920,3430,6750,2870:ACETATE=VAL(A$)
2940    ACETATE=ACETATE*WEIGHT
2950    IF NA=>ACETATE THEN NACTATE=ACETATE:NACL=NA-NACTATE:KCL=K
2960    IF NA<ACETATE THEN NACTATE=NA:KACTATE=ACETATE-NACTATE:KCL=K-KACTATE
2970    IF KCL<0 THEN PRINT"MORE ACETATE WAS REQUESTED THAN K & Na":PRINT:KACTATE=K:KCL=0
2980 INPUT "Mg [.25 - .5]  mEq/kg/day";A$:PRINT
2990 GOSUB 6770:ON EFLAG% GOTO 2980,3430,6750,2920:MG=VAL(A$)
3000    MG=MG*WEIGHT
3010 INPUT "Ca [200 - 500] mg/kg/day";A$:PRINT
3020 GOSUB 6770:ON EFLAG% GOTO 3010,3430,6750,2980:CA=VAL(A$)
3030    CA=CA*WEIGHT
3040 REM ******* test for CA & PO4 PPT ************
3050 GOSUB 7050:IF EFLAG%=0 GOTO 3060 ELSE GOTO 2730
3060 HEPARIN=.5
3070 PRINT "HEPARIN [.5 - 1] units/ml ";:GOSUB 6390:PRINT HEPARIN
3080 GOSUB 6400:ON EFLAG% GOTO 3070,3430,6750,3010
3090 IF FLAG%=0 THEN HEPARIN=VAL(A$)
3100 INSULIN=0
3110 PRINT "INSULIN [ .1 - .2] units/ml ";:GOSUB 6390:PRINT INSULIN
3120 GOSUB 6400:ON EFLAG% GOTO 3110,3430,6750,3070
3130 IF FLAG%=0 THEN INSULIN=VAL(A$)
3140 REM ******************************************
3150 REM * 'OTHER' constituents if needed
3160 REM ******************************************
3170 OTHER%=0
3180 PRINT CS$;DLF$;"How many additional CONSTITUENTS are needed";:INPUT A$
```

```
3190   GOSUB 6770:ON EFLAG% GOTO 3170,3430,6750,3110
3200   OTHER%=VAL(A$):PRINT
3210    IF OTHER%=0 GOTO 3430
3220   FOR I=1 TO OTHER%
3230    PRINT USING"Enter NAME of number #";I;:INPUT A$:PRINT
3240     GOSUB 6770:ON EFLAG% GOTO 3230,3430,6750,3170
3250     OTHER$(I)=A$
3260    PRINT "Enter UNITS per ml ie. mEq, mM, mg, mcgm";:INPUT A$:PRINT
3270     GOSUB 6770:ON EFLAG% GOTO 3260,3430,6750,3230
3280     OTHER.UNITS$(I)=A$
3290    PRINT "Enter STANDARD CONCENTRATON of ";OTHER$(I);" in ";OTHER.UNITS$(I);"/ml";
3300     INPUT A$:PRINT
3310     GOSUB 6770:ON EFLAG% GOTO 3290,3430,6750,3260
3320     OTHER.CNC(I)=VAL(A$)
3330    PRINT "Enter ";OTHER$(I);" in ";OTHER.UNITS$(I);"/kg/day";:INPUT A$:PRINT
3340     GOSUB 6770:ON EFLAG% GOTO 3330,3430,6750,3290
3350     OTHER.AMT(I)=VAL(A$)*WEIGHT
3360    PRINT
3370   NEXT I
3380   REM ****************************************
3390   REM * computation routines
3400   REM *        *******
3410   REM * determine bottle size
3420   REM ****************************************
3430   PRINT CS$:PRINT:PRINT USING "The TOTAL VOLUME is #### mls.";IVFLD:PRINT LF$
3440   EXTRABOT=0:BOTSIZE=250
3450   PRINT "Enter the CONTAINER VOLUME SIZE (mls) ";:GOSUB 6390:PRINT BOTSIZE
3460   GOSUB 6400:ON EFLAG% GOTO 3460,3430,6750,3180
3470   IF FLAG%=0 THEN BOTSIZE=VAL(A$)
3480   BOTVOL=BOTSIZE
3490   REM ****************************************
3500   REM * compute 'part of bottle' before flush
3510   REM ****************************************
3520   PARTOB=IVFLD-(INT(IVFLD/BOTVOL)*BOTVOL)
3530   REM ****************************************
3540   REM * determine flushing volume and
3550   REM * compute number of bottles
3560   REM ****************************************
3570   PRINT:PRINT "With this TOTAL VOLUME & BOTTLE SIZE, the last"
3580   PRINT USING "bottle will have#### mls in it before addition of";PARTOB
3590   PRINT "flushing volume.":PRINT
3600   EXTRAVOL=100
3610   PRINT "Enter EXTRA VOLUME needed for line flushing ";:GOSUB 6390:PRINT EXTRAVOL
3620   GOSUB 6400:ON EFLAG% GOTO 3620,3430,6750,3450.
3630   REM
3640   IF FLAG%=0 THEN EXTRAVOL=VAL(A$)
3650   TOTVOL=IVFLD+EXTRAVOL
3660   NOB=INT(TOTVOL/BOTVOL)
3670   PARTOB=TOTVOL-(NOB*BOTVOL)
3680   IF PARTOB>0 THEN EXTRABOT=1
3690   NOB=NOB+EXTRABOT
3700   REM ****************************************
3710   REM * compute component volumes
3720   REM ****************************************
3730   EXTRFCTR = 1
3740   IF IVFLD >= BOTVOL THEN GOTO 3760
3750   IF   TOTVOL <= BOTVOL THEN EXTRFCTR=TOTVOL/IVFLD ELSE EXTRFCTR = BOTVOL/IVFLD
3760   TEVOL=TRCELM*EXTRFCTR
3770   MVIVOL=MVTS*EXTRFCTR
3780   FOLVOL=(FOLATE/FOLCONC)*EXTRFCTR
3790   VB12VOL=(VITB12/VITB12CONC)*EXTRFCTR
3800   VITKVOL=(VITK/VITKCONC)*EXTRFCTR
3810   ADDITIVES=TEVOL+MVIVOL+FOLVOL+VB12VOL+VITKVOL
3820   TOTVOL=TOTVOL-ADDITIVES
3830   EXTRFCTR=TOTVOL/IVFLD
3840   ZINCVOL=(ZINC/ZINCONC)*EXTRFCTR
3850   NACTVOL=(NACTATE/NAACTCONC)*EXTRFCTR
```

```
3860 NACLVOL=(NACL/NACLCONC)*EXTRFCTR
3870 NAPO4VOL=(NAPO4/NAPO4CNC)*EXTRFCTR
3880 KACTVOL=(KACTATE/KACTCONC)*EXTRFCTR
3890 KCLVOL=(KCL/KCLCONC)*EXTRFCTR
3900 KPO4VOL=(KPO4/KPO4CNC)*EXTRFCTR
3910 MGVOL=(MG/MGCONC)*EXTRFCTR
3920 CAVOL=(CA/CACONC)*EXTRFCTR
3930 HEPVOL=(HEPARIN/HPRNCONC)*EXTRFCTR
3940 INSULINVOL=(INSULIN/INSULINCNC)*EXTRFCTR
3950 AAVOL=(AMNACD/AACONC)*EXTRFCTR
3960 IF OTHER%=0 THEN GOTO 4030
3970 FOR I=1 TO OTHER%
3980   OTHER.VOL(I)=(OTHER.AMT(I)/OTHER.CNC(I))*EXTRFCTR
3990 NEXT I
4000 REM *****************************************
4010 REM * sum up the individual volumes
4020 REM *****************************************
4030 VOLSUM=0
4040 VOLSUM=TEVOL+MVIVOL+FOLVOL+ZINCVOL+VB12VOL+VITKVOL+NACTVOL+NACLVOL+NAPO4VOL
4050 VOLSUM=VOLSUM+KACTVOL+KCLVOL+KPO4VOL+MGVOL+CAVOL+HEPVOL+AAVOL+INSULINVOL
4060 IF OTHER%=0 THEN GOTO 4100
4070 FOR I=1 TO OTHER%
4080   VOLSUM=VOLSUM+OTHER.VOL(I)
4090 NEXT I
4100 IF TOTVOL>VOLSUM GOTO 4170
4110 GOSUB 6530
4120 PRINT "IV fluid amount is too small for the solute load"
4130 PRINT DLF$:GOTO 1450
4140 REM *****************************************
4150 REM * FAT EMULSION bottle lable
4160 REM *****************************************
4170 IF FAT.EMULSION=0 THEN GOTO 4320
4180 PRINT "Printing FAT EMULSION BOTTLE LABEL"
4190 LPRINT "FAT EMULSION BOTTLE LABEL"
4200 LPRINT "Patient: ";LASTN$;", ";FIRSTN$;"  MED REC #";MEDREC$;"  Unit: ";UNITNUM$
4210 LPRINT USING "Date Ordered ##/##/##    Date/Time Due ##";MONTH;DAY;YEAR;MONTHDUE;
4220 LPRINT USING "/## @ ##:00 Hours";DAYDUE;HOURDUE
4230 LPRINT "DISCARD 24 HOURS AFTER HANGING !!!"
4240 LPRINT FATCONC;"% FAT EMULSION CONCENTRATION
4250 LPRINT USING "Patient to receive #### mls. FAT EMULSION";FAT.EMULSION
4260 LPRINT USING "TO RUN AT ##.# mls/hr.";FAT.EMULSION/24:LPRINT
4270 LPRINT:LPRINT
4280 REM *****************************************
4290 REM * TPN bottle labels
4300 REM *****************************************
4310 BOTNUM=BOTNUM-1
4320 HOLDBTNM=BOTNUM
4330 FOR I=1 TO NOB
4340 THISBOT=BOTNUM+I
4350 IF I=NOB AND PARTOB>0 THEN BOTVOL=PARTOB
4360 FACTOR=(IVFLD/BOTVOL)
4370 PRINT:PRINT "Printing TPN BOTTLE LABEL"
4380 LPRINT "TPN BOTTLE LABEL"
4390 LPRINT "Patient: ";LASTN$;", ";FIRSTN$;"  MED REC #";MEDREC$
4400 LPRINT "Unit: ";UNITNUM$;
4410 LPRINT USING "  Bottle ### which is ### of ###";THISBOT;I;NOB
4420 LPRINT USING "Date Ordered ##/##/##    Date/Time Due ##";MONTH;DAY;YEAR;MONTHDUE;
4430 LPRINT USING "/## @ ##:00 Hours";DAYDUE;HOURDUE
4440 LPRINT "DISCARD 24 HOURS AFTER HANGING !!!"
4450 LPRINT "KEEP REFRIGERATED UNTIL ONE HOUR BEFORE USE"
4460 LPRINT USING "Total bottle volume ##### mls";BOTVOL
4470 LPRINT USING "Patient to receive ##### mls to flow at ###.# mls/hr";IVFLD;IVFLD/24
4480 LPRINT USING "Dextrose ##.#% final concentration";DEXTROSE*100
4490 PLACE=10:GOSUB 6890:LPRINT "CONTENTS OF THIS BOTTLE"
4500 RT=25
4510 LPRINT USING "Sodium    ###.# mEq";(NACL+NACTATE+NAPO4)/FACTOR;
4520 GOSUB 6870: IF I<>1 THEN LPRINT: GOTO 4540
```

```
4530 LPRINT TE.TYPE$;:LPRINT USING " Trace Elements ###.# mls ";TRCELM/FACTOR
4540 LPRINT USING "Potassium ###.# mEq";(KCL+KACTATE+KPO4)/FACTOR;
4550 GOSUB 6870: IF I<>1 THEN LPRINT: GOTO 4570
4560 LPRINT USING "Multiple Vitamin ###.# mls";MVTS/FACTOR
4570 LPRINT USING "Chloride  ###.# mEq";(NACL+KCL)/FACTOR;
4580 GOSUB 6870: IF I<>1 THEN LPRINT: GOTO 4600
4590 LPRINT USING "Vitamin B12 ###.# mcgm";VITB12/FACTOR
4600 LPRINT USING "Acetate   ###.# mEq";(NACTATE+KACTATE)/FACTOR;
4610 GOSUB 6870: IF I<>1 THEN LPRINT: GOTO 4630
4620 LPRINT USING "Vitamin K ###.# mg";VITK/FACTOR
4630 LPRINT USING "Phosphate ###.# mM";((NAPO4*(3/NAPO4CNC))+(KPO4*(3/KPO4CNC)))/FACTOR;
4640 GOSUB 6870: IF I<>1 THEN LPRINT: GOTO 4660
4650 LPRINT USING "Folic Acid ###.# mcgm";FOLATE/FACTOR
4660 LPRINT USING "Magnesium ###.# mEq";MG/FACTOR;
4670 GOSUB 6870
4680 LPRINT USING "Heparin ###.# units";(HEPARIN/FACTOR)*IVFLD
4690 LPRINT USING "Calcium gluc ##### mg";CA/FACTOR;
4700 GOSUB 6870
4710 LPRINT USING "Zinc ####.# mcgm";ZINC/FACTOR
4720 LPRINT USING "Regular Insulin ### units";(INSULIN/FACTOR)*IVFLD
4730 LPRINT USING "Amino Acid ###.# gms";AMNACD/FACTOR
4740 IF OTHER%=0 GOTO 4790
4750 FOR J=1 TO OTHER%
4760   LPRINT OTHER$(J);:LPRINT USING" ####.# ";OTHER.AMT(J)/FACTOR;:
4770   LPRINT OTHER.UNITS$(J)
4780 NEXT J
4790 LPRINT "Screened by: _____  Made/Checked by: _____"
4800 LPRINT:LPRINT
4810 NEXT I
4820 REM ******************************************
4830 REM * produce TPN mixing instructions
4840 REM ******************************************
4850 BOTNUM=HOLDBTNM
4860 BOTVOL=BOTSIZE
4870 FOR I=1 TO NOB
4880 THISBOT=BOTNUM+I
4890 IF I=NOB AND PARTOB>0 THEN BOTVOL=PARTOB
4900 FACTOR=TOTVOL/BOTVOL
4910 PRINT:PRINT "Printing TPN MIXING INSTRUCTIONS"
4920 LPRINT "PEDIATRIC TPN MIXING INSTRUCTIONS"
4930 LPRINT "Patient: ";LASTN$;", ";FIRSTN$;"  MED REC #";MEDREC$
4940 LPRINT "Unit: ";UNITNUM$;
4950 LPRINT USING "  Bottle ## which is ## of ## bottles";THISBOT;I;NOB
4960 LPRINT USING "Date ordered ##/##/##   Date/Time Due ##";MONTH;DAY;YEAR;MONTHDUE;
4970 LPRINT USING "/## @ ##:00 Hours";DAYDUE;HOURDUE
4980 LPRINT USING "Total bottle Volume #####.# mls";BOTVOL
4990 DEXVOL=(DEXTROSE*BOTVOL)/(DEXCNC)
5000 LPRINT USING "Place ###.# mls of D ##.# in bottle";DEXVOL;DEXCNC
5010 PLACE=10:GOSUB 6890:LPRINT "PLACE THE FOLLOWING IN THE BOTTLE"
5020 RT=25
5030 LPRINT USING "NaCl  ###.# mls";NACLVOL/FACTOR;
5040 GOSUB 6870: IF I<>1 THEN LPRINT: GOTO 5060
5050 LPRINT TE.TYPE$;:LPRINT USING " Trace Elements ###.# mls ";TEVOL
5060 LPRINT USING "NaPO4 ###.# mls";NAPO4VOL/FACTOR;
5070 GOSUB 6870: IF I<>1 THEN LPRINT: GOTO 5090
5080 LPRINT USING "Multiple Vitamin ###.# mls";MVIVOL
5090 LPRINT USING "Na Acetate ###.# mls";NACTVOL/FACTOR;
5100 GOSUB 6870: IF I<>1 THEN LPRINT: GOTO 5120
5110 LPRINT USING "Vitamin B12 ###.# mls";VB12VOL
5120 LPRINT USING "KCl  ###.# mls";KCLVOL/FACTOR;
5130 GOSUB 6870: IF I<>1 THEN LPRINT: GOTO 5150
5140 LPRINT USING "Vitamin K  ###.# mls";VITKVOL
5150 LPRINT USING "KPO4 ###.# mls";KPO4VOL/FACTOR;
5160 GOSUB 6870: IF I<>1 THEN LPRINT: GOTO 5180
5170 LPRINT USING "Folic Acid ###.# mls";FOLVOL
5180 LPRINT USING "K Acetate ###.# mls";KACTVOL/FACTOR;
5190 GOSUB 6870
```

```
5200 LPRINT USING "Magnesium   ###.# mls";MGVOL/FACTOR
5210 LPRINT USING "Zinc ####.# mls";ZINCVOL/FACTOR;
5220 GOSUB 6870
5230 LPRINT USING "Heparin    ###.# mls";(HEPVOL/FACTOR)*IVFLD
5240 LPRINT USING "Calcium gluc ####.# mls";CAVOL/FACTOR;
5250 GOSUB 6870
5260 LPRINT USING "Regular Insulin ### mls";(INSULINVOL/FACTOR)*IVFLD
5270 LPRINT USING "Amino Acid ###.# mls";AAVOL/FACTOR
5280 IF OTHER%=0 THEN GOTO 5340
5290 TOT.OTHER.VOL=0
5300 FOR J=1 TO OTHER%
5310  LPRINT OTHER$(J);:LPRINT USING" ####.# mls";OTHER.VOL(J)/FACTOR
5320  TOT.OTHER.VOL=TOT.OTHER.VOL+OTHER.VOL(J)
5330 NEXT J
5340 IF I<>1 THEN ADDITIVES=0
5350 QS=BOTVOL-(ADDITIVES+DEXVOL+(NACLVOL+NAPO4VOL+NACTVOL+KCLVOL)/FACTOR)
5360 QS=QS-(KPO4VOL+KACTVOL+CAVOL+((HEPVOL+INSULINVOL)*IVFLD))/FACTOR
5370 QS=QS-(ZINCVOL+MGVOL+AAVOL+TOT.OTHER.VOL)/FACTOR
5380 LPRINT USING "Q.S. with ###.# mls sterile water to total volume ####.# mls";QS,BOTVOL
5390 LPRINT "Made by: _____ Checked by: _____ "
5400 LPRINT:LPRINT
5410 NEXT I
5420 REM *****************************************
5430 REM * overall description of what patient
5440 REM * received in TPN
5450 REM *****************************************
5460 FACTOR=WEIGHT
5470 BOTNUM=HOLDBTNM
5480 PRINT:PRINT "Printing CONTENTS OF PEDIATRIC TPN"
5490 FOR COUNT% = 1 TO 3
5500 IF COUNT%=2 OR COUNT%=3 THEN LPRINT:LPRINT
5510 LPRINT "CONTENT OF PEDIATRIC TPN"
5520 LPRINT "Patient: ";LASTN$;", ";FIRSTN$;"  MED REC #";MEDREC$
5530 LPRINT "Unit: ";UNITNUM$;
5540 LPRINT USING "  Bottle ## to ##";BOTNUM+1;BOTNUM+NOB
5550 LPRINT USING "Date Ordered ##/##/##   Date/Time Due ";MONTH;DAY;YEAR;
5560 LPRINT USING "##/## @ ##:00 Hours";MONTHDUE;DAYDUE;HOURDUE
5570 LPRINT USING "Total IV Volume ##### mls to flow at ###.# mls/hr";IVFLD;IVFLD/24
5580 LPRINT USING "Patient weighs ###.## kgs";WEIGHT;
5590 LPRINT USING " and will receive ### mls/kg/day";MLS.KG.DAY
5600 LPRINT USING "Dextrose ##.#% final concentration";DEXTROSE*100
5610 PLACE=14:GOSUB 6890:LPRINT "ADDITIVES Per (Units)/Day"
5620 RT=25
5630 LPRINT USING "Sodium    ###.# mEq/kg";(NACL+NACTATE+NAPO4+TOTIV.NACL)/FACTOR;
5640 GOSUB 6870
5650 IF TE.TYPE=1 THEN TE.FACTOR=FACTOR ELSE TE.FACTOR=1
5660 LPRINT TE.TYPE$;:LPRINT USING " Trace Elements ###.# ";TRCELM/TE.FACTOR;
5670  LPRINT TE.UNITS$
5680 LPRINT USING "Potassium ###.# mEq/kg";(KCL+KACTATE+KPO4)/FACTOR;
5690 GOSUB 6870
5700 LPRINT USING "Multiple Vitamin ###.# mls";MVTS
5710 LPRINT USING "Chloride  ###.# mEq/kg";(NACL+KCL+TOTIV.NACL)/FACTOR;
5720 GOSUB 6870
5730 LPRINT USING "Vitamin B12 ###.# mcgm";VITB12
5740 LPRINT USING "Acetate   ###.# mEq/kg";(NACTATE+KACTATE)/FACTOR;
5750 GOSUB 6870
5760 LPRINT USING "Vitamin K ###.# mg";VITK
5770 LPRINT USING "Phosphate ###.# mM/kg";((NAPO4*(3/NAPO4CNC))+(KPO4*(3/KPO4CNC)))/FACTOR;
5780 GOSUB 6870
5790 LPRINT USING "Folic Acid ###.# mcgm";FOLATE
5800 LPRINT USING "Magnesium ###.## mEq/kg";MG/FACTOR;
5810 GOSUB 6870
5820 LPRINT USING "Heparin ###.# units";HEPARIN*IVFLD
5830 LPRINT USING "Calcium gluc ##### mg/kg";CA/FACTOR;
5840 RT=28:GOSUB 6870
5850 LPRINT USING "Zinc ####.# mcgm/kg";ZINC/FACTOR
5860 LPRINT USING "Regular Insulin ### units";INSULIN*IVFLD
```

```
5870 LPRINT USING "Amino Acid ###.# gms/kg";AMNACD/FACTOR;:GOSUB 6870
5880 LPRINT USING #.# gms/kg";((FAT.EMULSION*(FATCONC/100))/FACTOR)
5890 IF OTHER%=0 GOTO 5940
5900 FOR J=1 TO OTHER%
5910   LPRINT OTHER$(J);:LPRINT USING " ####.# ";OTHER.AMT(J)/FACTOR;:
5920   LPRINT OTHER.UNITS$(J);"/kg"
5930 NEXT J
5940 IVCAL=((DEXTROSE*(IVFLD)*3.4)+(AMNACD*4)+(FAT.EMULSION*(FATCONC/10)*1.1))/WEIGHT
5950 LPRINT USING "TPN and FAT EMULSION provide ### calories/kg/day";IVCAL
5960 IF POFLD=0 GOTO 6050
5970 POCAL=POFLD*(CALOZ/30)/WEIGHT
5980 LPRINT USING"PO feeds of ## mls Q ## hours using ## cal/oz formula";AMOUNT;Q;CALOZ
5990 LPRINT USING "will provide ### calories/kg/day.  ";POCAL;
6000 ALL.PO=POCAL+((FAT.EMULSION*(FATCONC/10)*1.1)+(DEXTROSE * (IVFLD-POFLD) * 3.4))/WEIGHT
6010 ALL.PO=ALL.PO + (( AMNACD*4 )/WEIGHT)
6020 IF ORDER$="n" THEN LPRINT: GOTO 6050
6030 LPRINT "IV+PO Calories range from"
6040 LPRINT USING "### if all PO is given to ### if only IV is given.";ALL.PO;IVCAL
6050 IF LINES=0 GOTO 6140
6060 LPRINT USING "Please note that there are # other non-nutritional lines.";LINES
6070 IV.FLD=0
6080 FOR I=1 TO LINES
6090   LPRINT USING " Line # flows at ##.# mls/hr";I;IV(I)
6100   IV.FLD=IV.FLD+IV(I)*24
6110 NEXT I
6120 LPRINT USING "This will provide ###.# mls/kg/day ";IV.FLD/WEIGHT;
6130 LPRINT USING " and #.## mEq NaCl/kg/day";TOTIV.NACL/WEIGHT
6140 LPRINT "Screened by:_____"
6150 NEXT COUNT%
6160 SECTION%=7
6170 LPRINT:LPRINT:PRINT
6180 REM ********************************************
6190 REM * routine to allow for editing and re-
6200 REM * execution or computations
6210 REM ********************************************
6220 CMPTFLG%=1
6230 PRINT CS$;"If any of these results are incorrect because of"
6240 PRINT "incorrect input, you may now correct the values in"
6250 PRINT "error.  Once you have corrected those values, type"
6260 PRINT "COMPUTE.  This command will restart the computa-"
6270 PRINT "tions and printing.":PRINT
6280 PRINT "Do you wish to correct any section?";
6290 A$=INKEY$:IF A$="y" OR A$="Y" OR A$="n" OR A$="N" GOTO 6300 ELSE GOTO 6290
6300 IF A$="y" OR A$="Y" THEN PRINT CS$;"Which section do you wish to correct?":GOTO 6620
6310 PRINT:PRINT:PRINT "Want to compute another patient's TPN (y/n)?";
6320 GOSUB 6550
6330 IF C$="n" OR C$="N" THEN END ELSE CLEAR:CHAIN "TPN",540
6340 END
6350 REM ********************************************
6360 REM * subroutine section
6370 REM ********************************************
6380 REM * prompt with replacement routine
6390 P=POS(P)-2:RETURN
6400 PRINT SPACE$(P);:INPUT A$
6410 PRINT
6420 EFLAG%=0:IF A$="JUMP" OR A$="jump" THEN A$="":GOSUB 6600:GOTO 6440
6430   GOTO 6450
6440   IF EFLAG%=1 THEN RETURN ELSE GOTO 6420
6450 IF (A$="COMPUTE" OR A$="compute") AND CMPTFLG%=1 THEN EFLAG%=2:RETURN
6460 IF A$="BACKUP" OR A$="backup" THEN EFLAG%=4:RETURN
6470 IF A$="HELP" OR A$="help" THEN GOSUB 6910:EFLAG%=1:RETURN
6480 IF A$="RETURN" OR A$="return" THEN GOTO 6490 ELSE GOTO 6500
6490   IF RTNFLG%=1 THEN EFLAG%=3:RETURN ELSE GOTO 6750
6500 IF LEN(A$)=0 THEN FLAG%=1 ELSE FLAG%=0
6510 RETURN
6520 REM * error notification routine
6530 PRINT "****ERROR****":RETURN
```

```
6540 REM * routine to return a "y" or an "n"
6550 C$=INKEY$:IF C$="" GOTO 6550
6560 IF C$="Y" THEN C$="y"
6570 IF C$="N" THEN C$="n"
6580 IF C$="y" OR C$="n" THEN PRINT " ";C$:RETURN ELSE GOTO 6550
6590 REM * data entry modification routine
6600 RTNFLG%=1
6610 PRINT CS$;"Which section do you wish to JUMP to:
6620 PRINT
6630 PRINT "1 - Standard solution concentration."
6640 PRINT "2 - Name, Medical Record Number, Unit,"
6650 PRINT "    Bottle number, Dates."
6660 PRINT "3 - Fluid Input"
6670 PRINT "4 - Amino Acids and Dextrose"
6680 PRINT "5 - Trace elements & Vitamins"
6690 PRINT "6 - Electrolytes"
6700 IF SECTION%<>7 THEN PRINT:PRINT "You were in section";SECTION%
6710 PRINT:PRINT "Which section do you wish to return to?";
6720 SECTION$=INKEY$:IF SECTION$="" GOTO 6720
6730 IF VAL(SECTION$)<1 OR VAL(SECTION$)>6 GOTO 6720
6740 ON VAL(SECTION$) GOTO 170,970,1410,2160,2280,2730
6750 RTNFLG%=0:EFLAG%=1:RETURN
6760 REM * data entry routine
6770 EFLAG%=0:IF A$="jump" OR A$="JUMP" THEN A$="":GOSUB 6600:GOTO 6790
6780    GOTO 6800
6790    IF EFLAG%=1 THEN RETURN ELSE GOTO 6770
6800 IF (A$="COMPUTE" OR A$="compute") AND CMPTFLG%=1 THEN EFLAG%=2:RETURN
6810 IF A$="BACKUP" OR A$="backup" THEN EFLAG%=4:RETURN
6820 IF A$="HELP" OR A$="help" THEN GOSUB 6910:EFLAG%=1:RETURN
6830 IF A$="RETURN" OR A$="return" GOTO 6840 ELSE GOTO 6850
6840    IF RTNFLG%=1 THEN EFLAG%=3:RETURN ELSE GOTO 6750
6850 EFLAG%=0:RETURN
6860 REM * line printer 'tab' routine
6870 PLACE=LPOS(X)
6880 LPRINT LEFT$(BLANK$,RT-PLACE);:RETURN
6890 LPRINT LEFT$(BLANK$,PLACE);:RETURN
6900 REM * help menue for input
6910 PRINT:PRINT:PRINT:CMPTFLG%=1
6920 PRINT "You have two choices for editing previous entries:"
6930 PRINT "1 - Typing BACKUP returns you to the entry you have"
6940 PRINT "just passed. 2 - If you wish to 'jump' to a section"
6950 PRINT "of data entry questions which are more than a few"
6960 PRINT "entries away, then type JUMP."
6970 PRINT "    Once you have made the corrections, typing RETURN"
6980 PRINT "will cause resumption of program execution from the"
6990 PRINT "point where you decided to stop to correct errors."
7000 PRINT "    You will now be returned to the entry you were"
7010 PRINT "at when you typed HELP."
7020 PRINT:PRINT "Hit any key when ready!!":PRINT:PRINT:PRINT
7030 C$=INKEY$:IF C$="" GOTO 7030 ELSE CMPTFLG%=0:RETURN
7040 REM ****** CHECK FOR PPT OF CA AND PO4 ******
7050 IF CA/IVFLD> 4 AND PO4/IVFLD>.02 THEN GOSUB 6530 ELSE EFLAG%=0:RETURN
7060 PRINT "Precipitation will occur between Calcium and PO4"
7070 PRINT USING "at present concentrations of ###.# for Calcium";CALCIUM/IVFLD
7080 PRINT USING "##.# for PO4";PO4/IVFLD
7090 PRINT:PRINT "Hit any key when ready!!!";
7100 C$=INKEY$:IF C$="" GOTO 7100
7110 EFLAG%=4:RETURN
```

Index

359